FREE Study Skills

Dear Customer,

Thank you for your purchase from Mometrix! We consider it an honor and a privilege that you have purchased our product and we want to ensure your satisfaction.

As part of our ongoing effort to meet the needs of test takers, we have developed a set of Study Skills Videos that we would like to give you for FREE. These videos cover our *best practices* for getting ready for your exam, from how to use our study materials to how to best prepare for the day of the test.

All that we ask is that you email us with feedback that would describe your experience so far with our product. Good, bad, or indifferent, we want to know what you think!

To get your FREE Study Skills Videos, you can use the **QR code** below, or send us an **email** at studyvideos@mometrix.com with *FREE VIDEOS* in the subject line and the following information in the body of the email:

- The name of the product you purchased.
- Your product rating on a scale of 1-5, with 5 being the highest rating.
- Your feedback. It can be long, short, or anything in between. We just want to know your impressions and experience so far with our product. (Good feedback might include how our study material met your needs and ways we might be able to make it even better. You could highlight features that you found helpful or features that you think we should add.)

If you have any questions or concerns, please don't hesitate to contact me directly.

Thanks again!

Sincerely,

Jay Willis
Vice President
jay.willis@mometrix.com
1-800-673-8175

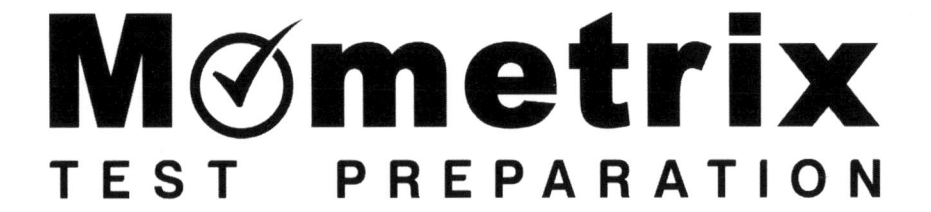

SCAN HERE

Mometrix
TEST PREPARATION

Mometrix
TEST PREPARATION

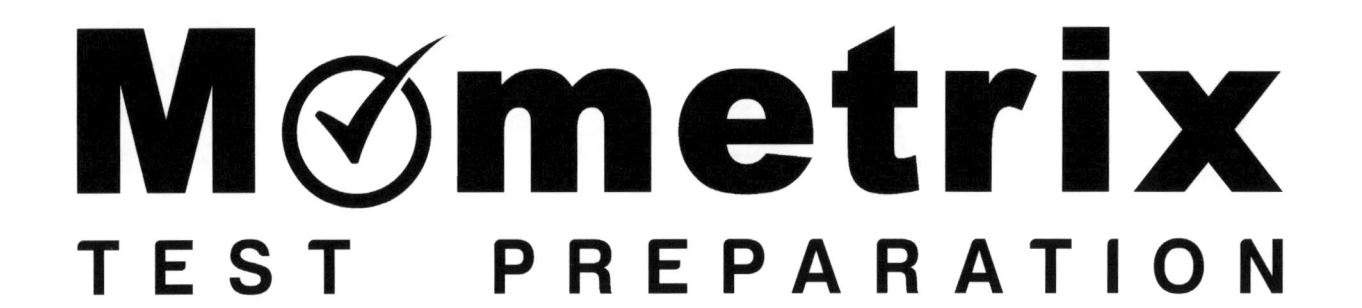

Athletic Training

Exam Secrets Study Guide

NATA® Test Review for the National Athletic Trainers' Association® Board of Certification Exam

Copyright © 2023 by Mometrix Media LLC

All rights reserved. This product, or parts thereof, may not be reproduced, stored in a retrieval system, or transmitted in any form or by any means—electronic, mechanical, photocopy, recording, scanning, or other—except for brief quotations in critical reviews or articles, without the prior written permission of the publisher.

Written and edited by Mometrix Test Prep

Printed in the United States of America

This paper meets the requirements of ANSI/NISO Z39.48-1992 (Permanence of Paper).

Mometrix offers volume discount pricing to institutions. For more information or a price quote, please contact our sales department at sales@mometrix.com or 888-248-1219.

Mometrix Media LLC is not affiliated with or endorsed by any official testing organization. All organizational and test names are trademarks of their respective owners.

Paperback
ISBN 13: 978-1-5167-1553-4
ISBN 10: 1-5167-1553-5

Ebook
ISBN 13: 978-1-5167-1537-4
ISBN 10: 1-5167-1537-3

Hardback
ISBN 13: 978-1-5167-1852-8
ISBN 10: 1-5167-1852-6

Dear Future Exam Success Story

First of all, **THANK YOU** for purchasing Mometrix study materials!

Second, congratulations! You are one of the few determined test-takers who are committed to doing whatever it takes to excel on your exam. **You have come to the right place.** We developed these study materials with one goal in mind: to deliver you the information you need in a format that's concise and easy to use.

In addition to optimizing your guide for the content of the test, we've outlined our recommended steps for breaking down the preparation process into small, attainable goals so you can make sure you stay on track.

We've also analyzed the entire test-taking process, identifying the most common pitfalls and showing how you can overcome them and be ready for any curveball the test throws you.

Standardized testing is one of the biggest obstacles on your road to success, which only increases the importance of doing well in the high-pressure, high-stakes environment of test day. Your results on this test could have a significant impact on your future, and this guide provides the information and practical advice to help you achieve your full potential on test day.

Your success is our success

We would love to hear from you! If you would like to share the story of your exam success or if you have any questions or comments in regard to our products, please contact us at **800-673-8175** or **support@mometrix.com**.

Thanks again for your business and we wish you continued success!

Sincerely,
The Mometrix Test Preparation Team

Need more help? Check out our flashcards at:
http://mometrixflashcards.com/NATA

Table of Contents

Introduction 1
Secret Key #1 – Plan Big, Study Small 2
Secret Key #2 – Make Your Studying Count 3
Secret Key #3 – Practice the Right Way 4
Secret Key #4 – Pace Yourself 6
Secret Key #5 – Have a Plan for Guessing 7
Test-Taking Strategies 10
Injury/Illness Prevention and Wellness Promotion 15
Examination, Assessment, and Diagnosis 53
Immediate and Emergency Care 90
Therapeutic Intervention 120
Healthcare Administration and Professional Responsibility 164
NATA Practice Test 197
Answer Key and Explanations 207
How to Overcome Test Anxiety 218
Additional Bonus Material 224

Introduction

Thank you for purchasing this resource! You have made the choice to prepare yourself for a test that could have a huge impact on your future, and this guide is designed to help you be fully ready for test day. Obviously, it's important to have a solid understanding of the test material, but you also need to be prepared for the unique environment and stressors of the test, so that you can perform to the best of your abilities.

For this purpose, the first section that appears in this guide is the **Secret Keys**. We've devoted countless hours to meticulously researching what works and what doesn't, and we've boiled down our findings to the five most impactful steps you can take to improve your performance on the test. We start at the beginning with study planning and move through the preparation process, all the way to the testing strategies that will help you get the most out of what you know when you're finally sitting in front of the test.

We recommend that you start preparing for your test as far in advance as possible. However, if you've bought this guide as a last-minute study resource and only have a few days before your test, we recommend that you skip over the first two Secret Keys since they address a long-term study plan.

If you struggle with **test anxiety**, we strongly encourage you to check out our recommendations for how you can overcome it. Test anxiety is a formidable foe, but it can be beaten, and we want to make sure you have the tools you need to defeat it.

Secret Key #1 – Plan Big, Study Small

There's a lot riding on your performance. If you want to ace this test, you're going to need to keep your skills sharp and the material fresh in your mind. You need a plan that lets you review everything you need to know while still fitting in your schedule. We'll break this strategy down into three categories.

Information Organization

Start with the information you already have: the official test outline. From this, you can make a complete list of all the concepts you need to cover before the test. Organize these concepts into groups that can be studied together, and create a list of any related vocabulary you need to learn so you can brush up on any difficult terms. You'll want to keep this vocabulary list handy once you actually start studying since you may need to add to it along the way.

Time Management

Once you have your set of study concepts, decide how to spread them out over the time you have left before the test. Break your study plan into small, clear goals so you have a manageable task for each day and know exactly what you're doing. Then just focus on one small step at a time. When you manage your time this way, you don't need to spend hours at a time studying. Studying a small block of content for a short period each day helps you retain information better and avoid stressing over how much you have left to do. You can relax knowing that you have a plan to cover everything in time. In order for this strategy to be effective though, you have to start studying early and stick to your schedule. Avoid the exhaustion and futility that comes from last-minute cramming!

Study Environment

The environment you study in has a big impact on your learning. Studying in a coffee shop, while probably more enjoyable, is not likely to be as fruitful as studying in a quiet room. It's important to keep distractions to a minimum. You're only planning to study for a short block of time, so make the most of it. Don't pause to check your phone or get up to find a snack. It's also important to **avoid multitasking**. Research has consistently shown that multitasking will make your studying dramatically less effective. Your study area should also be comfortable and well-lit so you don't have the distraction of straining your eyes or sitting on an uncomfortable chair.

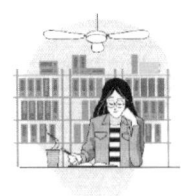

The time of day you study is also important. You want to be rested and alert. Don't wait until just before bedtime. Study when you'll be most likely to comprehend and remember. Even better, if you know what time of day your test will be, set that time aside for study. That way your brain will be used to working on that subject at that specific time and you'll have a better chance of recalling information.

Finally, it can be helpful to team up with others who are studying for the same test. Your actual studying should be done in as isolated an environment as possible, but the work of organizing the information and setting up the study plan can be divided up. In between study sessions, you can discuss with your teammates the concepts that you're all studying and quiz each other on the details. Just be sure that your teammates are as serious about the test as you are. If you find that your study time is being replaced with social time, you might need to find a new team.

Secret Key #2 – Make Your Studying Count

You're devoting a lot of time and effort to preparing for this test, so you want to be absolutely certain it will pay off. This means doing more than just reading the content and hoping you can remember it on test day. It's important to make every minute of study count. There are two main areas you can focus on to make your studying count.

Retention

It doesn't matter how much time you study if you can't remember the material. You need to make sure you are retaining the concepts. To check your retention of the information you're learning, try recalling it at later times with minimal prompting. Try carrying around flashcards and glance at one or two from time to time or ask a friend who's also studying for the test to quiz you.

To enhance your retention, look for ways to put the information into practice so that you can apply it rather than simply recalling it. If you're using the information in practical ways, it will be much easier to remember. Similarly, it helps to solidify a concept in your mind if you're not only reading it to yourself but also explaining it to someone else. Ask a friend to let you teach them about a concept you're a little shaky on (or speak aloud to an imaginary audience if necessary). As you try to summarize, define, give examples, and answer your friend's questions, you'll understand the concepts better and they will stay with you longer. Finally, step back for a big picture view and ask yourself how each piece of information fits with the whole subject. When you link the different concepts together and see them working together as a whole, it's easier to remember the individual components.

Finally, practice showing your work on any multi-step problems, even if you're just studying. Writing out each step you take to solve a problem will help solidify the process in your mind, and you'll be more likely to remember it during the test.

Modality

Modality simply refers to the means or method by which you study. Choosing a study modality that fits your own individual learning style is crucial. No two people learn best in exactly the same way, so it's important to know your strengths and use them to your advantage.

For example, if you learn best by visualization, focus on visualizing a concept in your mind and draw an image or a diagram. Try color-coding your notes, illustrating them, or creating symbols that will trigger your mind to recall a learned concept. If you learn best by hearing or discussing information, find a study partner who learns the same way or read aloud to yourself. Think about how to put the information in your own words. Imagine that you are giving a lecture on the topic and record yourself so you can listen to it later.

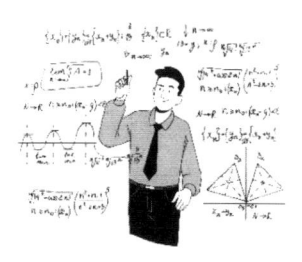

For any learning style, flashcards can be helpful. Organize the information so you can take advantage of spare moments to review. Underline key words or phrases. Use different colors for different categories. Mnemonic devices (such as creating a short list in which every item starts with the same letter) can also help with retention. Find what works best for you and use it to store the information in your mind most effectively and easily.

Secret Key #3 – Practice the Right Way

Your success on test day depends not only on how many hours you put into preparing, but also on whether you prepared the right way. It's good to check along the way to see if your studying is paying off. One of the most effective ways to do this is by taking practice tests to evaluate your progress. Practice tests are useful because they show exactly where you need to improve. Every time you take a practice test, pay special attention to these three groups of questions:

- The questions you got wrong
- The questions you had to guess on, even if you guessed right
- The questions you found difficult or slow to work through

This will show you exactly what your weak areas are, and where you need to devote more study time. Ask yourself why each of these questions gave you trouble. Was it because you didn't understand the material? Was it because you didn't remember the vocabulary? Do you need more repetitions on this type of question to build speed and confidence? Dig into those questions and figure out how you can strengthen your weak areas as you go back to review the material.

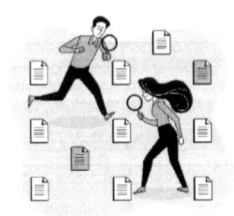

Additionally, many practice tests have a section explaining the answer choices. It can be tempting to read the explanation and think that you now have a good understanding of the concept. However, an explanation likely only covers part of the question's broader context. Even if the explanation makes perfect sense, **go back and investigate** every concept related to the question until you're positive you have a thorough understanding.

As you go along, keep in mind that the practice test is just that: practice. Memorizing these questions and answers will not be very helpful on the actual test because it is unlikely to have any of the same exact questions. If you only know the right answers to the sample questions, you won't be prepared for the real thing. **Study the concepts** until you understand them fully, and then you'll be able to answer any question that shows up on the test.

It's important to wait on the practice tests until you're ready. If you take a test on your first day of study, you may be overwhelmed by the amount of material covered and how much you need to learn. Work up to it gradually.

On test day, you'll need to be prepared for answering questions, managing your time, and using the test-taking strategies you've learned. It's a lot to balance, like a mental marathon that will have a big impact on your future. Like training for a marathon, you'll need to start slowly and work your way up. When test day arrives, you'll be ready.

Start with the strategies you've read in the first two Secret Keys—plan your course and study in the way that works best for you. If you have time, consider using multiple study resources to get different approaches to the same concepts. It can be helpful to see difficult concepts from more than one angle. Then find a good source for practice tests. Many times, the test website will suggest potential study resources or provide sample tests.

Practice Test Strategy

If you're able to find at least three practice tests, we recommend this strategy:

Untimed and Open-Book Practice

Take the first test with no time constraints and with your notes and study guide handy. Take your time and focus on applying the strategies you've learned.

Timed and Open-Book Practice

Take the second practice test open-book as well, but set a timer and practice pacing yourself to finish in time.

Timed and Closed-Book Practice

Take any other practice tests as if it were test day. Set a timer and put away your study materials. Sit at a table or desk in a quiet room, imagine yourself at the testing center, and answer questions as quickly and accurately as possible.

Keep repeating timed and closed-book tests on a regular basis until you run out of practice tests or it's time for the actual test. Your mind will be ready for the schedule and stress of test day, and you'll be able to focus on recalling the material you've learned.

Secret Key #4 – Pace Yourself

Once you're fully prepared for the material on the test, your biggest challenge on test day will be managing your time. Just knowing that the clock is ticking can make you panic even if you have plenty of time left. Work on pacing yourself so you can build confidence against the time constraints of the exam. Pacing is a difficult skill to master, especially in a high-pressure environment, so **practice is vital**.

Set time expectations for your pace based on how much time is available. For example, if a section has 60 questions and the time limit is 30 minutes, you know you have to average 30 seconds or less per question in order to answer them all. Although 30 seconds is the hard limit, set 25 seconds per question as your goal, so you reserve extra time to spend on harder questions. When you budget extra time for the harder questions, you no longer have any reason to stress when those questions take longer to answer.

Don't let this time expectation distract you from working through the test at a calm, steady pace, but keep it in mind so you don't spend too much time on any one question. Recognize that taking extra time on one question you don't understand may keep you from answering two that you do understand later in the test. If your time limit for a question is up and you're still not sure of the answer, mark it and move on, and come back to it later if the time and the test format allow. If the testing format doesn't allow you to return to earlier questions, just make an educated guess; then put it out of your mind and move on.

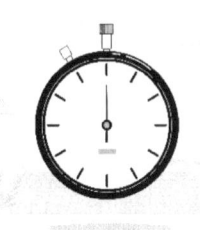

On the easier questions, be careful not to rush. It may seem wise to hurry through them so you have more time for the challenging ones, but it's not worth missing one if you know the concept and just didn't take the time to read the question fully. Work efficiently but make sure you understand the question and have looked at all of the answer choices, since more than one may seem right at first.

Even if you're paying attention to the time, you may find yourself a little behind at some point. You should speed up to get back on track, but do so wisely. Don't panic; just take a few seconds less on each question until you're caught up. Don't guess without thinking, but do look through the answer choices and eliminate any you know are wrong. If you can get down to two choices, it is often worthwhile to guess from those. Once you've chosen an answer, move on and don't dwell on any that you skipped or had to hurry through. If a question was taking too long, chances are it was one of the harder ones, so you weren't as likely to get it right anyway.

On the other hand, if you find yourself getting ahead of schedule, it may be beneficial to slow down a little. The more quickly you work, the more likely you are to make a careless mistake that will affect your score. You've budgeted time for each question, so don't be afraid to spend that time. Practice an efficient but careful pace to get the most out of the time you have.

Secret Key #5 – Have a Plan for Guessing

When you're taking the test, you may find yourself stuck on a question. Some of the answer choices seem better than others, but you don't see the one answer choice that is obviously correct. What do you do?

The scenario described above is very common, yet most test takers have not effectively prepared for it. Developing and practicing a plan for guessing may be one of the single most effective uses of your time as you get ready for the exam.

In developing your plan for guessing, there are three questions to address:

- When should you start the guessing process?
- How should you narrow down the choices?
- Which answer should you choose?

When to Start the Guessing Process

Unless your plan for guessing is to select C every time (which, despite its merits, is not what we recommend), you need to leave yourself enough time to apply your answer elimination strategies. Since you have a limited amount of time for each question, that means that if you're going to give yourself the best shot at guessing correctly, you have to decide quickly whether or not you will guess.

Of course, the best-case scenario is that you don't have to guess at all, so first, see if you can answer the question based on your knowledge of the subject and basic reasoning skills. Focus on the key words in the question and try to jog your memory of related topics. Give yourself a chance to bring the knowledge to mind, but once you realize that you don't have (or you can't access) the knowledge you need to answer the question, it's time to start the guessing process.

It's almost always better to start the guessing process too early than too late. It only takes a few seconds to remember something and answer the question from knowledge. Carefully eliminating wrong answer choices takes longer. Plus, going through the process of eliminating answer choices can actually help jog your memory.

Summary: Start the guessing process as soon as you decide that you can't answer the question based on your knowledge.

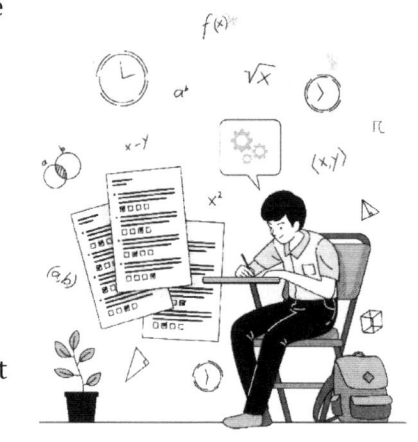

How to Narrow Down the Choices

The next chapter in this book (**Test-Taking Strategies**) includes a wide range of strategies for how to approach questions and how to look for answer choices to eliminate. You will definitely want to read those carefully, practice them, and figure out which ones work best for you. Here though, we're going to address a mindset rather than a particular strategy.

Your odds of guessing an answer correctly depend on how many options you are choosing from.

Number of options left	5	4	3	2	1
Odds of guessing correctly	20%	25%	33%	50%	100%

You can see from this chart just how valuable it is to be able to eliminate incorrect answers and make an educated guess, but there are two things that many test takers do that cause them to miss out on the benefits of guessing:

- Accidentally eliminating the correct answer
- Selecting an answer based on an impression

We'll look at the first one here, and the second one in the next section.

To avoid accidentally eliminating the correct answer, we recommend a thought exercise called **the $5 challenge**. In this challenge, you only eliminate an answer choice from contention if you are willing to bet $5 on it being wrong. Why $5? Five dollars is a small but not insignificant amount of money. It's an amount you could afford to lose but wouldn't want to throw away. And while losing $5 once might not hurt too much, doing it twenty times will set you back $100. In the same way, each small decision you make—eliminating a choice here, guessing on a question there—won't by itself impact your score very much, but when you put them all together, they can make a big difference. By holding each answer choice elimination decision to a higher standard, you can reduce the risk of accidentally eliminating the correct answer.

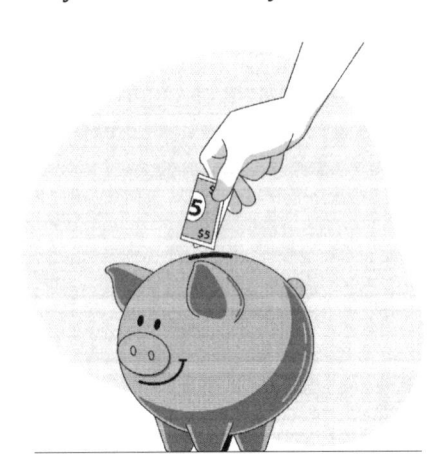

The $5 challenge can also be applied in a positive sense: If you are willing to bet $5 that an answer choice *is* correct, go ahead and mark it as correct.

Summary: Only eliminate an answer choice if you are willing to bet $5 that it is wrong.

Which Answer to Choose

You're taking the test. You've run into a hard question and decided you'll have to guess. You've eliminated all the answer choices you're willing to bet $5 on. Now you have to pick an answer. Why do we even need to talk about this? Why can't you just pick whichever one you feel like when the time comes?

The answer to these questions is that if you don't come into the test with a plan, you'll rely on your impression to select an answer choice, and if you do that, you risk falling into a trap. The test writers know that everyone who takes their test will be guessing on some of the questions, so they intentionally write wrong answer choices to seem plausible. You still have to pick an answer though, and if the wrong answer choices are designed to look right, how can you ever be sure that you're not falling for their trap? The best solution we've found to this dilemma is to take the decision out of your hands entirely. Here is the process we recommend:

Once you've eliminated any choices that you are confident (willing to bet $5) are wrong, select the first remaining choice as your answer.

Whether you choose to select the first remaining choice, the second, or the last, the important thing is that you use some preselected standard. Using this approach guarantees that you will not be enticed into selecting an answer choice that looks right, because you are not basing your decision on how the answer choices look.

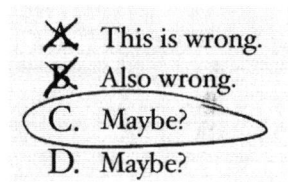

This is not meant to make you question your knowledge. Instead, it is to help you recognize the difference between your knowledge and your impressions. There's a huge difference between thinking an answer is right because of what you know, and thinking an answer is right because it looks or sounds like it should be right.

Summary: To ensure that your selection is appropriately random, make a predetermined selection from among all answer choices you have not eliminated.

Test-Taking Strategies

This section contains a list of test-taking strategies that you may find helpful as you work through the test. By taking what you know and applying logical thought, you can maximize your chances of answering any question correctly!

It is very important to realize that every question is different and every person is different: no single strategy will work on every question, and no single strategy will work for every person. That's why we've included all of them here, so you can try them out and determine which ones work best for different types of questions and which ones work best for you.

Question Strategies

ⓘ READ CAREFULLY

Read the question and the answer choices carefully. Don't miss the question because you misread the terms. You have plenty of time to read each question thoroughly and make sure you understand what is being asked. Yet a happy medium must be attained, so don't waste too much time. You must read carefully and efficiently.

ⓘ CONTEXTUAL CLUES

Look for contextual clues. If the question includes a word you are not familiar with, look at the immediate context for some indication of what the word might mean. Contextual clues can often give you all the information you need to decipher the meaning of an unfamiliar word. Even if you can't determine the meaning, you may be able to narrow down the possibilities enough to make a solid guess at the answer to the question.

ⓘ PREFIXES

If you're having trouble with a word in the question or answer choices, try dissecting it. Take advantage of every clue that the word might include. Prefixes can be a huge help. Usually, they allow you to determine a basic meaning. *Pre-* means before, *post-* means after, *pro-* is positive, *de-* is negative. From prefixes, you can get an idea of the general meaning of the word and try to put it into context.

ⓘ HEDGE WORDS

Watch out for critical hedge words, such as *likely, may, can, sometimes, often, almost, mostly, usually, generally, rarely,* and *sometimes*. Question writers insert these hedge phrases to cover every possibility. Often an answer choice will be wrong simply because it leaves no room for exception. Be on guard for answer choices that have definitive words such as *exactly* and *always*.

ⓘ SWITCHBACK WORDS

Stay alert for *switchbacks*. These are the words and phrases frequently used to alert you to shifts in thought. The most common switchback words are *but, although,* and *however*. Others include *nevertheless, on the other hand, even though, while, in spite of, despite,* and *regardless of*. Switchback words are important to catch because they can change the direction of the question or an answer choice.

⊘ Face Value

When in doubt, use common sense. Accept the situation in the problem at face value. Don't read too much into it. These problems will not require you to make wild assumptions. If you have to go beyond creativity and warp time or space in order to have an answer choice fit the question, then you should move on and consider the other answer choices. These are normal problems rooted in reality. The applicable relationship or explanation may not be readily apparent, but it is there for you to figure out. Use your common sense to interpret anything that isn't clear.

Answer Choice Strategies

⊘ Answer Selection

The most thorough way to pick an answer choice is to identify and eliminate wrong answers until only one is left, then confirm it is the correct answer. Sometimes an answer choice may immediately seem right, but be careful. The test writers will usually put more than one reasonable answer choice on each question, so take a second to read all of them and make sure that the other choices are not equally obvious. As long as you have time left, it is better to read every answer choice than to pick the first one that looks right without checking the others.

⊘ Answer Choice Families

An answer choice family consists of two (in rare cases, three) answer choices that are very similar in construction and cannot all be true at the same time. If you see two answer choices that are direct opposites or parallels, one of them is usually the correct answer. For instance, if one answer choice says that quantity *x* increases and another either says that quantity *x* decreases (opposite) or says that quantity *y* increases (parallel), then those answer choices would fall into the same family. An answer choice that doesn't match the construction of the answer choice family is more likely to be incorrect. Most questions will not have answer choice families, but when they do appear, you should be prepared to recognize them.

⊘ Eliminate Answers

Eliminate answer choices as soon as you realize they are wrong, but make sure you consider all possibilities. If you are eliminating answer choices and realize that the last one you are left with is also wrong, don't panic. Start over and consider each choice again. There may be something you missed the first time that you will realize on the second pass.

⊘ Avoid Fact Traps

Don't be distracted by an answer choice that is factually true but doesn't answer the question. You are looking for the choice that answers the question. Stay focused on what the question is asking for so you don't accidentally pick an answer that is true but incorrect. Always go back to the question and make sure the answer choice you've selected actually answers the question and is not merely a true statement.

⊘ Extreme Statements

In general, you should avoid answers that put forth extreme actions as standard practice or proclaim controversial ideas as established fact. An answer choice that states the "process should be used in certain situations, if…" is much more likely to be correct than one that states the "process should be discontinued completely." The first is a calm rational statement and doesn't even make a definitive, uncompromising stance, using a hedge word *if* to provide wiggle room, whereas the second choice is far more extreme.

☑ Benchmark

As you read through the answer choices and you come across one that seems to answer the question well, mentally select that answer choice. This is not your final answer, but it's the one that will help you evaluate the other answer choices. The one that you selected is your benchmark or standard for judging each of the other answer choices. Every other answer choice must be compared to your benchmark. That choice is correct until proven otherwise by another answer choice beating it. If you find a better answer, then that one becomes your new benchmark. Once you've decided that no other choice answers the question as well as your benchmark, you have your final answer.

☑ Predict the Answer

Before you even start looking at the answer choices, it is often best to try to predict the answer. When you come up with the answer on your own, it is easier to avoid distractions and traps because you will know exactly what to look for. The right answer choice is unlikely to be word-for-word what you came up with, but it should be a close match. Even if you are confident that you have the right answer, you should still take the time to read each option before moving on.

General Strategies

☑ Tough Questions

If you are stumped on a problem or it appears too hard or too difficult, don't waste time. Move on! Remember though, if you can quickly check for obviously incorrect answer choices, your chances of guessing correctly are greatly improved. Before you completely give up, at least try to knock out a couple of possible answers. Eliminate what you can and then guess at the remaining answer choices before moving on.

☑ Check Your Work

Since you will probably not know every term listed and the answer to every question, it is important that you get credit for the ones that you do know. Don't miss any questions through careless mistakes. If at all possible, try to take a second to look back over your answer selection and make sure you've selected the correct answer choice and haven't made a costly careless mistake (such as marking an answer choice that you didn't mean to mark). This quick double check should more than pay for itself in caught mistakes for the time it costs.

☑ Pace Yourself

It's easy to be overwhelmed when you're looking at a page full of questions; your mind is confused and full of random thoughts, and the clock is ticking down faster than you would like. Calm down and maintain the pace that you have set for yourself. Especially as you get down to the last few minutes of the test, don't let the small numbers on the clock make you panic. As long as you are on track by monitoring your pace, you are guaranteed to have time for each question.

☑ Don't Rush

It is very easy to make errors when you are in a hurry. Maintaining a fast pace in answering questions is pointless if it makes you miss questions that you would have gotten right otherwise. Test writers like to include distracting information and wrong answers that seem right. Taking a little extra time to avoid careless mistakes can make all the difference in your test score. Find a pace that allows you to be confident in the answers that you select.

⏱ Keep Moving

Panicking will not help you pass the test, so do your best to stay calm and keep moving. Taking deep breaths and going through the answer elimination steps you practiced can help to break through a stress barrier and keep your pace.

Final Notes

The combination of a solid foundation of content knowledge and the confidence that comes from practicing your plan for applying that knowledge is the key to maximizing your performance on test day. As your foundation of content knowledge is built up and strengthened, you'll find that the strategies included in this chapter become more and more effective in helping you quickly sift through the distractions and traps of the test to isolate the correct answer.

Now that you're preparing to move forward into the test content chapters of this book, be sure to keep your goal in mind. As you read, think about how you will be able to apply this information on the test. If you've already seen sample questions for the test and you have an idea of the question format and style, try to come up with questions of your own that you can answer based on what you're reading. This will give you valuable practice applying your knowledge in the same ways you can expect to on test day.

Good luck and good studying!

Injury/Illness Prevention and Wellness Promotion

IDENTIFYING RISK FACTORS

Identifying risks to the physically active population is beneficial because it provides the athletic trainer a way to recognize potential injuries before they occur and devise ways to prevent them. For example, assessments can identify biomechanical errors patients may be making such as lifting with straight legs and a bent back, which leads to back injuries. Pre-participation exams can identify patients' preexisting injuries, areas of weakness, and inflexibility. After recognition, the athletic trainer can address and correct these areas of concern with therapeutic exercises before the patient develops a new injury related to these biomechanical limitations. Reviewing injury surveillance data allows the athletic trainer to be cognizant of common injuries in different physical activities. Preventative actions can then be taken such as developing specific physical training and conditioning plans and ensuring a safe training environment to prevent those injuries from occurring.

WARM-UP EXERCISES

Warm-up exercises, performed for 15-30 minutes, should be the first part of any training exercise or participation in sports activities in order to increase circulation and muscle elasticity and prevent injury. Warm-up should begin slowly and then proceed systematically to involve all parts of the body. There are different types of warm-up activities:

- Passive: for example, massage and warm showers
- General body-wide: for example, jogging
- Specific stretching motions: While it's important to stretch and warm-up all muscles, special attention should be paid to the muscles most used in the sports activity, such as swinging the arm and throwing a ball in preparation for pitching. Stretching should be bilateral, held 10-30 seconds, and static rather than ballistic.

Warm-up activities often include a combination of exercise activities, such as slow running for 3-5 minutes to increase muscle circulation, 10 minutes of general stretching to improve muscle elasticity, and 10 minutes of specific pre-conditioning exercises for the particular sport. Athletes should be wearing proper clothing and footwear during warm-up exercises.

STRENGTH TRAINING AND WEIGHTLIFTING AND SAFETY HAZARDS

Strength training and weightlifting utilize the same equipment, such as free weights and weight machines, but the goals are different. Strength training aims to improve physical conditioning, while weightlifting (not recommended for children or adolescents) is a competitive sport that involves lifting maximal amounts of weight. There are a number of steps that should be taken to reduce safety hazards:

- Exercise equipment should be checked daily and cleaned to ensure it is safe.
- Instruction in lifting techniques and supervision should be provided.
- Athletes should be advised to do warm-up and stretching exercises before using equipment.
- Use of weights and equipment should be based on age- and size-appropriate standards to prevent injury.
- Weightlifting requires a spotter at all times.

- One or more spotters must assist with free-weight exercises in which the bar passes over the face or head, the athlete is positioned on his back, or the bar is racked in front of the shoulders.

BODY PLANES

Understanding the **planes** of the body is helpful when describing the motions and the body parts used by an athlete. Also, knowledge of body planes can help a trainer ensure that the athlete utilizes his or her body properly to avoid strain. The three major planes with examples are listed below:

- Frontal (coronal): Divides the body or parts into anterior (front) and posterior (rear) sections
- Arm during backstroke in swimming
- Transverse (horizontal): Divides the body or parts into superior (upper) and inferior (lower) sections
- Bat swing in baseball
- Movement of criterion arm in basketball jump shot
- Movement of criterion arm in forehand drive in tennis
- Median (Mid-sagittal/ lateral): Divides the body or parts into right and left sections.
    - Movement of criterion arm during serve in tennis
    - Pulling arms upward

MUSCLE CONTRACTIONS

Muscles usually contract (shorten) to create force, but there are a number of different types of **contractions** that must be understood by the athlete and by trainers:

- Isotonic (concentric and eccentric) contractions involve movement of the muscle as when pushing or pulling. Isotonic exercises usually balance concentric and eccentric contractions.
    - Concentric contractions cause the muscle to shorten, as occurs when the muscle is used to lift a weight, as with a bicep curl.
    - Eccentric contractions cause the muscle to lengthen, as occurs when lowering the weight.
- Isometric contractions occur without muscle movement, as when attempting to push or pull an immoveable object, tightening the muscle, or holding an object out in front of the body so that the weight pushes down but the muscle's opposing force keeps the object stable.
- "Passive stretch" contractions result in stretching when the muscle lengthens without stimulation to contract, such as the pull on the hamstrings when bending over to touch the toes.

RANGE OF MOVEMENT

Each part of the body has a **range of movement**. Exceeding the normal range can result in strains or sprains. The basic movements are as follows:

- *Flexion:* bending, as the back flexes bending forward
- *Extension:* movement drawing two ends of a jointed part or extensor in separate directions, as when the arms stretch straight
- *Abduction:* drawing away from the medial plane of the body, as when the arm lifts away from the side of the body
- *Adduction:* drawing toward the medial plane of the body, as when a leg crosses inward

- **Rotation:** turning around the medial line, as when standing still and turning the upper body from side to side
- **Pronation**: positioning face down while lying on the back or palms down
- **Supination**: positioning face up when lying on the back or palms up
- **Elevation**: raising upward, as in lifting shoulders forward
- **Depression**: lowering, as in pulling shoulders backward
- **Circumduction**: circular movement of limb or eye, as when moving arms in circles
- **Inversion**: turning inward
- **Eversion**: turning outward

ENDURANCE TRAINING
AEROBIC ENDURANCE TRAINING

The purpose of **endurance training** is to increase the production of energy to meet demands of athletic activities, such as running, swimming, and cycling. One of the goals of endurance training is to increase the maximal volume of oxygen uptake (VO2 max) and the lactate threshold. The VO2 max is primarily determined genetically, but with endurance training it can be increased about 20%. The lactate threshold level, at which aerobic activity becomes anaerobic and produces an abundance of lactate acid, is around 65% of maximum heart rate, but may be 80-90% in athletes:

- *Aerobic endurance activities*: Body's supply of oxygen and energy can keep pace with demands. Waste products are carbon dioxide (expelled through expiration) and water (expelled through sweating). Endurance activities may be short (2-8 minutes), medium (8-30 minutes), or long (30 minutes or longer). Exercises that increase aerobic endurance include continuous running (20-30 minutes) to increase oxygen uptake and interval training (three to five 10-minute periods with 2-3-minute rest intervals) to strengthen the heart muscle.

ANAEROBIC ENDURANCE TRAINING

While most activities are aerobic, building anaerobic endurance is an important part of fitness:

- *Anaerobic endurance activities*: During anaerobic activity, the demands for oxygen and energy exceed that available so the body burns stored energy and lactic acid begins to accumulate. As energy stores are depleted, usually within about 4 seconds, activity ceases and the muscles react with pain. Endurance activities are classified as short (<25 seconds), medium (25-60 seconds), or long (1-2 minutes). Short-distance running, such as 200 meters, is about 5% aerobic and 95% anaerobic. The longer the distance, the greater the shift to aerobic: a 5000-meter run is 80% aerobic and 20% anaerobic. Marathon running is only 2% anaerobic. The goal of anaerobic activity is to increase anaerobic endurance through high-intensity repetitive exercises with a short recovery period.

SPEED AND STRENGTH ENDURANCE TRAINING

- *Speed:* The goal of speed endurance is to increase the athlete's ability to run repeated high-speed sprints of short distances, improving coordination of muscle contractions. Repetitive running is used to increase endurance, including competitive running and participation in timed trials.

- *Strength:* The goal of strength endurance is to improve and maintain muscle contractions and force. Strength is essential for all athletes. Exercises to increase strength include weight training, hill and harness running, and Fartlek training, during which athletes run with varying the speed and intensity. For example, they may jog for 10 minutes, and then do a 2-mile hilly course, running up hills and jogging between, followed by a final 10-minute jog. Alternately, the coach may use a whistle to signal a change in pace.

NORMAL PULSE, RESPIRATION RATE, BLOOD PRESSURE, AND TEMPERATURE FOR ADULTS AND CHILDREN

The normal pulse for adults is between 60 to 100 beats per minute and 80 to 100 for children. Athletes may have a slower pulse rate due to physical conditioning. A faint, fast pulse could signify shock, heat exhaustion, bleeding, or a diabetic coma. A hard, slow pulse could signify stroke or a skull fracture.

The normal respiration rate for adults is between 12 to 20 breaths per minute and 15 to 30 for children. Shallow breathing could signify shock while coughing up blood signifies a chest injury such as a punctured lung.

The normal resting blood pressure is below 120mm mercury (Hg) for the systolic blood pressure and below 80mm Hg for the diastolic blood pressure. Females generally have a lower blood pressure than males of 8-10mm Hg for both systolic and diastolic measurements. A low blood pressure could signify bleeding, shock, organ injury or a heart attack.

The normal body temperature for both adults and children is between 98.2 and 98.6 degrees Fahrenheit. A rise in temperature could indicate an infection or a heat illness. A lowered body temperature could signify hypothermia.

USING PRE-PARTICIPATION EXAMINATIONS TO DETECT MEDICAL CONDITIONS DISQUALIFYING ATHLETES FROM PARTICIPATION IN SPORTS

The pre-participation examination screens athletes for potentially life-threatening conditions by asking pertinent medical questions and providing a thorough physical examination. Most conditions that warrant disqualification from sport participation should be identifiable during the pre-participation examination. The physician and organization have a legal basis to disqualify an athlete from participating in a sport if the decision to disqualify is specific to the patient, reasonable, and based on proficient medical evidence. This was determined by the case Knapp vs. Northwestern University.

The Committee on Sports Medicine recommends disqualifying an athlete from participation in contact sports if they have one of the following medical conditions; atlantoaxial instability, cardiovascular carditis, an enlarged liver, poorly controlled compulsive disorder, and an enlarged spleen. There are many other medical conditions that could be disqualifying based on the specific history of the patient.

The pre-participation examination consists of the following components:

- Medical history: Contains questions about medical conditions, family history, and is used to recognize conditions that may predispose athletes to injury. The medical history should be completed prior to the physical and orthopedic screenings and with assistance of parents if the athlete is a minor.
- Physical examination: Consists of height, weight, body composition, pulse, and blood pressure.

- Cardiovascular screening: The physician reviews the medical history as related to the heart and listens for abnormal heart sounds using auscultation.
- Orthopedic screening: An examination used to recognize musculoskeletal conditions in which the patient performs movements as instructed by the examiner while the examiner observes the quality of movements.
- General medical screening: A physical screening performed by the physician to include examination of the eyes, ears, nose, throat, abdomen, lymph nodes and skin. A maturity assessment should be performed as well as a review of all medications and supplements.
- Wellness screening: Contains questions that assess healthy behaviors related to nutrition, alcohol, drugs, stress control, and safety measures the patient takes.

Developing an Athletic Training Clinic's Policies and Procedures Manual

A policies and procedures manual should be developed in cooperation with all stakeholders and based the organization's vision and mission statements. The policies state rules and principles the organization abides by while the procedures articulate how processes will be done.

Policies and procedures manuals should be very thorough and include both program operations and human resources issues. Program operations that should be developed are objectives for the program, how the organizational structure will be laid out, the scope of practice, accepted referral procedures, documentation protocols, budget expectations, and emergency planning.

Human resources issues to include in the policies and procedures manual are job descriptions, how employee evaluations will be conducted, expected dress code, hiring procedures, and firing practices.

Behavioral Risks Involved with Physical Activity

There are many behavioral risks athletic trainers must be aware of to provide the best available care to the physically active population. Overtraining can occur when the physiological and psychological stresses placed on an individual outweigh their coping mechanisms, which can lead to staleness and burnout. Athletic trainers should be aware of signs and symptoms of each and be able to offer referrals and coping mechanisms as needed.

The nutritional needs of the physically active population must be met for patient safety and optimal performance. Athletic trainers must be aware of signs and symptoms of various eating disorders such as anorexia nervosa and refer patients as required. Athletic trainers must also be able to offer sound general nutritional advice as well as pre-game meal recommendations. Substance abuse is a concern athletic trainers must be aware of and be ready to provide immediate care and refer patients as required.

Catastrophic Risks Involved in Physical Activity

Various catastrophic risks exist when participating in physical activity. The athletic trainer must be cognizant of all catastrophic risks, work to prevent them, and be prepared to provide immediate and appropriate care should a patient suffer from a catastrophic injury or illness. Commotio cordis is a catastrophic injury that can occur to apparently healthy individuals and, unfortunately, about half of patients who suffer from commotio cordis suffer immediate death. The mechanism of injury for commotio cordis is a blow to the chest that occurs at a specific point in the repolarization phase of the cardiac cycle, 15 to 30 milliseconds before the peak of the T wave occurs. Usually, this blow results in ventricular fibrillation, making immediate defibrillation and resuscitation essential to reduce mortality rates.

Exertional heatstroke, caused by physical activity performed in a hot environment, is a serious heat illness that can lead to death. Exertional heatstroke requires immediate and appropriate care to increase patients' chances of survival. The patient's body temperature becomes extremely elevated, inhibiting the body's thermoregulatory system. If a patient is suspected to be suffering from exertional heatstroke, they should be immersed in a cold-water bath immediately until their body temperature is lowered to 102 degrees Fahrenheit. Once their body temperature is lowered, they must be transported for immediate, advanced medical care.

Musculoskeletal Risks Involved with Physical Activity

There are many types of musculoskeletal risks involved with participation in physical activity and athletic trainers must be able not only to recognize and treat these injuries, but also work to prevent them. Muscle strains occur when a muscle is stretched forcefully beyond its anatomical limits, or contracts against a resistance that is beyond its capabilities. These forces result in excessive stretching and tearing of the muscle fibers. Ligament sprains occur when a force is placed on a joint beyond its anatomical limits, resulting in excessive stretching and tearing of the ligaments. Sprains and strains can be prevented in many ways. A proper warm-up should always be incorporated with physical activity, flexibility exercises should be performed, strength training should be included, and athletes should be offered education on proper body positioning to prevent strains and sprains.

Referring Athletes for Further Evaluation Following a Pre-Participation Physical Examination

There are many possible reasons to refer an athlete for specialized care following a pre-participation physical examination. For example, patients with signs and symptoms of eating disorders should be referred to a mental health practitioner. Athletes with heart arrhythmias should be referred to a cardiologist. Athletes with body asymmetries or abnormalities that may lead to injuries should be referred to the appropriate healthcare provider who could work to correct the asymmetry. For example, athletes with flat feet or leg-length discrepancies could be referred to a podiatrist for orthotics. Athletes with a history of severe head traumas should be referred to a neurologist. Athletes who report symptoms of psychological concerns should be referred to a mental health provider.

Principles of Conditioning That Can Be Applied to Lower the Risk of Injury

- Safety: Ensure the area is free of safety hazards, and conditioning equipment is functioning properly. Athletes should be educated how to properly perform exercises and how to recognize normal and abnormal sensations when exercising.
- Warm-up and cool-down: Prior to the workout, the athlete's blood flow to working muscles should be gradually elevated by performing a dynamic warm-up routine. At the conclusion of the workout, exercise intensity should be gradually reduced and stretching should be incorporated.
- Motivation: Integrate variety into the training program using sport-specific periodization training to alleviate boredom and increase compliance.
- Overload: The body must be overloaded within a safe realm to respond to those demands and get stronger. The SAID (specific adaptations to imposed demands) principle is directly related to the overload principle.
- Consistency: Exercises must be done regularly and repeatedly to make and maintain improvements.
- Progression: Increasing demands should be placed on the body as appropriate to advance physically.

- Intensity: Exercise intensity should be stressed over an unnecessarily long workout.
- Specificity: Exercises should be chosen to improve athletes' specific sport and position performances.
- Individuality: Exercises should be selected based on the needs and preferences of the individual.
- Minimal stress: Be cognizant of stressors in athletes' lives and allow time away from conditioning as needed.

HEALTHY WEIGHT LOSS AND WEIGHT GAIN

Weight loss: For safe and effective weight loss, a combination of diet and exercise is recommended. Calories consumed may be reduced by 500 to 1,000 calories per day. However, females should consume at least 1,000-1,200 calories per day and males should consume at least 1,200 to 1,400 calories per day. Exercises should be performed for 30 to 45 minutes, 3 to 5 days a week. Weight loss goals should be 1-2 pounds per week and focus on long-term lifestyle changes.

Weight gain: The goal of a weight-gaining program is to increase lean muscle tissue, not body fat. This is achieved through an increase in muscle work with an increase in caloric intake. It is recommended to increase caloric consumption by 500-1,000 calories per day to gain 1 to 2 pounds of muscle tissue per week. Weight training must be included in the weight-gaining program, or the extra calories consumed will be stored as fat, not lean muscle tissue.

ERGONOMICS AND ERGONOMIC RISK ASSESSMENT (ERA)

Ergonomics combines knowledge of muscular activity and human measurement to design workplaces that increase functionality and decrease the risk of injury. An ergonomic risk assessment (ERA) reviews different jobs, identifies which jobs have the highest risk of injury, and address those first. This is done by reviewing the history of injuries, worker complaints, and performing a physical-demands analysis.

After performing an ERA, the athletic trainer would make appropriate adjustments to the workstation, educate about injury prevention techniques, and demonstrate appropriate stretches and strengthening exercises. Recommendations should be made to the worker, the supervisor, and the manager so that all involved parties know what preventative steps should be taken. Common factors that contribute to workplace injuries and are corrected during the ERA are repetitive movements, improper workplace setup, vibrations, twisting, reaching, bending, and other problematic body positions.

STRENGTH OF RECOMMENDATION TAXONOMY (SORT) RATINGS

Research of various qualities are available, so rating systems have been devised to help medical professionals more easily identify the quality of the research. The Strength of Recommendation Taxonomy (SORT) rating scale has been accepted for use by the NATA. The SORT rating scale evaluates research based on validity and the level of evidence the research provides. This scale gives grades of either A, B, or C to research. A SORT rating of an A means that the research is consistent, of good quality, and focuses on the needs of the patient. A rating of a B indicates research is inconsistent while still being focused on patient-outcomes. Finally, a rating of a C indicates that research is disease-oriented, based on expert opinion, or may be a case-study.

INJURY SURVEILLANCE DATA

Sports injury data is collected by multiple organizations and athletic trainers can use this information for many purposes. Injury surveillance data can be used to recognize injury trends and compare the injury statistics of the athletic trainer's organization against national statistical norms.

It can also be used to educate all stakeholders about the inherent risks in sports, and has been used to make rule changes to make sports safer.

There are many organizations that collect injury data but the ones most frequently used are the National Safety Council, the NCAA Injury Surveillance System, the National High School Sport-Related Injury Surveillance Study, the Annual Survey of Football Injury Research, the National Center for Catastrophic Sports Injury Research, and the National Electronic Injury Surveillance System. Athletic trainers are the primary reporters of injury data for both the NCAA Injury Surveillance System and the National High School Sports-Related Injury Surveillance Data.

HEAT-RELATED ILLNESS

There are 3 types of **heat-related illness**:

- *Heat stress:* Increased temperature causes dehydration. Athletes may develop swollen hands and feet, itchy skin, sunburn, heat syncope (pale moist skin, hypotension), and heat cramps. *Treatment* includes removing from heat, cooling, hydrating, and replacing sodium.
- *Heat exhaustion:* Involves water or sodium depletion; this condition is common in children and teenagers who are not acclimated to heat. Heat exhaustion can result in flu-like aching, nausea and vomiting, headaches, dizziness, and hypotension with cold clammy skin and diaphoresis. Temperature may be normal or elevated but less than 105°. *Treatment* to cool the body and replace sodium and fluids must be prompt in order to prevent heat stroke. Careful monitoring is important, as reactions may be delayed.
- *Heat stroke:* Involves failure of the thermoregulatory system with temperatures that may be greater than 105°F; may result in seizures, neurological damage, multiple organ failures and death. Exertional heat stroke often occurs in young athletes who engage in strenuous activities in high heat. *Treatment* includes evaporative cooling, rehydration, and immediate emergency transfer.

VULNERABILITIES OF HEAT-RELATED ILLNESS

Athletes are at particular risk of **heat-related illnesses** (hyperthermia) and must learn preventive steps and be advised to monitor other team members. About 65% of heat is lost through evaporation during exercise, but heat dissipates less readily in, hot humid environments and when the athlete is wearing wet, sweaty clothes. There are a number of steps to prevent heat loss:

- Utilize the wet bulb globe temperature index, which monitors the effects of humidity, temperature, and solar energy to determine risks.
- Identify athletes at high risk, such as those with diabetes mellitus or who are overweight.
- Provide adequate hydration: 16 oz of fluid (sports drink, not sodas) before activity and 8 oz every 20 minutes during activity to prevent thirst. Pre-and post-activity weight measurement, with 16 oz of fluid taken for every 1-pound loss of weight.
- Allow time for acclimatization (7-10 days).
- Monitor for signs of hyperthermia.
- Provide 10-minute breaks at least every hour.
- Promote evaporation: Change wet t-shirts.
- Provide shelter.

HYPOTHERMIA

Athletes who participate in sports or training during cold weather are at risk for frostbite and **hypothermia** and should be educated about signs of hypothermia and preventive safety measures. **Hypothermia** occurs with exposure to low temperatures that cause the core body temperature to fall below 95°F (35°C). Hypothermia may be associated with immersion in cold water, exposure to cold temperatures, metabolic disorders (hypothyroidism, hypoglycemia, hypoadrenalism), or central nervous system abnormalities (head trauma, Wernicke disease). Many patients with hypothermia are intoxicated with alcohol or drugs. *Symptoms* of hypothermia include pallor, cold skin, drowsiness, alteration in mental status, confusion, and severe shivering. Any numbness requires immediate attention. The patient can progress to shock, coma, cardiac abnormalities, and cardiac arrest. Frostbite occurs when the tissue begins to freeze, usually signaled by burning pain and numbness in the affected area, while hypothermia usually begins with shivering as the body's core temperature drops.

Safety measures to prevent **hypothermia** include:

- Wearing clothes that are appropriate for the environment, temperature, and chill index, as wind and humidity increase heat loss.
- Doing warm-up exercises to increase circulation.
- Beginning exercises slowly and avoiding slippery surfaces.
- Removing any wet clothes promptly and replacing with dry clothes.
- Avoiding accumulation of moisture in clothing by overheating.
- Wearing clothes in layers that allow for ventilation.
- Ensuring that the head and neck are well covered, as 50% of heat loss is from the head and neck.
- Wearing mittens or gloves appropriate for the temperature and conditions.
- Wearing moisture-wicking socks, such as those made of wool or polypropylene, to keep feet dry.
- Avoiding alcohol, which results in vasodilation, increased heat loss and impaired reasoning.

FROSTNIP AND FROSTBITE

Frostnip is a superficial freeze injury that is reversible. **Frostbite** is damage to tissue caused by exposure to freezing temperatures, most often affecting the nose, ears, and distal extremities. As frostbite develops, the affected part feels numb and aches or throbs, becoming hard and insensate as the tissue freezes, resulting in circulatory impairment, necrosis of tissue, and gangrene. There are 3 zones of injury:

- Coagulation (usually distal) is severe irreversible cellular damage.
- Hyperemia (usually proximal) is minimal cellular damage.
- Stasis (between other two zones) is severe, but damage is sometimes reversible.

Symptoms vary according to the degree of freezing:

- Partial freezing with erythema and mild edema, stinging, burning, throbbing pain
- Full thickness freezing with elevated edema in 3-4 hours; edema and clear blisters in 6-24 hours; desquamation with eschar formation and numbness; and then aching and throbbing pain

Prognosis is very good for 1st degree and good for 2nd degree frostbite.

Cold injuries, **frostnip and frostbite** (Part II):

- Full-thickness and into sub-dermal tissue freezing with cyanosis, hemorrhagic blisters, skin necrosis and "wooden" feeling, severe burning, throbbing, and shooting pains
- Freezing extends into subcutaneous tissue, including muscles, tendons, and bones, with mottled appearance, non-blanching cyanosis and eventual deep black eschar

Prognosis is poor for 3rd and 4th degree freeze injuries. Determining the degree of injury can be difficult because some degree of thawing may have occurred prior to hospital admission.

Treatment includes:

- Rapid rewarming with warm water bath (40-42°C, 104-107.6°F), 10-30 minutes or until the frostbitten area is erythematous (red) and pliable
- Treatment for generalized hypothermia

Treatment after warming and debridement of clear blisters:

- Aloe Vera cream every 6 hours to blistered areas
- Dressings, separation of digits
- Tetanus prophylaxis

NEAR DROWNING

Submersion asphyxiation caused by near drowning can cause profound damage to the central nervous system, pulmonary dysfunction related to aspiration, cardiac hypoxia with life-threatening arrhythmias, fluid and electrolyte imbalances, and multi-organ damage. Hypothermia related to near drowning has some protective effect, because blood is shunted to the brain and heart, but this is not likely to occur in a heated swimming pool. Preventive methods include:

- Forbidding roughhousing in the pool area.
- Never swimming or diving alone.
- Never swimming or driving while under the influence of drugs or alcohol.
- Securing pool facilities to prevent unauthorized access.

The person should be removed from the water and CPR begun immediately while awaiting emergency transfer. Even those who recover promptly and are breathing independently should be taken to an emergency department for evaluation, as physiological responses may be delayed.

Initial treatment includes:

- Establishment of airway, breathing and circulation (ABCs).
- High flow 100% oxygen with facemask.
- Monitoring for at least 72 hours for respiratory, cardiac, or neurological deterioration.

COMMUNITY-ACQUIRED METHICILLIN-RESISTANT *STAPHYLOCOCCUS AUREUS* INFECTIONS

Community-acquired methicillin-resistant *Staphylococcus aureus* (CA-MRSA) infections have markedly increased since 2002 and pose a particular risk for athletes, with a number of recorded outbreaks, especially related to football and wrestling. The risk factors for CA-MRSA are known as the 5 Cs:

- Crowding, such as in locker rooms
- Contact, such as occurs in contact sports
- Compromised skin, such as from cuts and scrapes
- Contaminated surfaces, such as equipment, and shared items, such as towels, clothing, razors, and bar soap
- Cleanliness (lack of), including environmental and personal lack of hygiene

Athletes and trainers should be educated to avoid risk factors and report signs of MRSA so that treatment with appropriate antibiotics can be initiated and the infected individual can be isolated from other team members until infection clears. MRSA infections may look like an insect bite initially. Symptoms include:

- Cellulitis or impetigo. Folliculitis, especially on the face, appearing like severe pustular acne. Furunculosis below the hairline. Carbuncles involving hair follicles. Fascitis with abscess formation.

PREPARTICIPATION EXAMINATION REGULATORY REQUIREMENTS

The **preparticipation examination** (PPE) is a procedure that allows the examiner to identify potential health problems related to an athlete's participation in sports. Utilizing national standards helps protect an organization against litigation. A number of organizations have published guidelines related to the need and schedule of PPEs:

- The American Academy of Family Physicians and other medical societies require that the examination be signed by a medical doctor or doctor of osteopathy, but regulations vary from one state to another.
- Athletes must have a PPE before participating in sports in middle school (junior high) and high school and when transferring to a new school, with annual updates and comprehensive exams repeated every 2-3 years.
- The National Collegiate Athletic Association (NCAA) also requires that college athletes have a PPE before participating in intercollegiate sports programs; also, annual updates are required.
- Federal regulations under the Health Information Portability and Accountability Act (HIPAA) allow healthcare providers to share information about an athlete's health condition after the patient or parent signs the permission waiver.

PURPOSE, COMMON CRITICISMS, AND OTHER SCREENING INFORMATION

National organizations, such as the American Medical Association (AMA) and the multi-organizational PPE Task force, have concluded that a **PPE** should perform the following functions:

- Identify athletes at risk of injury or death (especially from cardiac arrest) because of pre-existing medical conditions.
- Disqualify athletes from participation in sports only if there are compelling safety concerns or other reasons.
- Meet regulatory and insurance requirements in order to protect the organization from liability.

However, studies have indicated that the PPE is not always effective in meeting the requirements. The most common indicators of potential injury are a previous history of injury and a lack of physical maturity, so the healthcare provider conducting the PPE should spend adequate time obtaining a history of injury and assessing physical maturity. Only physicians and physician's assistants may assess for adenopathy and hernias.

MEDICAL HISTORY COMPONENT

The **medical history** is a critical component of the PPE, as the information contained within it can signal areas of concern or the need for further evaluation. The medical history should include:

- Previous hospitalizations or surgeries.
- Current or chronic illnesses and medical conditions.
- Current medications and history of illicit/illegal drug use, including steroids. Allergies, as well as the type of response (rash, anaphylaxis), and whether the person carries an Epi-pen.
- Any exercise-induced symptoms, such as dizziness, fainting, dyspnea, cough, or chest pain.
- History of hypertension.
- History of neurological disorders, pinched nerve, seizures, head injury. Cardiac abnormalities, such as palpitations or heart murmur. Vision abnormalities, such as color-blindness, need for prescription glasses or contacts.
- History of menses, including onset, last period, and frequency.
- Orthopedic injuries, past or present, such as fractures, sprains, strains. History of renal disorder including loss of kidney. Loss of eye or testicle. Current vaccinations, including tetanus. Need for accommodations.

CARDIAC ASSESSMENT COMPONENT

While the need for routine electrocardiograms and echocardiograms remains controversial, there is general agreement that athletes should have a thorough **cardiac assessment** to determine if they have cardiac abnormalities (such as hypertrophic cardiomyopathy or coronary artery abnormalities) that might put them at risk of complications or sudden death. Assessment should include:

- Blood pressure to determine if there is elevation of blood pressure,
- Pulse rate: Simultaneous assessment of radial and pulmonary pulses for evidence of delay that may indicate coarctation of aorta. Check for evidence of tachycardia, bradycardia or other abnormalities. Pulse rates less than 60 (sometimes as low as 48) are common in athletes who are physically fit and exercise regularly.
- Auscultation of the heart for evidence of murmurs or abnormal beats.

Athletes with any abnormalities should be referred to a specialist for further testing. Tall athletes (males over 6 feet and females over 5 feet, 10 inches) with two or more signs of Marfan's syndrome should have further evaluation.

Maturity Assessment Component

A **maturity assessment** should be part of the preparticipation examination for children and adolescents to determine their level of sexual, dental, and skeletal maturity. Only a physician or physician's assistant may assess an athlete for sexual maturity.

- Skeletal maturity is usually assessed by measurements of the hand and wrist as well as weight/height for age. Skeletal maturity and chronological age may differ. For example, if the chronological age is 14.3 and the skeletal age is 15.5, this would be expressed as 15.5-14.3 = SA + 1.2. Another method is to divide the skeletal age by the chronological age: a score greater than one indicates advanced skeletal maturity and a score less than one indicates a delay in skeletal maturity.
- The most common assessment tool for sexual maturity is Tanner's 5 stages of assessment. This tool assesses maturity for both males and females, based on direct observation of breasts and genitals:
    - Females: breast development, onset of menses, and pubic hair distribution.
    - Males: Penis and testes development and pubic hair distribution.

Vision Assessment Component

Vision is particularly important to athletes, and a thorough **vision assessment** should be done to determine if there are any abnormalities or disorders of the eye. The examination should include:

- Test for visual acuity.
- Pupillary response to light and accommodation.
- Extraocular muscle motility assessment.
- Test of peripheral vision.
- Ophthalmoscopic examination of inner eye.

Common refractive disorders of the eye include:

- Myopia: nearsightedness
- Hyperopia: farsightedness
- Astigmatism: Distortion of vision

Athletes with refractive disorders may require referral for corrective lenses, including contact lenses, which can be worn with protective goggles. Special sports contact lenses (both prescription and non-prescription) are now available and are used increasingly by athletes to block certain wavelengths and remove glare. These specialized lenses are intended primarily for outdoor use.

Q Angle Assessment Component

Females often differ biomechanically from males, putting them more at risk for injury. For example, females tend to have a wider pelvis than males, resulting in an increased **Q (quadriceps femoralis) angle**. When the athlete is standing, an imaginary straight line is drawn from the anterior superior iliac spine down the anterior thigh (femur), through and past the center point of the patella. A second line is drawn from the center point of the patella to the tibial tubercle, and then the angle between the two lines is measured at the point of the tibial tubercle. Normal angles:

- Male 13°
- Females 15°

An increased Q angle can result in increased knee stress. Female athletes experience 2-4 times the number of injuries to the anterior cruciate ligament (ACL) than male athletes. If an increased Q angle is found, the athlete may need flexible custom orthotics to prevent pronation of the foot, knee support, and a program of strength-building exercises for quadriceps and hamstrings.

BMI Assessment Component

The **Body Mass Index (BMI)** formula is a measurement that uses height and weight as an indicator of obesity/malnutrition. This can-not be used alone to diagnose obesity because body types differ. Women often have more body fat than men. Tables are available to make calculations simple, but the BMI can be calculated manually:

- BMI formula using pounds and inches:

$$BMI = \frac{(Weight\ in\ pounds) \times 703}{(Height\ in\ inches)^2}$$

- BMI formula using kilograms and meters:

$$BMI = \frac{Weight\ in\ kilograms}{(Height\ in\ meters)^2}$$

Resulting scores for adults age 20 and over are interpreted according to this chart:

Underweight	Normal weight	Overweight	Obese
Below 18.5	18.5-24.9	25.0-29.9	30 and above

BMI for those under age 20 uses age- and gender-specific charts provided by the CDC. These charts include a percentile curve. The criteria for obesity based on these charts and BMI for age are as follows:

<5th percentile	Underweight
85th-<95 percentile	At risk for overweight
≥95th percentile	Overweight

Skinfold Measurement Component

Skin-fold measurement using special calipers is a way to estimate body fat and may be performed on the triceps, biceps, suprailiac, and subscapular areas. For example, for the triceps skinfold thickness (TST) measure, the midpoint between the axilla and elbow of the non-dominant arm is measured, with the skin grasped between the thumb and index finger about 1 cm above the midpoint by grasping at the edges of the arm and moving the finger and thumb inward until a firm fold of tissue is observed. The calipers are placed around this fold at the midpoint (right below the fingers) and squeezed for 3 seconds, and then a measurement is taken to the nearest millimeter. Three readings are taken to achieve an average. The TST is a percentage of standard age-adjusted measurements for males and females:

- Males (Adult)
    - TST 12.5 mm
- Females (Adult)
    - TST 16.5 mm

The actual measurement is divided by the standard measurement and multiplied by 100. Thus, if a male's TST measured 11.8:

- 11.8 ÷ 12.5 = 0.944 x 100 = 94.4%

Marfan Syndrome Assessment

Marfan syndrome is a genetic disorder of the connective tissue that may put athletes at risk. Connective tissue, such as tendons, ligaments, heart valves, and blood vessels, are often defective and weak. Depending upon the severity of the disorder, athletes may be restricted from team sports, especially contact sports that may result in chest trauma, or isometric exercises, such as weightlifting. Symptoms of Marfan may be noted on the PPE and the athlete must be referred to a specialist. Traits can include:

- Tall, thin stature with loose joints, with the long bones disproportionately long.
- Scoliosis.
- Flat feet.
- Pectus carinatum (pigeon chest) or pectus excavatum (funnel chest).
- Long, narrow face with high-arched roof of mouth and crowding of teeth.
- Dislocation of lenses of eyes and sometimes retinal detachment, myopia.
- Aortic dilatation (with risk of dissection).
- Cardiac valve disorders with heart murmur.
- Stretch marks.
- Abdominal/inguinal hernia.
- Sleep apnea (rare).

Pediculosis Assessment

Pediculosis is infestation with lice, transmitted by direct contact with someone who is infested. It includes the following:

- Head lice (most common in children)
- Body lice (most common in transient populations). They feed on the body but live in clothing or bedding and are spread by sharing bedding, clothes, or towels.
- Pubic lice spread by sexual contact or, rarely, sharing clothes or bedding; may infest the genital area, eyebrows, eyelids, lower abdomen, and beard.

Symptoms include persistent itch (usually worse at night), irritation, excoriation, and sometimes secondary infection. *Diagnosis* is by clinical exam and finding of lice or nits. *Treatment* includes:

Permethrin 1% (Nix) (treatment of choice): This is a cream rinse applied after body or hair is washed with a non-conditioning shampoo and towel dried. It is left on for 10 minutes and then rinsed off, leaving residue designed to kill the nymphs emerging from eggs not killed with the first application. Treatment is often repeated in 7 to 10 days. Nits should be removed manually.

Exclusion from Sports

Based upon the finding of the preparticipation exam, an athlete may be excluded from participating in sports activities, as the purpose of the exam is to establish the athlete's fitness to play. **Exclusion** can be based on any of the following:

- Injuries.
- Latent conditions, such as cardiac abnormalities, which may cause harm.

- Physical disabilities that pose a danger to the person or others.
- Renal disease.
- Uncontrolled hypertension.
- Health conditions that pose a risk to others, such as an acute Staphylococcus aureus/MRSA infection and, in some cases, HIV and hepatitis infections.
- Disagreement among physicians regarding the safety of allowing the athlete to participate in sports activities.
- The failure of reasonable accommodations to eliminate risk.
- Contagious diseases that pose a risk to others.

In addition, athletes with one eye should be excluded from boxing, wrestling and full-contact martial arts, because adequate eye protection gear is unavailable.

IMPLEMENTING RISK MANAGEMENT PLANS

Implementing risk-reduction plans that follow current guidelines benefits the athletic trainer by ensuring that the best plans for injury risk reduction are utilized. This can be achieved by examining the risks in advance, researching best practices to reduce these risks, planning preventative strategies, and implementing steps to reduce the incidence of injuries. For example, to reduce the risk of cervical neck injuries in football, a preventative plan including education on proper tackling technique should be implemented to reduce the incidence of these potentially catastrophic injuries. Additionally, in sports with a high risk for ACL sprains, a risk-reducing conditioning program should be incorporated that works to strengthen appropriate musculature and teaches techniques to reduce the risk for ACL sprains such as proper jump-landing form. By studying the risks for injuries and guidelines to manage these risks, athletic trainers can implement sport-specific, injury risk reduction programs for all athletes for which they provide services.

COMPONENTS INCLUDED IN A RISK MANAGEMENT PLAN

When developing a risk management plan, the athletic trainer must include the following five elements:

- Security issues: Security of the athletic training clinic must be maintained for many reasons, one of those being to protect the privacy of medical records. Only those who need access to the clinic should have keys to the facility. Athletic trainers and team physicians should have access to the facility and any others with access must be determined by the needs of the organization.
- Fire safety: A fire evacuation plan must be developed and posted in the athletic training clinic. Smoke alarms should be present and tested systematically to ensure proper function.
- Electrical equipment safety: Ground fault interrupters (GFIs) must be installed in areas where water and electricity are used together such as whirlpools, electrical stimulation, and moist heat packs. Malfunctioning electrical equipment should be removed immediately and electrical equipment must be inspected annually.
- Emergency action plan: A plan to properly manage emergency situations must be developed in collaboration with emergency responders working in the community. The emergency action plan should detail procedures for calling advanced medical care, transportation considerations for all facilities, and proper management of patients wearing athletic equipment.
- Crisis management plan: A plan to properly manage potential crises that originate from weather, public health, or acts of terror must be developed. Crisis management plans must detail action steps all personnel will take in the event of these emergencies.

Functional Strength and Core Stability Training

Functional strength training is a technique to strengthen the body in functional movement patterns. It looks at the body as a kinetic chain, multiple body parts working together to create motion. For a proper movement pattern to occur, all the parts within the kinetic chain must be strong and functioning properly. With functional training, all the links in the kinetic chain are strengthened in ways that mimic the movements used in activity. For example, when a pitcher throws a pitch, he or she is not only using the strength of the shoulder, but also the core, hips, and legs. By using this strengthening technique, the athlete gains strength for the physical activities in which they participate in all three planes of motion. An example of a functional strengthening exercise is a standing diagonal rotation with TheraBand resistance.

Core stability training is a technique to improve the muscular strength, endurance, power, and neuromuscular control over the muscles of the abdomen, lower back, and hips. Strengthening of the core is essential for injury prevention as a weak core leads to improper movement patterns and injuries. Examples of exercises for core stability training are planks, bridging and various exercises performed on a stability ball.

Warm-Up and Cool-Down

A warm-up is performed to gradually increase muscle temperature, elasticity, and stimulate the cardiorespiratory system. A dynamic, sport-specific warm-up of five to twenty minutes in length should be performed. The warm-up can include bounding, footwork drills, active stretches, and should encourage continuous movement. The exercises selected and the intensity of the warm-up is dependent on the age and physical conditioning of the group. Right after the warm-up, activity should begin.

After the activity has concluded, a gradual cool-down should be performed to bring the body slowly back to its resting state. Cool-down should last five to ten minutes in length and can include light jogging followed by walking. After gradually slowing down the exercise intensity and heart rate, stretching exercises should be performed. Stretching should start with standing stretches, move to seated stretches, and can end with stretches performed while lying down.

Cardiorespiratory Endurance

Cardiorespiratory endurance is the ability to perform activities that require large-muscle movements of the entire body over an extended amount of time. Cardiorespiratory endurance is important because it enables oxygen to be effectively delivered throughout the body to the working tissues. If an individual has a low-level of cardiovascular endurance, they will be unable to sustain their activity, will be more likely to fatigue early on, and are at a greater risk of injury. To improve cardiorespiratory endurance, aerobic activities should be performed three to six times per week for a period of twenty to sixty minutes. Competitive athletes should perform aerobic exercises at least four times per week for a minimum of 45 minutes. Examples of aerobic activities include jogging, swimming, cycling, elliptical, and skipping rope.

Physiological Changes That Occur from Strength Training

Muscular strength training brings about in various physiological changes within the muscle tissue. Hypertrophy, an increase in muscle size, occurs in response to strength training as myofilaments within the individual muscle fibers increase in size and number. This results in an increased cross-sectional diameter of the muscle fibers which makes the muscles themselves appear larger. Strength training also improves neuromuscular control of muscles. This is achieved as more motor units are elicited to fire for muscular contraction which creates a more efficient and stronger contraction of the muscle.

Another physiological change resulting from strength training is non-contractile tissues such as ligaments and tendons are strengthened. Stronger ligaments and tendons will decrease the risk for sprains and strains respectively. Also, bone mineral density is increased making the bone stronger and therefore less likely to fracture. Finally, if the heart rate is elevated to a training level during strength training, the cardiorespiratory system simultaneously receives training and becomes more efficient as well.

SPOTTERS

A spotter is essential when performing free-weight exercises, especially when the weights are extremely heavy. Without proper spotting, weight lifters can lose control of heavy weights and put themselves at risk for injury. If this occurs without a spotter, the weights could fall on the lifter's head or neck causing severe injury or even death. The spotter should know their physical limitations and use a second spotter if the weight being lifted exceeds their capabilities. Not only should the spotter be able to protect the lifter from injury, they should also provide guidance on proper lifting form, and offer encouragement.

There are many techniques for proper spotting. The spotter should ensure the lifter knows how to get out of the way of a failed lifting attempt, especially when the weight is overhead. The spotter must ensure the lifter is in a stable and biomechanically correct position with a proper grip before attempting the lift. The spotter should stand behind the lifter and should always be in a position to protect the lifter and themselves. The spotter should monitor the lifting speed, range of motion of the lift, the lifter's breathing, and repetitions performed.

PLYOMETRIC EXERCISES

Plyometric exercises start with a quick, eccentric contraction followed immediately by a rapid, forceful concentric contraction. A box jump would be an example of a plyometric exercise. The athlete would quickly squat down prior to jumping, causing an eccentric contraction of the quadriceps muscle group. Then the athlete would jump up onto the box by quickly and powerfully producing a concentric contraction of the quadriceps muscle group. The speed of stretch during the eccentric phase is more important than the length of the stretch.

Plyometric exercises are used to improve muscular power, which is a combination of muscular strength and speed. They can also develop eccentric control during activity, which can prevent injuries. Plyometric exercises strengthen the muscles in biomechanically correct ways, and they also strengthen the tendons and ligaments. To keep athletes safe while performing plyometric exercises, it is important to teach and monitor proper form and tailor the exercises to the age of the athlete and their level of ability.

FLEXIBILITY

It is generally accepted that having good flexibility prevents injuries because there is more range-of-motion available to the muscle before it is at risk of strain. Further, any impedance of normal range-of-motion can produce altered movement patterns that may lead to injuries, especially overuse injuries.

There are many techniques to improve flexibility. Static stretching is a stretch-and-hold technique in which a muscle is held in a position of maximum stretch for an extended period. Dynamic stretching uses functional movements to stretch the muscle such as a butt-kick for stretching the quadriceps muscle group. Dynamic stretches are considered more functional as the movements performed for the stretches more closely mimic the movements required of the activities. Ballistic stretching uses a bouncing motion to stretch the muscle. Proprioceptive neuromuscular facilitation

(PNF) is a stretching technique that can achieve great gains in flexibility but requires a partner for the stretch. There are different variations of PNS stretching but all include an active contract phase and a passive relax phase. During the active contract phase the partner provides resistance as the person being stretched contracts the muscle. In the passive relax phase, the partner brings the athlete into a stretched position while they relax the muscle being stretched.

PERIODIZATION TRAINING

Periodization training is a technique that considers the entire training period and sets appropriate conditioning goals to meet the needs of athletes during different phases of the season. Specific training goals will be set for off-season, preseason, and in-season. Periodization allows for peak performance during the competitive season, reduces overuse injuries, and offers variety in conditioning.

A macrocycle is the complete training period. The length of a macrocycle depends on the sport. For a seasonal sport, such as basketball, the macrocycle would be one year. However, for Olympic competition, the macrocycle spans a four-year period. Macrocycles are broken down into mesocycles, smaller units such as off-season, preseason, and in-season.

The off-season is broken even further down depending on how far away the competitive season is. The goals and exercises of the off-season are then adjusted accordingly. The off-season starts with the transition period in which the athlete should perform recreational activities for their enjoyment to provide a mental and physical break from the stress of the season. Then endurance is achieved during the preparatory/hypertrophy phase, followed by the strength phase in which weight training focuses on sport-specific activities. During the preseason power is developed. During the competitive season the goals switch to maintenance of muscular strength and power already developed.

PROPER HAND HYGIENE

Proper hand hygiene is essential to preventing the spread of diseases and illnesses. To properly wash hands one must wet hands under running water, lather with soap being sure to scrub the back of the hands, between the fingers and under the fingernails. Hands should then be scrubbed together for at least twenty seconds, then rinsed under running water, and dried with a paper towel or air dried. Athletic trainers should wash their hands before and after caring for a patient with a wound, after treating each patient, and immediately after coming into contact with blood or bodily fluids. If it is not possible to wash hands right away, then an alcohol-based hand sanitizer should be used. To properly use hand sanitizer, apply the sanitizer to one hand and then rub both hands together until dry.

REMOVING GLOVES PROPERLY

Gloves protect the athletic trainer from possible exposure to bloodborne pathogens. The proper way to remove gloves is to take one glove off by turning it inside out. Once the first glove is removed, it is placed it in the gloved hand and the second glove is removed by turning it inside out. The ungloved hand must not touch the soiled surface of the glove. The gloves should then be thrown away and the athletic trainer should wash their hands immediately.

CLEANLINESS POLICIES

There are many rules that should be enforced in the athletic training clinic to protect the clinic from unnecessary exposure to dirt and germs. No cleated shoes should be allowed in the clinic and shoes should not be allowed on treatment or exam tables. Sports equipment should not be brought into the clinic and athletes should shower before receiving treatments.

Athletic trainers should work together with the custodial staff and equipment managers to ensure that all areas of the athletic environment are constantly maintained for cleanliness to prevent infection and injury. The athletic training clinic should be swept, sinks disinfected, and trash emptied daily. Athletic trainers should clean and disinfect treatment tables, hydrotherapy modalities, and equipment daily. Other areas that athletes are exposed to should be kept clean and sanitary as well as locker rooms, showers, water fountains, wrestling mats, and gear for practices and games.

PROTECTIVE EQUIPMENT

Standard **protective equipment** must be provided to athletes to minimize the risk of injury or death. Studies have shown that athletes who participate in high- risk sports often underuse protective equipment and engage in other high-risk activities, such as drinking and using tobacco, so educating athletes about the importance of safety equipment is important. Often athletes, especially young adolescents, do not understand the need for safety equipment, or they complain that the equipment is uncomfortable, so clear explanations and proper fitting of equipment may improve compliance. Additionally, the Certified Athletic Trainer and the organization/institution must establish clear inflexible guidelines for the use of safety equipment, and then check to ensure that the equipment is in use. Information about the need for safety equipment should be provided to parents to enable them to better reinforce the safety guidelines. A wide variety of protective equipment is available; the choice of equipment depends on the athlete's size, skill level, physical maturation, strength, and the activity.

APPROPRIATE USE OF PERSONAL EQUIPMENT

Providing education about the appropriate use of personal equipment benefits the athletic trainer because this helps to prevent injuries due to misuse of equipment. If protective equipment is misused it can cause injuries to the athlete, their teammates, and their opponents. For example, educating football players on proper use of helmets can prevent serious injuries. Avoiding helmet-to-helmet contact and spearing can prevent concussions and cervical spine injuries. Explaining the proper use of protective padding such as shoulder pads and shin guards can ensure that athletes understand the intended protective use of the equipment and wear it properly to avoid injury. Educating softball and baseball athletes about the dangers of batting without a proper helmet will increase compliance of the use of protective gear. Providing education on the proper use of braces and other protective devices will ensure that the protective equipment is used properly to protect the patient's injured area and will prevent the patient from reinjuring the area or causing a new injury due to misuse of the equipment.

SPORT-SPECIFIC PROTECTIVE EQUIPMENT

Each **sports activity** requires specific types of safety protective equipment, and students should be aware of necessary and discretionary equipment:

- **Baseball**: (Not always worn) batting helmets with mouth guards Catchers: mouth guard, shin guards, chest protector, and protective mitt.
- **Football**: Football helmet and mouth guard; shoulder, hip, and tailbone padding; and thigh guards
- **Basketball**: Basketball shoes (medium tops providing ankle support) and mouth guards
- **Gymnastics**: Wrist guards, handgrips, and soft gymnastic footwear; floor pads should be in use and equipment properly padded
- **Skateboarding**: Helmet, knee and elbow pads, and slip-resistant shoes with closed toes

- **Soccer**: Shin guards and special molded cleats or ribbed-sole shoes; goal posts should be padded to prevent head injuries
- **Volleyball**: Kneepads, protective pants, and shoes with ankle/arch support

Preventing Keratoderma

Athletes are prone to the development of **keratoderma** (callus formation), caused by hypertrophy of the stratum corneum layer of the epidermis, on the palms of the hands and on the bottom of the feet, depending upon the type of sports activity. Calluses on the feet are a particular problem if they become very thick and interfere with elasticity of the skin, because cracks may form, which may be quite painful, and blisters may form beneath the calluses. Preventive methods include:

- Soaking feet and using callus files to reduce the thickness of existing calluses.
- Wearing double socks to cushion the sole of the foot.
- Wearing properly fitted shoes.
- Applying emollients to feet and hands to prevent friction and keep skin supple.
- Wearing protective gloves, tape, or moleskin to protect the palms from friction.

Standard Protective Equipment

Lower Extremities

Injuries to the knees and ankles are the most common sports injuries of the **lower extremities.** Protective equipment may be required or discretionary. Equipment for the lower extremities includes kneepads, shin guards, knee and ankle braces, and shoes. Large-scale studies of high school athletes have shown that the use of discretionary equipment reduces injuries by about 9%, but the biggest advantage related to knee pads, which correlated with a 56% decrease in knee injuries. Interestingly, the use of ankle and knee braces markedly increased the incidence of injury, with knee injuries 61% more likely and ankle injury 75% more likely. Shoes should be fitted properly and should be the correct type for the sports activity.

Head and Face

The **National Operating Committee on Standards of Athletic Equipment** (NOCSAE) researches and establishes standards regarding protective equipment. Protective equipment for the head and face is especially important to prevent serious injuries:

- While batting face guards are rarely used, they can prevent many facial injuries and should be recommended, especially for younger athletes.
- Mouth guards should be made of flexible material by a dentist to fit the individual's jaw and upper teeth or fit-checked to make sure that they provide maximum protection and comfort.
- Helmets should fit snugly, so that they don't move if they are rotated, turned, or tilted. The helmet should be pressed down at the crown to check for fitting of the jaw pads and chin straps. Football helmets may be air/fluid-filled or padded.
- Flak jackets (padded vest-like snug protective gear) are intended to protect the thoracic area after rib injuries.

Eyes

The **American Society for Testing and Materials (ASTM)** sets the standards for eye protection for racquet sports as well non-racquet sports (like baseball, basketball, field hockey, and skiing) to reduce the risk of eye injury. Protective eye gear is intended to dissipate the force of impact from the eye/face to the skull without leading to intracranial injury and without interfering with the playing of the sport. Most eye protection is formed of polycarbonate plastic, which is very resistant to force. Lenses are 2mm for low-risk sports activities and 3-mm for higher risk activities. Eye protection can be made with prescription lenses if necessary. Protective eye gear must include both frames and lenses, and frames must meet impact-resistant standards. For some sports, such as hockey, a full-face cage of polycarbonate or wire is required. All athletes who have lost an eye should wear protective eye gear at all times.

FEET

Quality **athletic shoes** are made with proper cushioning and ankle support for specific types of sports activity, and guidelines about shoes should be provided to athletes. Additionally, athletes should be advised to wear the type of socks they will wear during the sports activity when fitting the shoes Additional supportive devices may be used as well:

- Insoles: These may be simple foam padding or rigid orthotics, which provide the best support.
- Arch supports: These are used to prevent pain in the arch or forefoot.
- Heel cups: One type of heel cup is firm plastic and essentially compresses fat in the heel to provide a cushion. Another type is padded and rubberized, compressing as the heel pushes downward and preventing the heel from contacting the shoe. Some padded heel cups have rubberized waffle-designs and others have cutouts (U-shaped) below the heel.
- Heel pads: These provide less support than heel cups but may relieve discomfort.

DEVICES THAT MINIMIZE THE RISK OF INJURY AND ILLNESS
RUNNING SHOES

Wearing improperly fitted or worn **running shoes** is a major cause of foot injuries. Running shoes should be constructed of breathable material with a soft but sturdy midsole, good forefoot flexibility, and a strong heel. Running shoes should be purchased from a reputable dealer who can advise the athlete. Most good quality running shoes support 350 to 550 miles of running, but shock absorption weakens with time, so shoes may need to be replaced before obvious wear occurs. Subtle changes in wear patterns may help to determine the need for a particular type of support, so the athlete should wear the old shoes so they can be examined when purchasing new ones. During the selection process, shoes should be worn for at least 10 minutes to ensure comfort, and some stores may allow the purchaser to do a trial run up and down the street if requested. New shoes should be broken in slowly (3-mile runs) and should never be worn in a marathon or other long race immediately after purchase.

ANKLE SUPPORTS

Ankle sprains are common in almost all sports. The **ankle** comprises 3 bones and 3 groups of ligaments that stabilize the joint. The talus bone connects in a hinge joint with the distal tibia and fibula, stabilized by anterior and posterior tibiofibular ligaments. The medial aspect of the ankle is stabilized by the deltoid ligament. Most sprints are inversion injuries with tearing of lateral ligaments. Because sprains may weaken the ankle, taping helps to stabilize the ankle and prevent further injury. However, studies of the effectiveness of taping vary from no results to decreased injury, and it's better to focus on strengthening exercises. A good program is as follows:

- Taping using 1.5-2-inch porous athletic tape or moleskin
- High-top shoes with inflatable support to protect the ankle
- Semi-rigid orthotic stabilizers that fit about the ankle
- Shoes with adjustable straps providing semi-rigid support to the ankle

BREAST SUPPORT DEVICES

Females engaged in sports are particularly vulnerable to **breast** injuries, with the nipple the most commonly injured because of sensory stimuli causing erection of the nipple tissue and subsequent friction from clothing, resulting in pain and bleeding. Breasts may also have contusions, abrasions, and lacerations from impact, especially in contact sports and sports in which balls or other items are hurled at high speeds. Breast injury has been shown to increase the risk of cancer. Breast protective devices should support Cooper's ligaments, which suspend the breasts:

- Polyurethane nipple and breast cups (worn under a sports bra)
- Seamless sports bras made of non-abrasive, hypoallergenic material. Compression sports bras are usually used for females with breast cup sizes of A or B. Encompassing sports bras are more appropriate for females with larger breasts, as they support each breast separately. Careful measuring should be done to ensure correct fitting.
- Polyurethane chest shields, usually placed over a sports bra and fitted snugly to the individual

MALE GENITAL PROTECTIVE DEVICES

Studies have indicated that about half of male athletes, especially in middle school and high school, do not routinely use **genital protection** while playing sports, sometimes because traditional cups are uncomfortable. Additionally, males often do not report painless testicular swelling, so educating athletes about the danger of injury to genitals is necessary to ensure compliance with safety guidelines, especially since about 20% of genital injuries result in permanent damage. Injuries include hematoma of a testis or of the scrotum; lacerations of the penis or scrotum; torsion; and hernia. Genital protection devices include:

- Genital cups, held by a jock strap: There is a wide variety of cups, from flat to contoured, designed to absorb impact. They must be large enough to comfortably fit over the genitals and minimize movement, or else they can be uncomfortable.
- Compression shorts made of nylon and spandex to limit movement and provide support.
- Running shorts combine shorts and briefs, but don't provide sufficient protection from cold.

MINIMIZING RISKS FROM THE PHYSICAL ENVIRONMENT AND EQUIPMENT

Designing and following plans to minimize risks from the physical environment and equipment benefits the athletic trainer by preventing a wide array of injuries from occurring. For example, following the standard operating procedures for weight training equipment can prevent many catastrophic injuries, minor injuries, and everything in between. Designing and implementing an education plan to teach and reinforce the proper utilization of football equipment can prevent death, paralysis, and many other injuries. Being aware of risks involved with athletes who compete on turf fields, and providing education and techniques to lower those risks can prevent various sprains and abrasions.

There are many different types of athletic equipment and multiple physical environments in which athletic trainers provide coverage. Therefore, athletic trainers should be well versed in the proper use and dangers of misuse for all equipment and physical environments in which their athletes compete. Further, athletic trainers should proactively design, implement, and reinforce injury prevention plans for all physical environments in which they provide coverage and all equipment their athletes use.

NOCSAE Certification and Warning

The National Operating Committee on Standards for Athletic Equipment (NOCSAE) has developed safety standards that football helmets must meet for certification. Football helmets must be NOSCAE certified for use and helmets must have the NOCSAE warning label affixed. The warning states that helmets cannot prevent all head injuries or neck injuries and must not be used to spear or ram an opponent. Failure to heed this warning could result in serious injury, paralysis, or death. Each player should read this warning aloud and sign a form stating that they understand the warning. Athletic trainers should educate athletes, parents, and coaches on the risks for concussion that still exist even when wearing helmets. Education should also be provided on the proper use of football helmets that prevents head-down contact, spearing, and helmet-to-helmet collisions. With proper education, many serious and potentially life-threatening injuries can be prevented.

Wellness Screening

A wellness screening is a tool athletic trainers can use to help gauge if participants are taking proper measures to ensure wellness in all areas of their lives. Wellness screenings can assist the athletic trainer in identifying individuals that may need education or a referral to other healthcare providers to develop and maintain a healthy lifestyle. Wellness screenings commonly include questions about proper diet, adequate exercise, and avoidance of drugs, alcohol, and tobacco. Other topics include safe practices in all areas of life such as driving, care when dealing with dangerous materials, and safe sexual behaviors. Stress-control habits are also addressed to ensure participants have adequate coping mechanisms so that they can effectively respond to stressors in life and in sport.

Minimizing the Risk of Heat and Cold Injuries and Illnesses

Athletic trainers must take many steps to minimize the risk of heat illnesses in the physically active population. Necessary steps include educating all stakeholders on prevention, ensuring a gradual acclimation is followed over a period of 7 to 14 days, proper hydration, unrestricted access to fluids, and selecting clothing for activity participation that is light-weight and light in color. High-risk individuals should be identified and closely observed and the heat index should be monitored and activities adjusted accordingly. Weight records should also be kept to ensure participants are rehydrating appropriately.

To prevent hypothermia, there are several steps the athletic trainer must take. Education should be provided to all stakeholders on proper attire, hydration, how to recognize and treat potential cold illnesses, along with education on the risks inherent with participation in cold weather. High-risk participants should be identified and monitored. Clothing selected should be lightweight, layered, waterproof, windproof, and allow for movement and sweat to evaporate. Wearing a hat should be encouraged and participants should properly warm-up prior to activity and wear warm-up suits when not competing. If the temperature falls below freezing, an extra layer of clothing should be added for every 5 mph of wind.

Minimizing the Risk of Lightning, Altitude, and Jet Lag

There are many steps the athletic trainer must take to ensure the safety of all participants and staff when there is a threat of lightning. An emergency action plan should be established that dictates how lightning will be monitored, who will monitor, and who makes the decision to suspend and resume activity. Weather should be closely monitored with the National Weather Service, commercial lightning detection services, or lightning detectors. If thunder is heard, a lightning strike is seen, or weather-monitoring services report a lightning strike within 5.75 miles, activity should be stopped and not resumed until 30 minutes has passed since the last thunder, lightning strike, or reported strike within 5.75 miles.

To prevent altitude sickness, acclimation to high altitudes should be achieved. The amount of time recommended for acclimation varies with some experts recommend 3 days, while others recommend 2 to 3 weeks. To prevent jet lag (circadian dysrhythmia), the participant should attempt to become adjusted to the new time zone before departing. They can do this by adjusting their sleeping, eating, and exercise schedules. Also, plenty of fluids should be consumed and alcohol should be avoided.

CATASTROPHIC NECK INJURIES IN TACKLE FOOTBALL

The most common mechanism for catastrophic cervical spine injuries (CSIs) is axial loading to the head. This can occur in tackle football with head-down contact, when the athlete leads with the crown of the head. It is this improper and illegal technique that causes CSIs, not football equipment worn. Therefore, proper education and rule enforcement is essential to prevent CSIs. All athletes participating in football must be taught the catastrophic risks of head-down contact, be instructed on proper tackling techniques, and have ample time to practice correct tackling form. Athletes should be taught to make contact with their chest and shoulders, while keeping their heads up so they can see their opponents. All stakeholders should reinforce safety rules that prohibit head-down contact to include coaches, officials, athletic trainers, administrators, parents, and athletes.

IMPLEMENTING SAFETY RULES, PROPER BIOMECHANICAL TECHNIQUES, AND HEALTHY NUTRITIONAL GUIDELINES

There are many strategies athletic trainers should take to prevent injuries. Implementing safety rules ensures that all standards developed for safety are followed. This includes safety rules for exercising in hot and cold temperatures, lightning safety rules, following manufacturers' guidelines for proper use of equipment, following protocols for head injury management, and obeying all sport-specific safety rules. Utilizing proper biomechanical techniques prevents many injuries from occurring. For example, teaching athletes to utilize a proper athletic stance enables them to elicit the stronger muscles of the body, generate force in a biomechanically correct manner, and protect the body from unnecessary strain. Following nutritional and hydration guidelines allows athletes to perform at an optimal capacity and reduces the risk of injuries due to fatigue and dehydration.

FOLLOWING MANUFACTURER GUIDELINES TO SELECT, INSPECT, AND MAINTAIN EQUIPMENT

Manufacturer guidelines should be followed when selecting, inspecting, and maintaining equipment. When purchasing equipment, reputable manufactures should be chosen and the safest possible equipment within budget should be bought. When purchasing helmets, only NOCSAE approved helmets should be selected. If assembly is required, manufacturer assembly guidelines should be followed and equipment should only be used for the purposes for which it was designed. Participants must be educated about the risks and proper use of the equipment. Routine inspections and cleanings should be performed and any broken equipment must be repaired or replaced immediately. Helmets must be recertified every two years by a NOCSAE-approved vendor. Finally, if an athletic trainer constructs a custom piece of equipment, this must be done with extreme caution and care to ensure patient safety.

PHYSICAL PROPERTIES OF MATERIALS USED IN PROTECTIVE SPORTS EQUIPMENT

The physical properties of materials used in sports protective equipment works to protect athletes in many ways. For example, the materials used in helmets work to lessen the impact transferred to athletes' heads by incorporating outer shells that flex, absorbing forces from blows to the head at strategic points on the helmets. Cantilevered shoulder pads arch above the tip of the shoulder, dissipating pressure throughout the shoulder pads, reducing impact to athletes' shoulder joints. Athletic trainers use a variety of foams for purposes such as injury protection. Foams vary in thickness and density making them easily customizable to the needs of the patient. Closed-cell foams rebound to their original shape more quickly after compression forces than open-cell foams, making them more desirable for protection during physical activity.

Scheduling Activities, Clothing, and Ensuring Proper Fluid Replacement

There are many steps the athletic trainer must take to decrease the risk of environmental injuries. The heat index must be monitored and activities adjusted accordingly. To determine the heat index, the athletic trainer can use a psychrometer, which accounts for heat, humidity, and the sun's radiation. The decision for practice and game clothing should take into account the heat and humidity. At the beginning of the season, lightweight t-shirts and shorts should be worn and participants should be gradually introduced to netted jerseys and pants. Dark-colored clothing should be avoided and rubberized clothing should never be used.

Participants should be educated on proper fluid replacement, be offered continuous access to fluids, and be closely monitored to ensure they are rehydrating. Two hours before practice they should consume 17-20 ounces of water or sports drink and ten to twenty minutes prior they should consume an additional 7-10 ounces. If a sports drink is used it should have 6% carbohydrates and not be carbonated.

Safety Hazards

Associated with Shower Facilities

Shower facilities pose a number of safety hazards resulting in falls, burns, and infections. Clear guidelines for showering and maintenance of the facilities should be established and supervised. Separate shower facilities should be available for males and females:

- Shower facilities, adjacent locker rooms, and environmental surfaces should be cleaned daily to prevent the spread of infection.
- Water temperature should be monitored and should not exceed 110° F to prevent burns.
- Shower areas should have non-slip floor surfaces.
- Liquid soap dispensers should be available at each shower and filled daily.
- Bar soap should not be used because it may harbor bacteria.
- Towels should not be shared and should be washed with soap and water at 160°F and dried with hot air.
- Athletes should wear foot protection, such as flip-flops or shower sandals, to prevent the spread of fungus infections.

Associated with Athletic Equipment

Athletic equipment, such as work benches or exercise machines, is often used by many different athletes and poses a number of safety hazards ranging from electric shock and infection to injury from incorrect use or damaged equipment. The following measures can minimize these risks:

- Electrical equipment should be checked regularly to ensure that cords are not frayed and that plugs are intact. Multiple adaptors and cords should be avoided.
- Electrical equipment should be shut off when not in use, and portable equipment, such as pitching machines, should be unplugged.
- Signs should be posted indicating that electrical equipment should not be used with wet hands or if the floor is wet.
- All environmental surfaces in contact with body fluids, including perspiration, should be cleaned daily or between uses with EPA-approved disinfectant.
- Athletes should wash hands before and after use of equipment.
- Prevent clutter or cords from blocking passageways, such as around equipment.

Associated with Buffer Zones

Buffer zones are the open spaces surrounding areas of sports activity within a sports facility. Buffer zones are needed because athletes often leave the playing area at a high speed (especially in sports like basketball) or may not be looking where they are going. There are standards for buffer zones for all sports, such as the distance from windows to prevent breaking glass from injuring athletes. Sometimes danger arises when coaches or trainers use "found" space for practice activities rather than the gymnasium. Buffer zones should always be adequate, and should not be used for any other purpose, such as equipment storage or scoring tables. Only spaces intended for athletic activities should be used for practice, and these areas should always be supervised.

Associated with Field Conditions

Many sports injuries (for example about 25% of soccer injuries) are caused by poor **field conditions,** such as holes in the field from poor maintenance, gophers, or other burrowing animals, or damage caused by sports activities. There may be pooled water, broken glass, rocks, raised sprinkler heads, or items that have been thrown onto the field, all of which pose a potential hazard. In many cases, there is no clear responsibility for checking the field prior to activities. Referees may be responsible at some institutions, but the reality is that they rarely walk the entire field and often arrive shortly before game time. Coaches are usually busy with the athletes. The athletic trainer should ensure that a procedure is in place to check the field before use. This may include groups of athletes walking the field before play or volunteers, such as athletic supporters or parents. Various approaches may be used: A group may walk from one end to another or the field may be divided into grids for inspection.

Associated with Pollution

Pollution can pose a considerable risk to the health of athletes. In many areas, especially urban or industrial, playing areas or fields are located in high traffic areas, increasing the risk of exposure to particulate matter (fumes and soot) from automobile exhaust. Additionally, in some areas ozone levels and pollen counts are of concern:

- Practices/games should be held after rush hour, usually in the late afternoon.
- Pollen counts and ozone levels should be checked daily and outdoor activities should be cancelled or delayed when appropriate.
- Exercises may be done in the early AM when it is cooler and ozone pollution levels ore lower, because heat combines with some compounds to produce ozone.
- Aerobic exercise, such as jogging, increases the use of mouth breathing and the intake of particulate matter and may require modification, movement to a less polluted area, or to an indoor facility.

Associated with Floor Mats

Floor mats pose a potential hazard to athletes, such as wrestlers, who come in skin contact with the mat. Mats should meet the standards and specifications of the particular sport so that they provide adequate cushioning to prevent injury. Mats should be:

- Examined regularly and replaced if cushioning deteriorates.
- Checked to ensure they are smooth, without surface cracks, prior to each event.
- Cleaned thoroughly, following manufacturer's guidelines, and disinfected before each session.
- Protected from people walking on them without proper footwear, as this may damage the cushioning and the surface of the mat.

- Installed away from walls or protrusions that might injure the athlete during activities.
- If not left in place, stored according to manufacturer's guidelines to prevent damage to the mat.

ASSOCIATED WITH LIGHTNING

Lightning, which kills about 100 people a year in the United States and injures 400-500, poses a serious safety hazard for athletes. Storms can arise and become dangerous in a very short time, less than 30 minutes, especially in areas of the country with frequent thunderstorms. While lightning often accompanies rainstorms, it can occur without rain as well. The athletic trainer usually monitors weather conditions and advises the coaches and other staff when hazardous conditions arise, or when changes in weather conditions suggest a potential hazard may occur. There are a number of steps that should be followed to minimize risk:

- Check weather report daily.
- Use portable (*SkyScan* or *Thorguard*) detection system if possible to detect lightning, and use the Internet to check weather changes.
- Identify safe shelters prior to sports activities and gauge the length of time needed to access the shelter: Buildings grounded with electrical wiring or plumbing OR vehicles with hard metal roofs and windows closed. Avoid sheds, which are usually not secure or grounded.
- Utilize "flash-to-bang" method to estimate the proximity of lighting: count the seconds from the flash to the bang of thunder and divide by 5 to arrive at the distance in miles.
- Stop all activity when "flash-to-bang" nears 30 seconds or lightning detection system indicates increasing storm activity.
- Advise spectators to seek shelter and exit metal bleachers.
- Seek shelter away from lone objects, tall trees, standing water, or open fields, avoiding metal structures. Avoid the locker room, showers, and indoor pools or tubs.
- Open area: crouch low with only feet touching the ground.
- Avoid the use of telephone landlines, which can transmit electrical charges.
- Ensure that CPR-certified individuals are available.

MAINTENANCE OF CLINICAL AND TREATMENT AREAS

Depending upon the size of the organization or facility, the **clinical and treatment area** may be shared by a number of different staff and athletes. The area may include office space, examining rooms, taping area, wound care area, rehabilitation area, electrotherapy (ultrasound, diathermy) and hydrotherapy tubs and pools. The clinical and treatment areas are ideally located within close proximity to training areas, such as adjacent to locker rooms or gymnasiums. Not only the space but also the equipment within must be maintained in accordance with accepted standards:

- A schedule for use should be maintained and updated weekly to avoid conflicts.
- Athletic trainers are usually responsible for cleaning equipment and maintaining floors and environmental surfaces.
- Treatment tables should be cleaned daily and after each use.
- Hydrotherapy equipment should be disinfected daily following manufacturer guidelines and using EPA-approved disinfectants.
- Treatment areas should have access to a clean and functioning ice machine in case cold packs are needed.
- Hydrotherapy area should have elevated outlets (5 feet) to prevent splashing of outlets and/or electric shock.
- Athletes should be required to shower before non-emergency treatment.

- Equipment, including cleats, should be left outside treatment area.
- Shoes should not touch treatment tables.
- Telephones must be accessible in case emergency assistance is required.
- Smoke detectors and fire safety information must be available.
- The athletic trainer should be sure at all times to operate within the scope of practice when supervising and providing treatment to athletes.

Observing and Acting in Response to Environment Conditions

When the athletic trainer ensures the safety of all people involved in athletic events by monitoring and responding appropriately to environmental conditions, many injuries and illnesses are prevented, of which several are life threatening. The athletic trainer must be able to recognize various environmental conditions that pose threats to the physically active population and can readily offer safety recommendations to prevent those from occurring.

There are many examples of environmental conditions that threaten the health and wellbeing of those exposed to these elements. For example, lightening poses great risk for catastrophic injuries and the athletic trainer must be prepared to immediately respond to protect all involved parties from risk of injury. Heat, especially when combined with high humidity, poses a risk for heat illnesses. Cold weather poses a risk for hypothermia, high altitude poses risks for multiple injuries and illnesses, and air pollution is another environmental condition that athletic trainers must be cognizant of and be ready to offer injury-preventing advice.

Jet Lag

Jet lag is caused by a disturbance in the Circadian rhythm of waking and sleeping when traveling from one time zone to another, especially over multiple time zones. Jet lag may result in lethargy, dizziness, insomnia, dehydration, drowsiness, and impaired athletic performance. Travel from west to east seems to cause more problems than travel from east to west. Some believe that it takes one day to compensate for each time zone crossed. There are some steps an athlete can take to minimize the effects of travel:

- Sleep well the night before.
- Hydrate well prior to boarding the plane, avoiding alcohol.
- Avoid drinking juices, sodas, caffeinated beverages, and alcohol during the flight.
- Try to eat and sleep on a schedule that coincides with home time if possible, when an extended period of adjustment is not possible.
- Remove shoes, stretch, and walk about periodically to improve circulation.
- Schedule rest time during the day if necessary.

High-Altitude Sickness

When ascending to high elevations, most people experience some degree of shortness of breath from the change in altitude. While air is still 21% oxygen, the atmospheric pressure is lower, so the oxygen molecules are further apart, so people take in less oxygen with each breath. There is a 17% decrease in oxygen at 5000 feet and a 31% decrease at 10,000 feet. Between 20 and 30% of the population develop a degree of **high-altitude sickness** when ascending above 8000 feet, and 75% gets sick when above 14,000. Athletes training or competing at high altitudes must be aware of the dangers of high-altitude sickness and preventive measures. There are 3 main types of high-altitude sickness:

- Acute mountain sickness (AMS), which indicates failure to acclimatize; may be mild to severe and often presents with headache, lethargy, nausea, confusion, unsteady gait, and dyspnea. Occurs 6-24 hours after ascent.
- High-altitude cerebral edema (HACE), which can lead to acute neurological damage, causing seizures, coma, and death.
- High-altitude pulmonary edema (HAPE), which can lead to acute respiratory distress and death.

Typical changes that occur during acclimatization include:

- Hyperventilation to increase oxygen uptake (hypoxic ventilatory response).
- Increased urination and dehydration.
- Increased heart rate.
- Frequent awakening during the night and Cheyne-Stokes respirations.
- Increased blood pressure.

Preventive methods should begin below 10,000 feet, but a gradual ascent with a few days of planned rest before exertion is optimal:

- Immediately stop ascent with any signs of AMS until symptoms subside.
- Always descend immediately for emergency treatment when signs of HACE or HAPE emerge.
- Increase elevations above 10,000 feet at the rate of 1000 feet daily, with one day rest for each 1000 feet.
- If flying/driving to high elevation, avoid exertion or more ascents for 24 hours. Drink copious (4-6 liters/day) amounts of to keep urine clear or pale. Avoid exercises and over-exertion until acclimatized, and sleep only at night.
- Eat a 70% carbohydrate diet. Avoid use of alcohol, tobacco, or depressant drugs.

PRIORITIZING WELLNESS FOR INDIVIDUALS AND GROUPS

Prioritizing wellness for individuals and groups helps the athletic trainer by promoting overall well-being for all involved parties and preventing a multitude of injuries and illnesses that may occur because of various aspects in the lives of the individuals. Promoting wellness goes beyond the field of play and athletic performance. It addresses and promotes healthy lifestyle behaviors in all aspects of the athlete's life such as good nutritional choices, stress management, getting adequate amounts of sleep, proper exercise, implementing safety practices, and avoidance of drugs, alcohol, and tobacco. Athletic trainers can use wellness screenings to monitor the wellness of individuals and groups and detect possible areas of concern. If an area of concern is noted, the athletic trainer can offer assistance either through referral, education, or encouragement depending on the type of wellness concern and the needs of the individual.

EFFECT OF EMOTIONAL STRESSORS ON THE RISK OF INJURY

There are many emotional stressors that can increase athletes' risks for injury. Unrealistic expectations, worry, anger, discouragement, and frustration all lead to an increased state of negative stress, predisposing an athlete to injury. Negative stressors decrease focus, flexibility, coordination, and efficiency of movement patterns. Negative stress also increases muscle tension and activates the fight-or-flight response. Without appropriate coping mechanisms, negative stress can become a chronic condition. Athletic trainers can offer many techniques to help patients manage stress such as imagery, negative thought stoppage, and cognitive restructuring. Athletic trainers must also refer patients to psychologists and psychiatrists as needed.

Referring Athletes for Psychological Concerns

There are many psychological concerns athletic trainers should be aware of that require referral to mental health professionals for proper care. These include the following:

Depression: Signs and symptoms include feelings of helplessness, alterations in eating and sleeping habits, and thoughts of hurting oneself.

Paranoia: Individuals suffering from paranoia are extremely suspicious about certain things and over time develop bitterness and rage towards the object or person of their paranoia.

Posttraumatic stress disorder: After a psychologically traumatic event such as abuse or surviving a life-threatening situation, some develop posttraumatic stress disorder. Individuals may relive the traumatic experience in nightmares or be easily startled.

Eating disorders: There are various eating disorders such as bulimia nervosa, anorexia nervosa, and anorexia athletica. All evidence of eating disorders is reason for referral to a mental health provider. They have various signs and symptoms such as a distorted body image, purging one's food, starving oneself, and participating in overly excessive physical activity.

Signs and Symptoms of Anxiety Disorders

Anxiety disorders account for about 20% of all medical conditions for which Americans seek care. Panic attacks and phobias are both classified as anxiety disorders. A panic attack is characterized by unanticipated feelings of terror with a physiological reaction similar to one who feels their life is in danger. Around 30% of young adults experience panic attacks. Panic attacks are more likely to be experienced at night and can be genetic. A patient who suffers from suspected panic attacks should be referred to a mental health provider. Treatments include behavioral modifications and medications that repress fear.

A phobia is an unfounded fear that persists over time and leads to the person avoiding the situation or object that causes them fear. Common phobias are fear of heights, social interactions, and fear of flying. Symptoms of this condition can include an elevated heart rate and troubles breathing. A patient who suffers from a suspected phobia should be referred to a mental health provider. Treatments can include antianxiety or antidepressant medications, behavioral modifications, and desensitization, which is a technique in which the patient is gradually exposed to their phobia to overcome it.

Importance of Diet
Basic Elements

A basic understanding of the elements of a good **diet** is necessary for the athlete. The energy for the body is supplied by:

- Fats = 9 calories per gram. Fats provide the slowest but most efficient form of energy, requiring 5 hours to metabolize. Fats should comprise 30% of the diet.
- Carbohydrates = 4 calories per gram. Simple carbohydrates (sugars, fruits, dairy products) are the fastest source of energy, requiring about 30 minutes to metabolize. Complex carbohydrates (whole grains, vegetables) convert more slowly to energy, taking about 2 hours. Carbohydrates should comprise about 55% of the diet. Carbohydrates provide more energy per unit of oxygen expended than other food components.
- Proteins = 4 calories per gram. Protein, including meat and fish, metabolizes more slowly (3 hours) but provides a longer-lasting source of energy. Protein should comprise about 15% of the diet.

Athletes expend 2200-4400 calories daily. In order to prevent dehydration, athletes must also consume adequate amounts of water, approximately 2 1/2 liters per 2400-calorie energy output.

Modifications for Exercise

Carbohydrate loading and protein **diet modifications** are often used to increase the storage of glycogen before endurance sports, and to prevent energy loss and anemia:

- Intake of simple carbohydrates immediately before an event may increase dehydration and cause an increase in insulin, thus lowering blood sugar. If activities last longer than 90 minutes, then stored glycogen is adequate. If activities last more than 2 hours, then sports drinks that are 6-8% glucose may be used during the event.
- While high carbohydrate diets (70%) should not be used for prolonged periods, carbohydrate loading diets are often used for 3 days before endurance events. Shorter durations (1 day) may cause water retention and muscular stiffness.
- Exercise increases the need for protein, and insufficient intake may result in anemia. Endurance activities require 1.2-1.4 g protein/kg of body weight. Resistance and strength activities require 1.6-1.7 g protein/kg. Protein supplements should be avoided.
- Pre-event meals should be 500-1000 calories 3-4 hours before the event.

Concerns for Female Athletes

Female athletes often believe that they should lose weight to compete better, but they run the risk of inadequate nutrition, which can impair performance instead. At least 1200-1500 calories/day are usually required for most girls and women, but female athletes may require many more calories. Female athletes often require increased iron in their diets because they lose iron through menses. Many female athletes develop amenorrhea as their bodies attempt to conserve stores of iron. Amenorrhea or excessive exercise can lead to bone loss and osteoporosis, so a diet with sufficient iron, from sources like red meat and pork, is advised. Adequate calcium intake may counteract the bone loss, but calcium supplements of 1500 mg/day may be required to avoid stress fractures, especially for participants in activities that require running and jumping. Additionally, vitamin C, which helps with the absorption of iron, is necessary.

Ways Overweight Athletes Can Prevent Injury

Overweight athletes are often engaged in sports that require large size and mass, as for instance football, basketball, and wrestling. These athletes should be carefully assessed for risks. In addition, these athletes should have their body masses double-checked, since individuals with extreme muscle mass are often inaccurately categorized as overweight. The overweight athlete is more likely to suffer from injury. Overweight athletes should be advised to:

- Avoid any use of performance-enhancing supplements, steroids or stimulants in trying to lose weight or convert fat to muscle, because these may result in hypertension, cardiac abnormalities, or other health problems.
- Avoid high-volume, high-intensity plyometric exercises, which can result in joint damage.
- Acclimatize to heat and to exercise by staying hydrated and staying alert for signs of heat-related illness.
- Maintain a nutritious diet.

Eating Disorders

There are eating disorders that the athletic trainer should cognizant of to provide proper care to patients. Bulimia nervosa is characterized by the consuming of extreme amounts of food in a very short amount of time after a period of self-starvation. After consumption, the individual then attempts to purge the calories consumed with self-induced vomiting, laxatives, or diuretics. This cycle goes on repeatedly and can cause damage to the stomach, heart, liver, teeth, throat, and mouth. All individuals with suspected eating disorders should be approached early on, empathetically, and referred to mental health professionals.

Anorexia nervosa is characterized by an extremely thin individual who believes they are overweight and is very concerned about weight gain. The individual denies their hunger and may participate in excessive amounts of exercise. As many as 15-21% of people diagnosed with anorexia nervosa die from this disease. Early detection, referral, and the patient's ability to recognize their need for help is essential for treatment to be effective.

Anorexia athletica is an eating disorder specific to athletes. Signs and symptoms include a disordered body image, worries about weight gain, amenorrhea, and weight loss greater than 5% of total body weight. The individual does not self-starve but may binge, purge, or significantly restrict their caloric intake.

Dangers of Eating Disorders for Athletes

Eating disorders are a health risk for athletes, especially females although males sometimes also have eating disorders, often presenting as excessive exercise. Different types include:

- ***Anorexia nervosa*** affects 0.5-3.7% of females; it is characterized by profound fear of weight gain and severe restriction of food intake, often accompanied by abuse of diuretics and laxatives, which can cause electrolyte imbalances, kidney and bowel disorders, and delay or cessation of menses. Anorexics may become emaciated and die.
- ***Bulimia nervosa*** affects 1.1-4.2% of females and includes binge eating followed by vomiting, often along with use of diuretics, enemas, and laxatives. Gastric acids can damage the throat and teeth. While bulimics may maintain a normal weight, they are at risk for severe electrolyte imbalances that can be life threatening.
- ***Binge eating*** affects 2-5% of females and includes grossly overeating, often resulting in obesity, depression, and shame.

Early intervention can prevent physical damage, but hospitalization and intense therapy for long periods of time may be required.

Dangers of Alcohol

Ethanol is the form of alcohol found in alcoholic beverages, flavorings, and some medications. It is a multisystem toxin and central nervous system depressant. Teenagers and young adults frequently use ethanol as the drug of choice, but binge drinking can lead to serious morbidity or death. Ethanol has direct effects on the central nervous system, myocardium, thyroid, and hepatic tissue. Ethanol is absorbed through the mucosa of the mouth, stomach, and intestines, with concentrations peaking about 30-60 minutes after ingestion. About 90% of ethanol is metabolized in the liver, and the rest excreted through the pulmonary and renal systems. **Ethanol overdose** affects the central nervous system as well as other organs in the body. If people are easily aroused, they can usually safely sleep off the effects of ingesting too much alcohol, but if the person exhibits an altered mental status, nausea and vomiting, or is semi-conscious or unconscious, emergency medical treatment should be initiated.

Syphilis

Syphilis is caused by the spirochete *Treponema pallidum* and has increased in incidence over the last ten years, associated with risk-taking behavior such as drug use. There are 3 phases to the disease, with an incubation period of about 3 weeks:

- *Primary*: chancre (painless) in areas of sexual contact, persisting 3-6 weeks.
- *Secondary*: General flu-like symptoms (sore throat, fever, and headaches) and red papular rash on trunk, flexor surfaces, palms, and soles; lymphadenopathy occurs about 3-6 weeks after end of primary phase and eventually resolves.
- *Tertiary (latent):* Affects about 30% and includes CNS and cardiovascular symptoms 3-20 years after initial infection.

Athletes with evidence of syphilis should be referred for diagnosis and treatment. *Diagnosis* is by dark-field microscopy (primary or secondary) or serologic testing. The CDC provides treatment protocol for different populations.

Treatment includes:

- Primary, secondary, early tertiary: Benzathine penicillin G 104 million units IM in one dose.
- Tertiary: Benzathine penicillin G 2.4 million units IM weekly for 3 weeks.

Chlamydia

Chlamydia is a sexually-transmitted disease (STD) caused by *Chlamydia trachomatis* and is often co-infected with gonorrhea. It may be transmitted by oral, anal, and vaginal sex. It is the most common STD in the United States. *Symptoms* of chlamydia include:

- Males: urethritis, epididymitis, proctitis, or Reiter's syndrome (urethritis, rash, conjunctivitis). Many cases are asymptomatic.
- Females: Mild cervicitis with vaginal discharge and dysuria, but complications can lead to infertility and pelvic inflammatory disease (PID).

Any athlete presenting with evidence of chlamydia should be referred for diagnostic testing and treatment. *Diagnosis* is most reliable from nucleic acid amplification test (NAAT) (Amplicor®, Probe TEC®). *Treatment* includes:

- Azithromycin 1 g orally in one dose OR
- Doxycycline 100 mg orally twice daily for 1 week.
- Avoidance of sexual contact for 1 week.

Treatment of the infected person's sexual partner is very important to avoid reinfection after treatment.

Gonorrhea

Gonorrhea is caused by *Neisseria gonorrhoeae* and should be suspected with urinary infections. *Symptoms* include:

- Males: Dysuria and purulent discharge from the urethra, epididymitis, and prostatitis.
- Females: Many women are asymptomatic or may have lower abdominal pain, cystitis, or mucopurulent cervicitis; if untreated it can result in PID and chronic pain.

Rectal infections are common in women and homosexual males. Untreated, gonorrhea can become a systemic infection, resulting in petechial or pustular skin lesions, arthralgias, tenosynovitis, fever and malaise, and septic arthritis. Athletes with urinary infections or other signs of gonorrhea should be referred for diagnosis and treatment. *Diagnosis* is by cervical or urethral culture or NAAT. Gram stains of urethral smears are more accurate for males than females. Cultures of multiple sites may be needed to confirm disseminated disease. *Treatment* includes:

- Cefixime 400 mg orally in one dose OR
- Ceftriaxone 125 mg Im in one dose OR
- Ciprofloxacin 500 mg orally in one dose OR
- Levofloxacin 250mg orally in one dose.

Safe Sex Practices

While abstinence is the only sure way to avoid sexually-transmitted diseases and pregnancy, the reality is that many teenagers and most adults are sexually active. Athletes should be advised of safe sex practices in order to prevent unwanted pregnancies and sexually-transmitted diseases.

There are a number of safety guidelines.

- Males should use a latex condom for each sex act, and females should demand that their partners use condoms.
- Females should practice appropriate birth control, including the use of a female condom, IUD, diaphragm or birth control pills or patch.
- Males and females should avoid multiple sex partners and sex with people they don't know well.
- Males having sex with males and others who have engaged in unsafe sex practices should be tested for HIV and hepatitis before engaging in sex with new partners.
- Males and females should seek medical advice after any sign of pain, difficulty urinating, discharge, or lesions.

Amphetamines and Cocaine Use

Amphetamine toxicity: may be caused by intravenous injection, inhalation, or sniffing of various substances (methamphetamine, methylphenidate), and ephedrine and phenylpropanolamine. Cocaine may be ingested orally, IV or by sniffing, while crack cocaine is smoked. Amphetamines and cocaine are CNS stimulants that can cause multi-system abnormalities. *Symptoms* may include chest pain, dysrhythmias, myocardial ischemia, myocardial infarction, seizures, intracranial infarction, hypertension, dystonia, repetitive movements, unilateral blindness, lethargy, rhabdomyolysis with acute kidney failure, perforated nasal septum (cocaine), and paranoid psychosis (amphetamines). Crack cocaine may cause pulmonary hemorrhage, asthma, pulmonary edema, barotrauma, and pneumothorax. Swallowing packs of cocaine can cause intestinal ischemia, colitis, necrosis, and perforation. Athletes should be referred for immediate diagnosis and treatment. *Diagnosis* includes clinical findings, CBC, chemistry panel, toxicology screening, ECG, and radiograph. *Treatment* includes:

- Gastric emptying (1 hour or more) and charcoal administration. IV access and supplemental oxygen.
- Sedation for seizures. Haloperidol for agitation.
- Hypertension: Nitroprusside, phentolamine 2.5-5mg IV.
- Cocaine quinidine-like effects: Sodium bicarbonate.

ROHYPNOL

Rohypnol (flunitrazepam) is a type of benzodiazepine, commonly referred to as the "date rape drug" or "roofie" because it causes anterograde amnesia. Rohypnol is popular with teens and young adults and is often taken with alcohol, which potentiates its effects. Rohypnol is a CNS depressant that causes muscle relaxation, slurs speech and reduces inhibitions. The effects occur within 20-30 minutes of ingestion but may persist for 8 to 12 hours. Repeated use can result in aggressiveness, and withdrawal may cause hallucinations and seizures. Overdoses cause hypotension, altered mental status, vomiting, hallucinations, dyspnea, and coma. Females are the most common victims, and may not remember the event except for a perception of lost time or physical discomfort. *Diagnosis* is by history and clinical examination.

Treatment includes:

- Assessment for rape and STDs.
- Gastric emptying (less than 1 hour).
- Charcoal.
- Monitoring for CNS/respiratory depression.
- Supportive care.
- Counseling referral for rape.

MONONUCLEOSIS

Mononucleosis is an infectious disorder caused by the Epstein-Barr virus. It is spread through saliva and airborne droplets and occurs most often in teenagers and young adults. The incubation period is 4-6 weeks. *Symptoms* are usually similar to an upper respiratory infection or flu, with adults affected more than children. The following symptoms may persist for weeks:

- Weakness.
- Headaches.
- Fever.
- Persistent sore throat.
- Enlarged lymph nodes in neck and axillae.
- Enlarged tonsils.
- Generalized red macular rash.
- Enlarged spleen (rupture may occur in rare cases).

Diagnosis may include clinical examination, antibody tests (such as Monospot®), and CBC. *Treatment* is primarily supportive, as there is no treatment for the virus, and includes:

- Rest and restricted activity to avoid spleen rupture.
- Acetaminophen or ibuprofen.
- Adequate fluid intake.

TINEA CRURIS AND TINEA PEDIS

Tinea cruris (jock itch) is a fungal infection of the perineal area, penis, inner thighs, and inguinal creases, but may also occur under breasts in women and beneath abdominal folds where skin is warm and moist. It rarely occurs before adolescence. *Symptoms* include:

- Scaly, itching, erythematous rash that may contain papules or vesicle and is usually bilateral and symmetrical.

Treatment: Selenium sulfide shampoo wash of area before applying medication. Topical antifungal (clotrimazole, miconazole, tolnaftate, naftifine, terbinafine) 2 times daily for 4 weeks.

Tinea pedis (athlete's foot) is a fungal infection of the feet and toes. It is rare before adolescence and more common in males. Symptoms include:

- Severe itching with vesicles or erosion of instep and with peeling maceration and fissures between toes.
- Dry, scaly, mildly erythematous patches on plantar and lateral foot surfaces.

Treatment:

- Same as tinea cruris. Keep feet dry with absorbent talc.
- Allow feet to air dry and use 100% cotton socks, changed twice daily.

ANABOLIC STEROIDS

Athletic organizations must take a firm no-use stand on **anabolic steroids** as they have been widely used among athletes. Athletes must be educated about the dangers of the drugs. Anabolic steroids, such as cypionate and testosterone enanthate, are used to increase muscle mass and improve athletic performance, but they have serious side effects and have no place in sports:

- Liver disorders (especially oral anabolic steroids).
- Cardiovascular disorders.
- Increased aggressiveness and libido.
- Males:
  - Decreased sperm count, atrophy of testes, and erectile dysfunction.
  - Gynecomastia (breast development) in males.
- Females:
  - Inhibition of formation of follicles and irregularities of menstrual cycle, including amenorrhea.
  - Hypertrophy of clitoris.
  - Acne.
  - Hair loss and male pattern balding with increased facial hair.
  - Breast atrophy.
  - Masculinization of body, features, and lowering of voice.

Tobacco Use

While the use of **tobacco** has decreased to about 21% of the population in the United States, it is still the leading preventable cause of death. Teenagers and young adults often experiment with both cigarettes and chewing tobacco and should be apprised of the risk these substances pose to their health and the potential for addiction to nicotine. All facilities and vehicles used by athletes should be non-smoking environments:

- Cigarettes are directly implicated in the development of respiratory and cardiovascular disorders.
- Smoking can worsen asthma or other respiratory disorders.
- Secondhand smoke poses risks similar to actually smoking.
- Chewing tobacco can cause pre-cancerous lesions in the mucous membranes (leukoplakia) that can progress to cancer of the mouth or throat, halitosis, gum disease, and tooth damage.
- Smoking may impair athletic performance.
- Cigarettes age and yellow the skin and teeth.

Examination, Assessment, and Diagnosis

Taking a Thorough History During the Physical Evaluation

Taking a thorough history during the physical evaluation helps the athletic trainer accurately assess injuries because the history portion of an evaluation reveals many indications as to the cause and nature of the injury. This assists the athletic trainer to differentiate between possible diagnoses for injuries that present in similar ways but require very different treatment for appropriate care. Because of this, the history portion of an evaluation is often considered one of the most important aspects.

Asking the patient to describe vital information about the injury such as the mechanism of injury, the location of pain, the type of pain, sounds or sensations felt during the injury, and any preexisting injuries can guide the athletic trainer through the rest of the evaluation in determining the diagnosis. Special tests can be focused on testing for injuries that match the history of the injury that the patient reports. Therefore, the patient can be more efficiently evaluated and not exposed to excessive special tests that may further aggravate the injury.

The history-taking portion of a physical examination must be very thorough as it can prove to be the most important phase of the evaluation. Findings from the history can guide the evaluation, provide clues to the proper diagnosis, and help determine immediate and follow-up actions. When asking the patient about the history of their injury, the athletic trainer should reassure the patient, ask open-ended questions, maintain eye contact, actively listen, and record exactly what the patient reports. No palpation should be performed during this part of the evaluation but observation is acceptable.

The athletic trainer should to determine the mechanism of injury by asking the patient to describe exactly what happened during the injury, how the body moved, and any sensations felt or heard. The precise location of the injury should be determined by asking the patient to point to the pain using only one finger. The patient should be asked to describe the pain they are experiencing. For example, they should be asked if the pain is a dull ache, piercing, or burning. Questions about the structural integrity of the joint should be asked. To accomplish this, the athletic trainer should ask the patient if the effected joint feels like it is going to give out or if it locks up. The length of time the injury has been affecting the patient should be determined and if the injury has happened before.

Sociological Responses to Injuries and Providing Social Support

There are many possible sociological responses patients may experience when injured. They may feel excluded from the team from which they previously found belonging and identity leaving them feeling isolated and questioning their self-worth. The athletic trainer should take steps to ensure social support is provided to patients to help them cope with injuries. Patients should be included in team functions as much as they are physically able. Support groups are beneficial for patients, especially when the group include athletes with similar injuries who have successfully completed rehabilitation.

When interacting with the patient, the athletic trainer should actively listen, show authentic concern, build rapport, explain the injury in a way the patient understands, include the patient in decisions made about rehabilitation, and recommend stress-reducing techniques such as imagery and negative thought stoppage. Finally, when return-to-play for the patient is near, the athletic trainer should help the patient reenter competition by designing sport-specific rehabilitative drills that can be performed during normal practice times on the team's field of play.

CRANIAL NERVES

The twelve pairs of cranial nerves control neurologic functions of the head and are labeled by Roman numerals. Their names and functions are as follows:

- Olfactory: sense of smell
- Optic: responsible for vision
- Oculomotor: pupil's reactivity to light, eyelid opening, and eye movement
- Trochlear: lateral and downward eye movement
- Trigeminal: facial feeling and chewing
- Abducens: lateral eye movement
- Facial: expressions of the face
- Vestibulocochlear: balance and hearing
- Glossopharyngeal: swallowing
- Vagus: swallowing and speech
- Accessory: swallowing and neuromuscular control of the sternocleidomastoid muscle
- Hypoglossal: moves the tongue and controls speech

The function of the cranial nerves must be assessed following head injuries as impairment indicates possible serious injury that requires referral for immediate advanced medical care. To evaluate cranial nerve function, check the patient's sense of smell (I), vision (II), eye tracking (III, IV, VI), and pupil's reaction to light (III). Instruct the patient to bite down (V), mimic facial expressions (VII), check their hearing (VIII), and tell them to swallow (IX, X, XI). Finally, have the patient shrug their shoulders against resistance (XI), and stick out their tongue (XII).

PERFORMING DEEP TENDON REFLEX TESTING

Deep tendon reflex testing can be performed by having the patient relax and hitting the tendon of the muscle to be tested with a reflex hammer. An example of this is the knee jerk reflex that occurs when the patellar tendon is hit with a reflex hammer. Deep tendon reflexes result in an involuntary muscular contraction elicited by a placing a quick stretching force on a muscle's tendon. The grading system that rates deep tendon reflexes gives grades of zero to four. A grade of a zero indicates no reflex can be elicited, a one indicates a diminished reflex is present, a grade of a two indicates a normal reflex, a three indicates and exaggerated reflex, while a grade of a four is given for a markedly hyperactive reflex and is often associated with clonus muscular contractions. The athletic trainer can perform deep tendon reflex testing on the biceps (C5), brachioradialis (C6), extensor digitorum (C6), triceps (C7), adductor (L2), patella (L4), Achilles (S1), and hamstring (S2).

DERMATOMES AND TESTING SENSORY FUNCTIONS

A dermatome is an area of the skin innervated by the sensory nerve fibers of a single spinal or cranial nerve. To perform sensory testing of the dermatomes, the athletic trainer applies varying sensory stimuli to the dermatomes and compares the sensation the patient experiences bilaterally. Touching the dermatomes with a cotton ball can assess superficial sensation. Touching dermatomes with a pin can assess superficial pain. Squeezing muscles within the dermatomes can assess deep pain. Touching the dermatomes with an ice cube can test sensation of temperature. Touching a vibrating tuning fork to the dermatomes can assess the ability to sense vibration. The patient's sense of position can be determined by passively moving the patient's fingers or toes and asking them to identify the movement.

Determining a Patient's Mechanism of Injury

Determining the mechanism of injury (MOI) is crucial to be able to accurately assess various injuries seen in the field of athletic training. Some different injuries have similar signs and symptoms and to accurately differentiate between them, determining the MOI is essential. Many times, patients may not be able to effectively communicate how the injury occurred without the athletic trainer asking pertinent questions. Therefore, the athletic trainer should ask open-ended questions and allow the patient to thoroughly describe how they were injured. The athletic trainer should ask follow-up questions as needed such as when the injury occurred, the direction the injured body part moved, how the patient landed, and if they heard or felt any sensations during the injury. The athletic trainer should also ask if there is anything the patient wants to add that the athletic trainer did not ask about. After asking all the questions the athletic trainer should restate what they heard to check with the patient for accuracy.

Risks of Injury When Playing on a Turf Field

Participating in physical activity on a turf field increases the risks for certain injuries and athletic trainers should take measures to prevent these injuries. Abrasions and turf toe are two common injuries patients suffer when participating on a turf field. Advising athletes to wear pads on their knees and elbows for protection can reduce the occurrence of abrasions. Turf toe, a hyperextension injury to the great toe, occurs more often on turf due to the increased dorsiflexion allowed by athletic shoes made for participation on turf fields. To prevent turf toe injuries, shoes with a stiff forefoot should be selected. Insoles can be added that have steel under the forefoot or a thermo-moldable plastic can be made to limit excessive dorsiflexion.

Iron-Deficiency Anemia

Iron-deficiency anemia is a condition in which the body does not have enough iron and therefore the red blood cells' ability to carry oxygen to working muscles is inhibited. This leaves the patient feeling fatigued and unable to compete at maximum potential. Three conditions occur with iron-deficiency anemia, the red blood cells are smaller than normal, hemoglobin is reduced, and the concentration of ferritin is too low. Populations most at risk of suffering from iron-deficiency anemia are menstruating females and males aged 11 to 14.

There are multiple causes of iron-deficiency anemia such as a lack of nutritional iron intake, improper absorption of iron, and gastrointestinal losses of iron. In females, menstruation also results in a loss of iron. The most accurate way to check for iron-deficiency anemia is by evaluating serum ferritin levels. Proper treatment includes consuming a nutritionally balanced diet which includes more red and dark meat, consuming vitamin C for increased absorption of iron, and avoiding coffee and tea as they reduce proper iron absorption. Finally, iron supplementation may be warranted.

Dietary Calcium

Calcium is needed for various functions in the human body such as strengthening the teeth and bones, muscular contraction, and nerve-impulse conduction. If enough calcium is not consumed, the body will remove calcium stores from the bones, which can lead to osteoporosis. When a patient suffers from osteoporosis their bones become excessively porous and frail making their bones at higher risk of fracture. Osteoporosis is eight times more likely to occur in women than men.

Young adults need 1,300 mg of calcium daily. However, 25% of females in America consume less than 300 mg of calcium daily. Calcium is found most reliably in milk sources such as milk, cheese, and yogurt. Kale, broccoli, and calcium-fortified foods such as juices and bread with calcium added are also great sources. The most effective types of calcium supplementation are calcium carbonate and calcium citrate.

AMPHETAMINES

Amphetamines are very hazardous stimulant drugs that are banned by both the NCAA and US Olympic Committee. They are one of the most abused drugs for performance enhancement. Amphetamines can be taken by tablet, inhaled, or injected. Patients may use amphetamines because they believe their athletic performance is improved with increased quickness, energy levels, and confidence. However, studies show there is no performance improvement with amphetamine use, and patients are at increased risk for a circulatory system collapse, more prone to injure themselves and others, and more likely to become fatigued.

Physiological side effects of amphetamine use include abnormal pupil dilation (mydriasis), hyperthermia, increased reflex reaction (hyperreflexia), and increased blood pressure. The psychological side effects of amphetamine use include irrational behavior, amphetamine psychosis, hallucinations, and paranoia.

APPROPRIATE PHARMACOLOGICAL PRACTICES

The pharmacological practices allowed in the field of athletic training vary greatly from state-to-state as well as setting-to-setting. Therefore, athletic trainers must research and follow the guidelines set in place by their state for the population in which they serve. For example, in secondary-school settings the pharmacological practices are generally more restrictive than in a collegiate setting. If the state in which an athletic trainer practices allows him or her to administer a drug, certain steps must be followed to ensure patient safety. Over-the-counter drugs must be clearly labeled to include the name of the product, active and inactive ingredients, directions for use, purpose, and warnings. Athletic trainers must keep accurate records of all medicines administered and always make sensible and careful decisions concerning pharmacological practices.

ETIOLOGY, PATHOLOGY, DIAGNOSIS, DIFFERENTIAL DIAGNOSIS, AND PROGNOSIS

Etiology: The source of an injury or illness. The etiology of a concussion could be a blow to the head.

Pathology: Structural and functional changes that occur to the body as a result of an injury. After a severe ankle sprain, the ankle joint may be pathologically unstable.

Diagnosis: The identification of a disorder that is determined after a thorough evaluation. A bone scan can be used to diagnose a stress fracture.

Differential diagnosis: When insufficient evidence exists to properly reach a diagnosis, a differential diagnosis is used. This is a list of possible conditions that cannot be ruled out until further information is acquired.

Prognosis: The patient's expected outcome following and injury or illness. The prognosis for a hamstring strain may be full-recovery after several weeks of rehabilitation.

SOAP

The acronym SOAP stands for subjective, objective, assessment, and plan. A SOAP note is a way to document injury evaluations and the plan of care. The subjective section should contain all the subjective information the patient reports about the injury. For example, a patient suffering from a knee injury may report pain, knee locking, and hearing a pop at the time of the injury. These pieces of information belong in the subjective section. The objective section contains all the physical signs that the athletic trainer can physically observe related to the injury as well as results of special testing. For example, the same patient may display edema, ecchymosis, and crepitus. They may also have positive findings for the anterior drawer test and McMurray's test. These pieces of information belong in the objective section.

In the assessment section the athletic trainer states what they believe the diagnosis of the injury to be. Possible differential diagnoses could be included here as well if applicable. The plan section is where the athletic trainer would dictate the course of action for the injury. If necessary, this may include a referral, a plan for treatment, and rehabilitation.

MEDICAL DOCUMENTATION ABBREVIATIONS

AC: Refers to the acromioclavicular joint in the shoulder or an acute condition. The acromioclavicular joint is the joint where the acromion of the scapula and the clavicle meet.

ADL: Stands for activities of daily living, which are things that patients do in their everyday lives such as prepare meals and walk

ASIS: An acronym for the anterior superior iliac spine which is a bony projection on the ilium

B: Stands for bilateral which refers to both sides of the body

C/O: Stands for complained of which can be used when dictating symptoms a patient reports. It also stands for under care of such as identifying medical professionals who are providing care for a patient

D/C: Stands for discharge, when a patient no longer needs treatment they are discharged.

Dx: Stands for diagnosis, which is the naming of a specific condition after a thorough evaluation.

ES: An acronym for electrical stimulation, which is an electrical therapeutic modality commonly used for pain treatment, education of edema, and muscular reeducation.

FWB: An acronym meaning full weight bearing which denotes that a patient is able to bear full weight on a body part following and injury

Fx: Stands for fracture of a bone, an x-ray is the most common diagnostic tool for a possible fracture.

NKA: An acronym meaning no know allergies that signifies that a patient has no allergies they are aware of.

PRE: An acronym for progressive resistance exercises, which are strengthening exercises that progress in difficulty as the patient progresses through rehabilitation.

R/O: Stands for rule out, such as a specific diagnosis must be ruled out. For example, in a severe ankle sprain many times a possible fibular fracture must be ruled out.

RTP: An acronym for return to play such as a patient has completed rehabilitation and is ready for full sport participation

US: An acronym for ultrasound, a sound energy therapeutic modality that is commonly used for heating tissues.

Obtaining a Medical History

A complete **medical history** is necessary in order to assess current or potential injuries or health-related conditions. The Certified Athletic Trainer must use good communication skills to elicit information. The history should be obtained in a private, quiet area. Guidelines for questioning include:

- Avoid questions that require "yes" or "no," such as "Have you injured your ankle?"
- Request descriptions, such as, "Describe any ankle injury you have had."
- Ask content questions, such as, "When and how did you injure your ankle?"
- Clarify all reports of injury or illness by asking information about duration and symptoms: "What type of problems did you have from your injury and how long did they persist?"

Allow the athlete time to respond and provide summaries: "I understand you to say that you sprained your ankle playing baseball." The athlete should be questioned about any changes, such as weight loss/gain, new medications, bowel or bladder habits, diet, sleep, or stress.

Using Physical Examinations When Determining a Differential Diagnosis

Performing a physical examination that includes diagnostic testing helps the athletic trainer in determining a differential diagnosis because the diagnostic testing can help to rule-out possible injuries or illnesses that have similar signs, symptoms, and mechanisms of injury. For example, when performing a physical examination for a patient who reports inverting their ankle and feeling a pop, it is important to determine if the injury is a fractured bone, a torn ligament, or both. All of these are possible diagnoses for this injury. Requesting an x-ray would either rule-out or confirm the diagnosis of a fractured bone and would lead towards the correct diagnosis. Determining a correct diagnosis leads to a proper plan of care and best possible patient outcomes.

Inspection of Soft-Tissue Injuries

Soft-tissue injuries may be closed or open. Closed wounds occur with the skin intact, while open wounds expose tissues beneath the skin, posing a threat of infection. There are a number of different types of tissue injury:

- *Abrasion*: damage to superficial layers of skin, such as with road burn or ligature marks.
- *Contusion*: occurs when friction or pressure causes damage to underlying vessels, resulting in bruising. Contusions that are bright red/purple with clear margins have occurred within 48 hours and those with receding edges or yellow-brown discoloration are older than 48 hours.
- *Laceration*: a tear in the skin resulting from blunt force, often from falls on protuberances, such as elbows, or other blunt trauma. Lacerations may be partial to full-thickness.
- *Avulsion*: tissue that is separated from its base and lost or without adequate base for attachment.

Auscultation, Palpation, and Percussion

There are a number of **examination techniques** that are part of physical evaluation and should be used consistently when completing a physical examination or assessing injury or illness:

- *Auscultation:* using a stethoscope to listen to movement of air or fluid within the body and characterizing the sound according to intensity (loudness), frequency (pitch), and quality. Auscultation is commonly used to assess heart and lung function, circulatory impairment (bruit), and bowel sounds.

- **Palpation:** using the touch of the fingertips to evaluate characteristics, such as hardness, temperature, swelling, size, and mobility. In some cases, sound may be felt as vibration.
- **Percussion:** a technique in which the fingers of one hand are laid flat against the skin and tapped with the fingertips of the other hand, causing sound to resonate. This is most commonly used to assess organ size or changes in tissue density.

BALANCE AND THE TANDEM GAIT TEST

Balance is the ability to stand or sit upright without falling. Balance is controlled by three sensory systems that send signals to the brain stem and cerebellum, which coordinate the information to achieve balance. Two out of the three systems must function correctly to maintain balance:

- Vestibular system (inner ear), which senses the direction of motion
- Eye movement, which senses position in space and direction
- Proprioceptive system, which senses position and movement of the muscles and joints

Tandem gait is one test to assess balance:

The person stands upright and places one foot directly in front of the other and then walks, maintaining heel-to-toe placement. The trainer must walk with the athlete and provide support when necessary. Patients with damage to the cerebellar vermis (the area that receives proprioceptive sensory information between the two cerebellar hemispheres) or associated neural pathways will usually lose balance and require a wide-legged stance. Other conditions can also cause loss of balance, such as ethanol intoxication.

BALANCE AND THE ROMBERG TEST

The ***Romberg test*** evaluates balance; in it, the trainer stands behind the athlete with arms reaching around the shoulders (not touching), in case the athlete loses balance. The athlete stands with heels and feet together and eyes open for 15-20 seconds. Then, this same procedure is repeated with the eyes closed. If there is a minor problem with the vestibular or proprioceptive systems, the athlete is usually able to compensate and maintain balance when his eyes are open; but if his eyes are closed, he loses balance. For more serious injury, the athlete is unable to maintain balance even with his eyes open. The inability to remain balanced is a positive finding for the Romberg test, and the athlete should be referred for evaluation.

GLASGOW COMA SCALE

The **Glasgow coma scale** (GCS) measures the depth and duration of coma or impaired consciousness and is used for postoperative assessment. The GCS measures three parameters: best eye response, best verbal response, and best motor response, with a total possible score ranging from 3 to 15:

- **Eye opening**
    - 4: Spontaneous, 3: To verbal stimuli
    - 2: To pain (not of face), 1: No response
- **Verbal**
    - 5: Oriented, 4: Conversation confused, but can answer questions
    - 3: Uses inappropriate words, 2: Speech incomprehensible
    - 1: No response

- **Motor**
    - 6: Moves on command, 5: Moves purposefully in response to pain
    - 4: Withdraws in response to pain, 3: Decorticate posturing (flexion) in response to pain
    - 2: Decerebrate posturing (extension) in response to pain,
    - 1: No response

Injuries/conditions are classified according to the total score: 3-8: Coma; 8: Severe head injury; 9-12: Moderate head injury; 13-15: Mild head injury.

CRANIAL NERVE ASSESSMENT

The athletic trainer should be familiar with **cranial nerve assessment** as part of evaluation for suspected head injury:

- *Olfactory* (smell): The athlete is asked to smell and identify a substance, such as coffee or soap, with first one nostril held closed, and then the other.
- *Optic* (vision): Test of visual acuity and the ability to recognize color. Test each eye separately. Red desaturation is tested by having the athlete look at a red object with first one eye and then the next to determine if the color looks the same with both eyes or is dull with one eye.
- *Oculomotor* (eye muscles and pupil response): Using a penlight, the examiner checks eyes for size, shape, reaction to light and accommodation. Eyes are checked for rotation and conjugate movements. The lids should be examined for ptosis.
- *Trochlear* (eye muscles—upward movement): Eye movement is checked by having the person follow a moving finger with the eyes on the vertical plane.
- *Trigeminal* (chewing muscles, sensory): The person closes eyes for the sensory examination and is instructed to indicate when part of the face is stroked (light stroke with cotton). The forehead, cheek, and jaw are stroked. The same areas are then examined for sharp or dull sensations. The eye should be observed for blinking and tearing, but touching the cornea with cotton or other items should be avoided, as it can cause abrasion. The jaw muscles are assessed by having the person hold the mouth open, as well as by palpating the muscles on each side to determine if they are equal in size and strength.
- *Abducens* (eye muscles—lateral movement): The person is also asked to follow the finger from the 1 o'clock position clockwise to the 11 o'clock position. At the horizontal and vertical axes, the eyes should be checked for deviation or nystagmus, which normally occur only in the extreme lateral position.
- *Facial nerve* (facial expression, tears, taste, and saliva): Usually, only the motor portion is evaluated for nerve VII, and taste is examined by testing cranial nerve IX, but one can test the ability to discriminate between salt and sugar. Motor functions are assessed by asking the person to frown, smile, puff out the cheeks, and wrinkle the forehead. The muscles are observed for symmetry. The person is asked to hold his eyes tightly closed while the examiner attempts to open his lids with the thumb on the lower lid and the index finger on the upper lid, using care not to apply pressure to the eye.

- **Vestibulocochlear** (balance and hearing): Balance is checked with tandem gait and Romberg's test. Hearing is checked (with the person's eyes closed) by rubbing fingers together or holding a ticking watch next to one ear and then the other. Weber's test may be done to evaluate lateralization, and the Rinne test may be performed to evaluate bone and air conduction.
    - **Weber's test:** A vibrating tuning fork is touched to the top of the head or the forehead, and the person is asked if sound is equal in both ears. Hearing deficit in one ear suggests sensorineural hearing loss.
    - **Rinne's test:** A vibrating tuning fork is held on the mastoid bone and the time is measured until sound ceases. Then, the vibrating tuning fork is held at the external ear. Sound is normally heard twice as long through air as through bone. If there is conductive hearing loss, the sound is heard longer through the bone. If there is sensorineural hearing loss, the sound is heard longer through the air.
- **Glossopharyngeal** (taste, mouth sensation): This test is not usually performed unless the person complains of lack of taste or abnormalities of taste. The mouth must be moist for accurate assessment, so the person should drink water if possible before the test, and the testing substance should be in solution. The person is tested for recognition of sweet, sour, bitter, and salt.
- **Vagus** (swallowing, gag reflex): The examiner has the person open his mouth and say "aw." The uvula and palate should elevate equally on both sides. The gag reflex is usually tested if the person reports difficulty swallowing or changes in speech. Gag reflex is tested by lightly touching the tongue blade to the soft palate. Some people are hyper-responsive, so accurate testing of the gag reflex may be difficult.
- **Spinal accessory** (muscle movement—sternocleidomastoid, trapezius): These muscular movements are tested by the examiner placing the hands along the side of the face and asking the person to turn the face first to one side and then the other against resistance to determine if strength is normal and equal. Then, the examiner places his hands on the person's shoulders and asks the person to shrug his shoulders, elevating them upward against resistance to determine if the strength is normal and equal.
- **Hypoglossal** (tongue): The examiner asks the person to stick out the tongue to determine if it deviates to one side, indicating a lesion on that side of the brain. To determine if there is equal strength on both sides of the tongue, a tongue blade is held against the side of the tongue and the person is asked to push against it with his tongue. Both sides are checked to determine if strength is normal and equal.

Peripheral Nerve Assessment

A musculoskeletal evaluation should include **peripheral nerve assessment** to determine if injury has impaired nerve function. Nerve function should be assessed for both sensation and movement. Assessment of sensation is done with a sharp or pointed instrument, using care not to prick the skin. The person should feel a slight prick if the sensory function is intact:

- **Median:** The median nerve branches from the brachial plexus, which arises from C5, C6, C7, C8, and T1. The median nerve travels down the arm and forearm, through the carpal tunnel. Sensation is evaluated by pricking the top or distal surface of the index finger. Movement is evaluated by having the person touch the ends of the thumb and little finger together and flex the wrist.

- **Peroneal:** The peroneal nerve branches from the sciatic nerve, which arises from the L4, L4 and S1, S2, and S3 dorsal nerves and travels down the leg. The peroneal nerve enervates the lower leg, foot, and toes. Sensation is evaluated by pricking the webbed area between the great and second toe. Movement is evaluated by having the person dorsiflex and extend the foot.
- **Radial:** The radial nerve branches from the brachial plexus and enervates the dorsal surface of the arm and hand, including the thumb and fingers 2, 3, and 4. Sensation is evaluated by pricking the skin in the webbed area between the thumb and the index finger. Movement is evaluated by having the person extend his thumb, wrist, and fingers at the metacarpal joint.
- **Tibial:** The tibial nerve branches from the sciatic nerve. The tibial nerve travels down the back of the leg, through the popliteal fossa at the back of the knee, and terminates at the plantar side of the foot. Sensation is evaluated by pricking the medial and lateral aspects of the plantar surface of the foot. Movement is evaluated by having the person plantar flex the toes and then the ankle.
- **Ulnar:** The ulnar nerve branches from the brachial plexus and travels down the arm from the shoulder, traveling along the anterior forearm beside the ulna, to the palm of the hand. Sensation is evaluated by pricking the distal fat pad at the end of the small finger. Movement is evaluated by having the person extend and spread all fingers.

CARPEL TUNNEL SYNDROME ASSESSMENT

Carpel tunnel syndrome occurs when the median nerve is compressed within the carpel tunnel, formed from ligaments and bones, between the forearm and the hand. The carpal tunnel also contains tendons. Initial symptoms include numbness, tingling, or burning in the hand (especially the palm, thumb, index, and middle fingers) with eventual weakening and inability to grip. Compression increases when the wrist is flexed, so the symptoms may worsen during sleep. Carpal tunnel syndrome may result from subluxation of the carpal bones from trauma, scar tissue, or fluid. Positive tests include:

- **Tinel's sign:** Percussion or pressure directly over the carpal tunnel elicits thumb and first 3 fingers, but this test is not always reliable.
- **Phalen's test:** Placing the dorsum (backs) of the hands together and flexing the wrist to the full extent; holding light pressure for 1 minute elicits symptoms.
- **Oriental prayer test:** Palms of hands are placed together with fingers and thumb fully abducted, and thumbs don't touch.

LATERAL COLLATERAL LIGAMENT ASSESSMENT

The **lateral collateral ligament** connects the femur to the fibula and bands about the lateral knee, providing stability to the joint during movement. The ligament may be injured by direct blunt trauma or repetitive stress, as may occur in sports that require quick stops and twisting of the joint, such as basketball and soccer. Symptoms include instability of the joint, locking or catching, pain, swelling, and stiffness. A positive **varus stress test** can indicate a tear:

- Note: Test the uninjured leg first for comparison.
- Place the athlete in a supine position on a table, with the knee extended and the leg hanging over the side of the table.
- Hold the ankle with one hand and the knee with the fingers to the medial aspect with the other hand.
- Flex the knee to 30°.
- Push the knee in a varus movement (away from the center) while holding the ankle stable.
- Pain in the lateral joint and increased varus movement are positive findings.

Gluteus Medius Muscle Assessment

The **gluteus medius** muscle originates below the iliac crest and inserts at the top of the greater trochanter. It controls abduction of the thigh and allows the hip to rotate internally and externally; during running, it also stabilizes the pelvis, so injuries to this muscle and subsequent weakness are common among runners. The ***Trendelenburg test*** is used to evaluate for weakness of the gluteus medius:

- Note: This test may be done by having the athlete hold onto a table or bar for support and observing from behind, or by kneeling in front of the athlete, placing the hands on his or her hips, and having the athlete hold onto the examiner's shoulders.
- The athlete stands on one foot, with the opposite knee flexed for 10 seconds, and then repeats for the other foot.
- If the non-standing hip elevates, it is a negative sign. If the non-standing hip drops, this is positive and indicates weakness of the gluteus medius.

Achilles Tendon Assessment

A **ruptured Achilles tendon** can be caused by blunt trauma to the tendon, excessive forced dorsiflexion of the ankle, or injury to a taut tendon. The injury occurs about 2-3 cm above the area where the tendon attaches the gastrocnemius (calf muscle) to the calcaneus (heel bone). The area of injury is usually tender to palpation, edematous, and bruised, with a palpable gap where the tendon ruptured. ***Thompson's test*** is used to evaluate the injury:

- Place the person in a prone position (face down) with the knee of the uninjured leg flexed to 90° and the foot relaxed.
- Squeeze the gastrocnemius muscle of the uninjured leg, causing it to contract and the foot to flex, noting the degree of response for comparison.
- Repeat test for the injured leg.
- If the Achilles tendon is partially or completely intact, plantar flexion of the foot occurs (negative finding).
- If plantar flexion is absent (positive finding), this is indicative of a ruptured tendon.

Deep Vein Thrombophlebitis of Calf Assessment

Deep vein thrombophlebitis (DVT) is usually related to poor circulation or damage to vessels, and is more common in those over age 40. It can be induced by sitting for long periods without activity, as for instance when flying long distances. Symptoms include pain or aching in the calf, especially on activity, and swelling. DVT should be differentiated from other injuries when athletes complain of calf pain. ***Homan's sign*** may be used to identify DVT:

- Person is lying in prone position with lower shin and foot extending over the edge of the table.
- The examiner passively dorsiflexes the ankle while palpating the proximal calf.
- Positive findings are pain in the calf on dorsiflexion of the ankle or pain during the palpation.

Trochanteric Bursitis Assessment

Bursitis is inflammation of the bursa (fluid-filled spaces or sacs that form in tissues to reduce friction) causing thickening of the lining of the bursal walls. Common types of bursitis include shoulder, olecranon (elbow), trochanteric (hip) and prepatellar (front of knee). **Trochanteric bursitis** in the hip is the most common running-induced bursitis, and is characterized by pain in the greater trochanteric area of the lateral hip, radiating down the lateral thigh. Bursitis may result from direct trauma, such as when an athlete is tackled and falls on the lateral hip, or overuse of muscles and tendons, such as may occur with repetitive exercises like running. Palpation shows point tenderness over the area and causes pain to radiate down the lateral hip. Pain increases when lying on the injured side. Pain may be elicited by passive external hip rotation. Pain usually also occurs with hip flexion and hip abduction with resistance. Treatment may include physical therapy, rest, restricted activity, and corticosteroid injections to reduce inflammation.

ILIOTIBIAL BAND SYNDROME ASSESSMENT

The iliotibial band is a wide band of fascia extending from the iliac crest to the patella and tibia along the lateral thigh. The band moves over the lateral epicondyle of the femur during knee flexion and extension. The band may be too tight, or poor technique or overuse related to running and cycling can cause friction, resulting in **iliotibial band syndrome,** inflammation of the bursa between the band and the epicondyle. Symptoms include diffuse burning pain at the lateral knee, usually after running/cycling for a few minutes or after completing the activity. Pain occurs earlier when inflammation increases.

Ober's test is performed to evaluate iliotibial band syndrome:

- Person lies on uninjured side with hip and knee flexed to 90°.
- The examiner stabilizes the person's pelvis and then abducts and extends the affected knee until it is on a straight line with the trunk.
- The affected leg is lowered into adduction.
- A positive finding is failure to adduct and pain in the lateral knee.

BICEPS TENDINITIS ASSESSMENT

Tendinitis (or tendonitis) is inflammation of the long, tubular tendons and tendon sheaths, adjacent to bursa. The causes of tendinitis are similar to those of bursitis. Frequently, both bursa and tendons are inflamed. Athletes participating in water sports, baseball, football, and other throwing sports often develop tendinitis in the upper extremities. Poor conditioning may contribute to tendinitis. Common types of tendinitis include wrist and rotator cuff in the arm and Achilles and patellar in the leg. **Biceps tendinitis** (bicipital tenosynovitis) occurs from repetitive throwing motions made while playing tennis or pitching. *Speed's test* is commonly used to assess biceps tendonitis, although studies suggest it's only about 50% effective in diagnosis:

The person stands, holding his arm out at 60° angle, and attempts to flex the arm while the examiner applies isometric resistance. Pain at the bicipital groove is positive, indicating the presence of inflammation.

- The person stands, holding his arm out at 60° angle, and attempts to flex the arm while the examiner applies isometric resistance. Pain at the bicipital groove is positive, indicating the presence of inflammation.

The symptoms of tendinitis typically include pain with movement, edema, dysfunction, and decreased range of motion. Treatment is similar to the program for bursitis. *Yergason's test* (also known as the supination test) is another test performed to evaluate biceps tendinitis:

- Standing or sitting, the person holds the arm tightly against the side of the body with the arm flexed to 90° and the arm pronated.
- The trainer palpates the bicipital groove with one hand and holds the wrist firmly with the other hand while the person attempts to supinate and externally rotate the arm against resistance.

If this maneuver elicits pain in the proximal bicipital groove, then the test is positive for tendinitis. It is also considered positive if the examiner feels the tendon move out of the groove during the test.

GOLFER'S ELBOW ASSESSMENT

Golfer's elbow (or thrower's elbow) is the common name for inflammation of the medial epicondyle on the inside of the elbow. The inflammation causes tenderness at the site of tendon insertion, but the pain may also radiate down the forearm or up to the upper arm, so in some cases the pain may be more generalized. The cause of the inflammation is repetitive muscle strain, so this injury is not limited to golfers but is common in others, such as construction workers.

The *golfer's elbow test* can help to evaluate the injury:

- With the individual seated, the affected arm is pronated with the elbow flexed at 90° and the fingers forming a fist.
- The arm (supported at the elbow and wrist by the examiner) is extended fully and supinated.
- A positive finding is pain at the medial epicondyle.

TENNIS ELBOW ASSESSMENT

Tennis elbow is inflammation of the lateral epicondyle, affecting the tendon of the extensor carpi brevis muscle. This injury occurs in sports and activities that involve repetitive wrist extension against resistance, such as badminton and squash, and often relates to poor technique or incorrect grip size. It is more common in those over the age of 30. Symptoms include lateral elbow pain, stiffness, and forearm pain. Tests include the ***Tennis elbow test:***

- With the individual seated, the elbow on the affected arm is extended (with severe pain, flexed to 90°), wrist flexed and hand in a fist.
- The examiner supports the elbow with one hand.
- The forearm is pronated, and the wrist is extended and deviated radially against resistance.
- A positive finding is pain at the lateral epicondyle on the outside of the elbow.

GLENOID LABRUM TEAR ASSESSMENT

The **glenoid labrum** is the fibrocartilaginous support of the shoulder socket (the glenoid). Tears can result from trauma, such as may occur when extending the arm with a sudden overhead reach in order to break a fall, or from repetitive shoulder motion, such as is made while throwing or lifting weights. Usual symptoms include pain (especially when reaching overhead); catching or locking of the joint; the sensation of popping or grinding at the joint; shoulder instability; stiffness; and decrease in range of motion. The ***Clunk test*** is used to evaluate a tear of the glenoid labrum:

- The person is in supine position, with the examiner behind the person's head.
- The examiner places one hand under the posterior aspect of the affected shoulder and the other hand on the distal humerus above the elbow.
- The examiner applies anterior pressure to the head of the humerus while passively abducting and laterally rotating the arm.
- A positive finding is a clunking/grinding sensation at the joint.

THORACIC OUTLET SYNDROME

Thoracic outlet syndrome comprises a number of disorders affecting the nerves of the brachial plexus as well as the nerves and vessels that travel from the neck to the axilla. Traumatic thoracic outlet syndrome most commonly affects the athlete and relates to repetitive hyperextension of the arm. Muscle weakness causes narrowing of the thoracic outlet, which is between the clavicle and the first rib, resulting in pressure on both the nerves and vessels. Symptoms include lack of sensation; tingling; burning; pain in neck, shoulder, and arm; and decreased circulation to arms and hands. The collateral circulation of the hand also may be impaired by other types of injuries or occlusion of arteries from thrombophlebitis. The Allen test and Adson test may be performed to evaluate thoracic outlet syndrome and circulation in the radial and ulnar arteries.

The **Allen test** is done to evaluate circulation of the radial and ulnar arteries at the wrist:

- The person is sitting with his shoulder abducted (90°) and externally rotated (90°) and elbow flexed (90°).
- The person makes a tight fist and maintains it for at least 20 seconds before testing.
- The examiner grasps the hand, applying pressure against both the radial and ulnar arteries at the wrist.
- The person opens his hand, which should immediately blanche.
- The ulnar artery is released first, and if circulation is normal, color will return within 5-7 seconds. If there is ulnar blockage, the palm will remain blanched until the radial artery is released.
- The test is repeated, releasing the radial artery first.

The **Adson test**: The person takes a deep breath, hyperextends his neck, and turns his head to the right while the examiner palpates the left radial pulse. A positive finding is a reduction of pulse strength. Test is repeated on opposite side.

SCOLIOSIS SCREENING

Scoliosis is the lateral curvature ≥11° of the spine, usually occurring (in 2-3% of adolescents) during the period between the ages of 10 and 15 when the child goes through a growth spurt, so screening should be done at least twice during this period. Scoliosis is more common in girls than boys. Screening includes:

- Child stands upright as shoulders, waist, and hips are assessed.
- Adams forward bending test, in which the child bends over at the waist (as in toe touching) and the screener observes the hips to determine if there is a difference in height.
- Scoliometer measures the curvature of the spine in the thoracic and lumbar area when the child bends over.
- Moire topography uses a grating positioned near the child, which casts shadows indicating contour lines.
- X-rays confirm positive screenings.

Positive findings may include one shoulder that is lower than another; uneven waistline; prominence of shoulder blade(s); one hip higher than another; or lateral leaning when standing upright.

MENISCUS ASSESSMENT

The **medial and lateral menisci** are the protective sections of cartilage between the distal femur and proximal head of the tibia; they absorb about a third of the impact on a joint and provide some stability. Only the periphery of the menisci is vascular and enervated, so a tear usually lacks nutrition to mend itself and may not be accompanied by pain. The menisci are divided according to location: anterior horn (front), body (middle section), and posterior horn (back). Sports injuries result from twisting or blunt trauma (most notably in football and skiing). Symptoms of tears include stiffness, locking, pain, and swelling. **McMurray's test** is performed to evaluate meniscal tears: With the individual supine, the hip and knee are fully flexed, with the foot flat and as close to the hip as possible.

Medial meniscus: The examiner externally rotates the foot with one hand and places the other hand over the knee, palpating the medial joint line while externally rotating the tibia, and applying valgus pressure while extending the knee.

Lateral Meniscus: (Similar to medial) The examiner palpates the lateral joint line while internally rotating the tibia, applying various pressure while extending the knee.

A positive finding for lateral or medial tears is popping or pain at the associated joint line.

Another test that may be used to evaluate for a tear of the meniscus is the *Apley's compression test:*

- With the individual prone, the affected knee is flexed to 90°.
- The examiner holds the foot with both hands and applies downward pressure while rotating the lower leg laterally.
- Pain is positive for injury of the lateral or medial meniscus.

TIBIAL STRESS FRACTURE ASSESSMENT

One of the most common sports injuries is the **tibial stress fracture**, which may result from overtraining or training beyond the level of strength and endurance. Symptoms may be non-specific but may involve point tenderness or increasing pain during activity. Stress fractures may not be evident on an X-ray, and may require a bone scan for diagnosis. Stress fractures may be difficult to differentiate from other injuries. The *Talar bump test (heel percussion test)* is performed to differentiate tibial stress fracture (talus or calcaneus) from medial tibial stress syndrome:

- The person is in supine position with his knee and proximal calf on the table and the rest of his leg extending over the edge.
- The examiner holds the foot in neutral position with one hand.
- With the other open palm, the examiner applies percussive force (slapping) against the plantar surface of the foot.
- A positive sign of fracture is pain at the point of injury during percussion.

ANKLE JOINT INJURY ASSESSMENT

The **ankle joint** is stabilized medially by the deltoid ligament, which runs from the tibial malleolus to the calcaneus and talus, and laterally by the calcaneofibular ligament, which runs from the fibular malleolus to the lateral calcaneus. These ligaments are commonly injured during athletic activities that stress the joint. The *Talar tilt test* is performed to test for injury of the deltoid ligament and the calcaneofibular ligament:

- The person is sitting or lying supine on the table with the distal part of the calf and foot extending over the table.
- Deltoid: Foot is in neutral position. Examiner holds foot. Examiner grasps the foot and abducts and everts the calcaneus to a valgus position.
- Calcaneofibular: Foot is in neutral position. Examiner grasps the foot and adducts and inverts the calcaneus to varus position.
- Positive findings for either ligament include laxity of joint or pain.

Patellar Tendinitis Assessment

Patellar tendinitis/tendinopathy (also known as "jumper's knee") is a stress injury to the quadriceps and patellar tendons that join the patella to the tibia, allowing the quadriceps to straighten the leg. Repetitive stress tendinitis is typically related to jumping sports (such as basketball, volleyball, and the high jump), although the injury actually results from landing rather than jumping. The condition may be exacerbated by overtraining and jumping on hard surfaces. Symptoms increase in stages:

- First, good function but pain after exercise.
- Next, good function but pain both during and after exercise.
- Then, function deteriorates and pain is prolonged during and after exercise.
- Finally, poor function and increased pain as the tear becomes complete.

Symptoms usually include pain in the anterior and posterior areas of the patella on palpation, stiffness, and pain on contraction of the quadriceps. The hamstring and quadriceps muscles are often taut, but the range of motion of the knee remains intact. Therapy includes modification of activities; icing the knee 4-6 times daily; stretching exercises; and strengthening exercises.

Rotator Cuff Injury

The **rotator cuff** comprises the muscles and ligaments of the shoulder joint. The bones in the joint include the scapula and humerus. Muscles (subscapularis, supraspinatus, infraspinatus, and spines minor) and tendons anchor to the head of the humerus so that the arm can move in all directions, while ligaments connect the bones. Part of the rotator cuff is under the scapula. The bursa is between the rotator cuff and shoulder joint, providing protection. Injury may result from trauma, such as a fall, forced external rotation (often while playing football) or repetitive stress, such as from pitching a baseball. Tears, tendinitis, and bursitis may occur in the ligaments and muscles. Symptoms include pain in the shoulder, weakness, and limited range of movement. Bone spurs may cause inflammation and pain. Most injuries respond to physical therapy (including strengthening and range of motion exercises), although in some cases NSAIDS, corticosteroid injections, or surgical repair may be indicated.

Rotator Cuff/Supraspinatus Tendon Injury Assessment

The most common injury to the rotator cuff is a **tear in the supraspinatus tendon**, so that the tendon is separated from its attachment. Typically, the athlete complains of pain in the lateral shoulder, increasing at night and with movement, such as lifting the arm. There may be weakness both while lifting the arm and while externally rotating it. The following tests can be performed sitting or standing:

- **Drop arm test**
  - Arm is abducted (90°) and slowly lowered.
  - Positive findings for tear/pathology are if arm drops or lowering is jerky.
  - If trainer lightly taps on abducted arm, the arm may drop suddenly.
- **"Empty can" or supraspinatus strength test**
  - The arms are held in scaption (30° horizontal adduction with the shoulder abducted to 90°), so the arms are out straight in front.
  - The trainer applies downward pressure to the arms while the person tries to hold the arms stable, resisting pressure.
  - If the person cannot resist the pressure and the affected arm falls, this positive result indicates supraspinatus damage.

- **Painful arc**
  - Person stands with arm resting at the side of the body. Arm is passively and/or actively abducted (raised from the side to straight overhead in a half-circle arc). Positive for supraspinatus pathology: Pain between 120-170°. Note: external rotation during abduction may relieve pain by decreasing pressure, so close observation is necessary. Positive for AC joint pathology: Pain between 140-180°.
- **Apley's scratch test**
  - Person sits for testing. Person reaches with injured arm behind head and tries to touch the outer rim of the superior medial scapula. Pathology of the rotator cuff (usually the supraspinatus) is indicated by pain or failure to reach target area.
- **Ludington sign**
  - Person sits for test. Person is directed to place both hands behind his neck.
  - A tear in the rotator cuff is indicated by failure to carry out action with the affected arm or the need for compensatory movement to carry out action.

ACROMIOCLAVICULAR JOINT INJURY ASSESSMENT

The **acromioclavicular (AC) joint** connects the scapula and the clavicle, providing shoulder support. The joint is stabilized by the conoid and trapezoid ligaments and the capsuloligamentous complex. Injuries to this joint often occur during football or other contact sports. Injury may cause separation of the ligaments. Pain is usually in the anterior/superior aspect of the shoulder. The crossover test is performed to evaluate for pathology. The **crossover test** (also called the crossover impingement test) is usually performed with the athlete in the sitting position:

- The trainer places one hand on the posterior shoulder of the affected side of the person to provide support.
- The trainer holds the person's elbow with the other hand.
- The trainer applies pressure against the elbow toward the opposite side to maximally adduct the shoulder, pushing the arm across the chest.
- A positive finding occurs when pain is felt in the superior shoulder at the AC joint.
- Pain in the posterior or anterior areas suggests rotator cuff injury.

UNSTABLE SHOULDER ASSESSMENT

Subluxation of the shoulder may result in an unstable shoulder; however, symptoms may be non-specific with complaints of discomfort or pain in the shoulder area. Subluxation usually occurs during sports that involve intense or repetitive use of the shoulder. The **apprehension test** is used to evaluate shoulder instability (both sides checked for comparison):

- The person is sitting or supine with his arm over the side of the table.
- The shoulder is abducted to 90° and the elbow is flexed at 90° initially.
- The examiner holds the head of the humerus with one hand and places the other hand behind the shoulder.
- The examiner externally rotates the shoulder, applying pressure anteriorly and inferiorly at 60°, 90°, and 120° of abduction.
- A positive indication of subluxation is pain in the shoulder area and/or tensing of the muscles.

ANTERIOR CRUCIATE LIGAMENT INJURY ASSESSMENT

The **anterior cruciate ligament** is one of the 4 ligaments that support the knee. It provides stability, prevents the tibia from moving anterior to the femur, and limits rotation. A tear or partial tear can result from marked twisting of the joint or blunt trauma. Symptoms usually include pain and swelling of the joint as well as instability of the knee, depending upon the degree of damage. The *Anterior drawer test* is used to evaluate stability of the knee:

- The person lies supine on an examining table with his foot on the affected side at the side of the table, his hip flexed to 45° and his knee at 90°.
- An assistant stabilizes the foot, or (alternately) the examiner sits on the foot, using his buttocks to stabilize the foot.
- The test is performed with the foot in 3 positions: neutral and externally rotated 15° and 30°.
- The examiner places both hands on the upper calf at the head of the tibia and pulls anteriorly with even pressure.
- A positive sign of damage to the anterior cruciate ligament is palpable anterior tibial displacement.

This technique should be used with care in acute or multiple knee injuries, as it can cause further damage. In acute injuries, the muscles may contract reflexively to protect the joint, which may result in false positive results because the knee appears stable. Additionally, pain may restrict flexion. In acute injuries, the *supine Lachman test* may be used:

- The person lies in supine position with his hip flexed to 45° and his knee flexed 20-30°.
- The examiner uses one hand to grasp and stabilize the distal thigh above the knee, and the other hand to grasp the upper calf at the head of the tibia, which is then pulled anteriorly to evaluate for displacement.

POSTERIOR CRUCIATE LIGAMENT INJURY ASSESSMENT

The posterior cruciate ligament (back of the knee joint) is one of the 4 ligaments supporting the knee. It provides support to the knee, preventing hyperextension, side to side movement, and rotational movement. The injury may result from blunt trauma to the knee while the knee is flexed, forcing the tibia posteriorly and stretching or tearing the ligament. There is usually less swelling than with an anterior cruciate tear, but the knee may be stiff and somewhat unstable. The **posterior drawer test** is the most sensitive test for evaluation:

- Note: The person's position is similar to that of the anterior drawer test: supine with hip flexed at 45°, knee at 80°, and foot in neutral position.
- The examiner anchors the person's foot and palpates the hamstrings to ensure they are relaxed.
- The examiner places both hands immediately below the knee and applies pressure posteriorly to the tibial head.
- Subluxation of the tibia posterior to the femur is positive for posterior cruciate defect.

RECTUS FEMORIS MUSCLE INJURY ASSESSMENT

The **rectus femoris** muscle is the most commonly injured part of the quadriceps; it extends along the anterior thigh from the hip to the knee. Contusions to the muscle can result from blunt trauma, such as a helmet hitting the leg during football. Symptoms usually include pain, stiffness, and bruising, but in severe trauma compartment syndrome can occur. The muscle may be strained or ruptured, most often related to overuse of the muscle during kicking or sprinting. Symptoms include a muscle bulge at the proximal anterior thigh, with pain radiating the length of the muscle. The muscle damage restricts extension, because the muscle cannot contract. In some cases, the rectus femoris tendon may strain or rupture at the knee, but this is most common in those over 40. Symptoms of tendon sprain or rupture include pain during flexion or ambulation. Rupture prevents extension of the knee.

Concussion Assessment

Concussions are biomechanical injuries to the brain and are usually transient, causing no permanent neurological damage. Symptoms may last a few minutes or several hours. Concussion can occur in almost any sport, but is especially common in contact sports. Concussions are most often caused by blunt trauma to the head or face, although trauma to other areas may cause force to the head resulting in concussion. Typical symptoms of concussion are:

- Alterations in consciousness or loss of consciousness, confusion.
- Impaired coordination.
- Disorientation and vision disturbances.
- Headache and dizziness.
- Nausea.

Concussions usually don't involve structural damage, and impairment is rapid but brief. At the Prague Conference in 2004, concussions were categorized as follows:

- Simple: Symptoms subside quickly, with complete resolution in 5-10 days and no residual effects. A simple concussion can usually be managed by an athletic trainer with medical supervision.
- Complex: Symptoms persist, including some evidence of cognitive impairment. This is most common with more severe injuries or repeated concussions, and should be managed by a physician.

Cantu Guidelines for Concussions

There are a number of sets of guidelines regarding the return to play for an athlete who has experienced a concussion, and there is no current consensus as to which set is the safest: The **Cantu (2001) guidelines** are as follows:

- *Grade I:* These are mild concussions that involve no loss of consciousness, but the athlete may exhibit post-traumatic amnesia (memory disruption after injury) or other mild symptoms that last 30 minutes or longer.
- *Grade II:* These are moderate concussions with loss of consciousness less than 1 minute accompanied by post-traumatic amnesia or other symptoms lasting 30 minutes or more but not more than 24 hours.
- *Grade II:* These severe concussions include loss of consciousness for more than 1 minute or post post-traumatic amnesia persisting longer than 24 hours or general symptoms of concussion persisting more than 7 days.

Return to play guidelines:

- After 1st concussion: When symptoms subside
- After 2nd concussion: In 2 weeks if asymptomatic for one week
- After 3rd concussion: No return to play for the current season

Colorado Medical Society Guidelines for Concussions

Guidelines regarding concussions were established by the **Colorado Medical Society** in 1991, and these guidelines remain in use. The grades are more restrictive than the Cantu guidelines in regard to loss of consciousness, but the return to play guidelines are similar:

- *Grade I:* These are mild concussions that involve only temporary confusion but not loss of consciousness or post-traumatic amnesia.
- *Grade II:* These are moderate concussions with no loss of consciousness, but there is confusion associated with post-traumatic amnesia.
- *Grade III:* These are severe concussions with loss of consciousness, even momentary.

Return to play guidelines:

- After 1st concussion: After 20 minutes of no symptoms
- After 2nd concussion: After 1 week of no symptoms
- After 3rd concussion: No return to play for 3 months

American Academy of Neurology Guidelines for Concussions

Guidelines regarding concussions were established by the **American Academy of Neurology** in 1997, and these guidelines are still in use. These guidelines are similar to the Colorado Medical Society guidelines and more restrictive than Cantu, but are more specific in regard to the duration of symptoms and more restrictive in regard to the return to play:

- *Grade I:* These are mild concussions with only short-term concussion symptoms lasting less than 15 minutes but no loss of consciousness.
- *Grade II:* These are moderate concussions with symptoms lasting longer than 15 minutes but no loss of consciousness.
- *Grade III:* These are severe concussions that include a loss of consciousness, even momentary.

Return to play guidelines:

- After 1st concussion: Return to play after 1 week of no symptoms
- After 2nd concussion: Return to play after 2 weeks of no symptoms
- After 3rd concussion: No specific guideline was provided, but a 3rd concussion generally results in termination of play for the season

Maddocks' Questions for Cognitive Evaluation

While loss of consciousness is a clear sign of concussion, it is important to assess the cognitive state of an athlete who has suffered a brain injury of any type. **Maddock's questions** are a field assessment tool that is frequently used to determine if the athlete is disoriented. The questions may be modified, depending upon the sport or event. These questions include:

- What field/place are we playing at?
- What is the name of the team/school/institution we are playing for?
- What is the name of your opponent?
- Which session/quarter/half of the game/tournament/trial are we in at present?
- Who/what team did we play last week?

These questions should not be used to the exclusion of other evaluation, because the athlete may be well-oriented but still have other symptoms of head injury, such as headache or nausea.

Sports Concussion Assessment Tool

The **Sports Concussion Assessment Tool (SCAT)** was developed from the findings of the Prague Conference of 2004. This is more restrictive and specific than other methods of assessment, based on evidence that even mild concussions may cause persistent injury. Under these guidelines, athletes who exhibit any sign of concussion are to be removed from play and referred for a medical evaluation. The SCAT card is a list of symptoms with a scale of 0-6 (none to severe); the athlete is asked to score each symptom immediately after the injury. There are 18 symptoms to be scored, including headache; neck pain; hearing difficulties or ringing in the ear; and confusion. A low score may not necessarily mean that there is little injury. Others who know the athlete may be queried. In addition, there are a number of follow-up symptoms, such as insomnia and feeling sad. These guidelines recommend that the person should be observed for 24-48 hours, as delayed symptoms may occur.

Dermatomes

Each spinal nerve has both motor and sensory functions. **Dermatomes** are areas of skin associated with particular dorsal root spinal nerves. Each dermatome has points used for testing. Pain in a certain area of a dermatome may be evidence of injury, and can help to isolate the point of injury. The shape and size of the dermatome may change with injury to the dorsal roots.

- *C2-C4* includes the top of the head to below the clavicle.
- *C5-T1* includes the arms and hands.
- *T2-T12* includes the axillary, chest, and back to the hip girdle.
- *L1-L5* includes the hips, groins, anterior thighs and medial and lateral lower legs.
- *S1-S5* includes the medial buttocks, perineal and perianal areas, posterior thighs, lower legs, and heels.

Manual Muscle Grading

Manual muscle grading is done by an athletic trainer to assess muscle strength and endurance, and requires experience to determine the amount of resistance required to assess normal muscle force in different positions. Observation of the muscles for size and shape should precede testing, and the trainer should test muscles on both sides to assess the difference. There are a number of different scales, but the most commonly used is *Janda's 0-5 scale:*

- **0:** The muscle shows no contractility.
- **1:** The muscle contracts slightly, but there is no effective movement.
- **2:** The muscle contracts slightly and range of motion is complete if the effects of gravity are eliminated.
- **3:** The muscle can go through the complete range of motion against gravity without resistance.
- **4:** The muscle has good strength and complete range of motion against moderate resistance.
- **5:** The muscle has good strength and complete range of motion against strong resistance.

ImPACT

The **Immediate Post-Concussion Assessment and Cognitive Testing** (ImPACT®) computer program is an excellent resource both for assessing an athletes' readiness to resume activity after a concussion and for educating athletes about the effects of concussion on cognitive abilities. This program is currently in use at many high school and universities, especially for sports with risk of concussion, such as football. Athletes establish baseline scores in memory and reaction time before participating in sports activities. If the athlete suffers a concussion, he or she then takes the

ImPACT® test again and repeats it as needed until scores approximate those of the baseline. This test allows for more objective assessment and provides immediate feedback to the athlete. It prevents over-eager athletes from ignoring or failing to report symptoms related to the concussion. Athletic trainers must be trained to administer and interpret the test results. Participation helps to make athletes aware of the dangers of concussions.

SELECTING THE BEST AVAILABLE CARE USING THE PATIENT'S HISTORY AND PHYSICAL EXAMINATION

Formulating a clinical diagnosis using the patient's history and physical examination helps the athletic trainer to select the best available care for the patient because there are multiple injuries and illnesses that have similar signs and symptoms but require completely different courses of action for proper care. Using the history and the results of the physical examination will assist the athletic trainer in determining the appropriate clinical diagnosis, which will guide the athletic trainer in selecting the best care to achieve best patient outcomes. For example, a patient that complains of lateral knee pain may be suffering from a multitude of injuries, two of which could be a lateral collateral ligament (LCL) sprain or iliotibial band syndrome (ITBS). The appropriate care for a LCL sprain and ITBS are very different, so to achieve best care for the patient, it is imperative to formulate an accurate clinical diagnosis through interpretation of findings from the history and physical examination.

CLASSIFICATIONS OF INJURIES

Injuries may be classified according to the type and extent of injury. Some common **classifications** include:

- *Signs*: what are observable and to some degree measurable. These may include the extent of edema, ecchymosis (bruising), erythema (redness), lacerations, abrasions, and deformity, such as might occur with a fracture.
- *Symptoms*: what the athlete reports, such as the degree of pain, headache, nausea, and inability to walk. Symptoms may occur with signs, especially if the injury is orthopedic in nature, but other types of health problems, such as diabetes, may not be obvious from observation.
- *Acute* illnesses occur suddenly and are usually of limited duration, such as acute appendicitis or fracture. The athlete is usually aware when an acute injury or illness has occurred.
- *Chronic* illnesses develop over time and have an extended duration; examples include diabetes mellitus and hypertension. With chronic illnesses, the athlete may not be aware of the duration, or even that the illness exists.

CONTACT DERMATITIS

Contact dermatitis is a localized response to contact with an allergen, resulting in a rash that may blister and itch. Common allergens include poison oak, poison ivy, latex, benzocaine, nickel, and preservatives, but there is a wide range of substances to which people may react.

Treatment includes:

- Identifying the causative agent by evaluating the area of the body affected, taking a careful history, or performing skin-patch testing to determine allergic responses.
- Soothing oatmeal baths and Caladryl® lotion to relieve itching.
- Topical corticosteroid cream.
- Antihistamines to reduce allergic response.

- Lesions should be gently cleaned and observed for signs of secondary infection. Rash is usually left open to dry.
- Referral for antibiotics is necessary only if secondary infection occurs.

Avoidance of allergen will prevent recurrence. Some people develop chemical trauma from chemicals applied to the skin, as from lotions or adhesives. Rash and itching are similar to contact dermatitis. Skin must be cleansed and the irritant must be identified and eliminated.

FOLLICULITIS AND IMPETIGO

Folliculitis is bacterial infection of the hair follicles, often on the face, resulting in pustules, erythema, and crusts that are painful and itchy. Recently, there has been an increase in cases of community-acquired methicillin-resistant *Staphylococcus aureus* folliculitis infections among football players and wrestlers. Folliculitis may result from chronic nasal colonization of *MRSA*.

Treatment includes antibacterial soaps and topical and oral antibiotics.

Impetigo is a contagious itchy bacterial infection of the skin, commonly on the face or hands, causing clusters of blisters or sores. Impetigo is prevalent among wrestlers. Group A Streptococcus usually causes small blisters that crust over. Staphylococcus aureus usually causes larger blisters that may be bullous and cause lesions 2-8 cm large that persist for months. Treatment includes:

- Avoidance of itching.
- Gently cleanse area with soap and water.
- Oral and/or topical antibiotics.

Athletes with signs of folliculitis or impetigo should be referred for treatment and returned to competition only on the advice of the physician to prevent spread.

STRAINS

A **strain** is an overstretching of a part of the musculature ("pulled muscle") that causes microscopic tears in the muscle or tendon, usually resulting from excess stress or overuse of the muscle. Strains may be caused by blunt trauma to a muscle or overstretching related to sports activities, such as field events, football, and soccer. Common sites for strains include the ankle, back, and hamstrings. Neglect of warm-up routines and fatigues may increase the risk of strains. Onset of pain is usually sudden, with local tenderness on use of the muscle.

Strains are classified according to the severity of injury:

- **1st degree:** This injury is relatively mild and symptoms, such as slight discomfort and tenderness to palpation, may be delayed until the following day, as the athlete may be unaware of the injury. Range of motion remains intact.
- **2nd degree:** This injury comprises a wide range of symptoms resulting from stretching or partial tearing of the muscle or tendon. Pain is usually felt on injury, with tenderness on palpation and decreased passive and active range of motion, depending upon the site of injury. There may be signs of injury, such as edema and bruising. Pain increases with passive stretching or active contraction of injured muscles.
- **3rd degree:** The muscle or tendon is completely ruptured and pain occurs with injury. A defect may be palpable. Often there is extensive edema and bruising from injury to vasculature. While loss of function in affected muscle occurs, strength and loss of range of motion varies according to the site of injury.

Sprains

A **sprain** is damage to a joint, with a partial rupture of the supporting ligaments, usually caused by wrenching or twisting related to a fall. The rupture can damage blood vessels, resulting in edema, tenderness at the joint, and pain on movement, with pain increasing over 2-3 hours after injury. An avulsion fracture (in which a bone fragment is pulled away by a ligament) may occur with strain, so x-rays rule out fractures. Sprains may be classified according to severity:

- **1st degree:** This is a relatively mild degree of injury, usually associated with good range of motion and mild pain. Swelling may vary considerably, depending upon whether vessels are disrupted by the sprain.
- **2nd degree:** This comprises a wide range of signs and symptoms, as there is further injury and partial rupture of the ligaments. Usually range of motion is limited by pain. Edema and bruising are usually present but vary in degree. The joint may be somewhat unstable.
- **3rd degree:** This involves total rupture of the ligament with immediate marked pain (although sometimes less than with 2nd degree), bruising, edema, and decreased range of motion. The joint is usually markedly unstable.

Fractures and Dislocations

Fractures and dislocations usually occur as the result of trauma, such as from falls. Fractures are caused by repetitive trauma, such as from forced marching. *Salter* fractures involve the cartilaginous epiphyseal plate near the ends of long bones in children who are growing. Damage to this area can impair bone growth. Orthopedic injuries of special concern include:

- Open fractures with soft tissue injury overlying the fracture, including puncture wounds from external forces or bone fragments, can result in osteomyelitis.
- Subluxation (partial dislocation of a joint) and luxation (complete dislocation) can cause neurovascular compromise, which can be permanent if reduction is delayed. Dislocation of the hip can result in avascular necrosis of the femoral head.

Careful inspection and observation of range of motion, palpation and observation of abnormalities is important because pain may be referred. Neurovascular assessment should be performed immediately to prevent vascular compromise.

Maxillary and Orbital Fractures

Maxillary fractures of the face are uncommon in sports, but can occur as the result of collisions and contact sports. Three primary types are:

- Le Fort I: horizontal (low downward force)
- Le Fort II: pyramidal (low or mid maxilla force)
- Le Fort II: transverse (force to bridge of nose or upper maxilla)

However, many injuries are a combination with more than one type of fracture.

Symptoms may include malocclusion and open bite, apparent lengthening of face, CSF rhinorrhea (clear nasal discharge), and periorbital ecchymosis.

Orbital fractures most often occur with blunt force against the globe causing a rupture through the floor of the orbital bone or a direct blow to the orbital rim, often related to high velocity impact, as from tennis or racquetball. Injuries are most common in adolescents and young adults. *Symptoms* include ecchymosis and edema of eyelid, numbness at site, decreased sensation of cheek and upper gum, diplopia, and enophthalmos.

Turf Toe

Turf toe is a condition in which the great toe has damage to the joint capsule and/or ligaments at the base of the toe, caused by forcefully bending the toe upward. This injury may occur in runners who push off the foot or athletes who jump frequently, engage in martial arts, or play on artificial turfs. Symptoms include stiffness, pain, and swelling at the site of injury, the base of the great toe. Pain can be elicited by passively flexing and extending the great toe. Because these symptoms are similar to those of a fracture, the athlete should be referred for an x-ray. If there is no fracture, then the athlete should avoid pressure to the area for 2-4 days (usually using crutches) and avoid activities that stress the joint for 3 weeks. Upon resumption of athletic activities, the athlete may need to wear a support for the large toe or wear hard-soled shoes to prevent further hyperextension.

Pes Cavus

Pes cavus (claw foot) is a condition characterized by a very high arch, which can be genetic or acquired through trauma or neuromuscular diseases, such as muscular dystrophy. A sudden onset should trigger testing for spinal tumor. Pes cavus is not a sports injury, but activities that stress the foot, such as running, can put pressure on the ball of the foot, causing pain in the metatarsals as well as callus formation. Contraction of the plantar fascia, clawed toes, and cock-up deformity of the great toe are common symptoms. The muscles of the calf often become very taut because of the awkward position of the foot. Many people compensate for the high arch by shifting weight to the lateral foot, increasing ankle instability. A simple test is to have the athlete step on concrete with wet feet to create an imprint. Athletes may need orthotic arch supports, special shoes, and stretching to relax taut muscles. In severe cases, surgical repair may be needed.

Anterior Ankle Impingement

Anterior ankle impingement (footballer's ankle) is caused by overstretching of the ankle or bone spurs in the joint capsule at the anterior ankle, usually resulting from dorsiflexion or repeated ankle sprains. It is a common injury for football players but can affect others who hold the foot in dorsiflexion, such as baseball catchers, basketball players, and dancers. Repeated kicking actions, such as from football or soccer, can cause bone spurs to develop on the talus or tibia. Symptoms of anterior ankle impingement include edema, pain, and pressure in the joint when the foot is placed flat on the floor with the knee extended over the ankle, causing the tendons and ligaments to become impinged between the bones. Some may experience clicking of the joint and/or instability of the ankle. X-rays to be done to check for bone spurs, which may require surgical repair. Treatment includes rest and stretching and strengthening exercises.

Plantar Fasciitis

Plantar fasciitis is inflammation of the fascia along the bottom of the foot, extending from the heel to the toes. This can result from overuse and excess pressure on the heel (especially for those engaged in running, jogging, and ballet dancing). It may also result from poorly-fitting shoes, high arch, or flat feet, causing the weight to be distributed unevenly on the foot. Symptoms usually include acute pain in the heel, often first thing in the morning, localized to the anterior medial aspect of the heel. Untreated, the condition may progress to tears and the development of bone spurs. Treatment includes rest until symptoms subside, night splints, orthotics (such as arch supports and heel cups) if indicated, stretching exercises for the Achilles tendon and the plantar fascia, and strengthening exercises for the lower leg to help stabilize the ankle and foot.

Suspected Concussion/Head Injury

A **field neurological exam** should be conducted if there is suspicion of concussion or other head injury. The exam includes:

- Assessment of airway, breathing, and cardiac status (ABCs).
- Assessment of cognitive status (such as Maddock's questions).
- Glasgow coma scale assessment.
- Questioning athlete about neck pain. Neck should be immobilized if the athlete is unconscious or complaining of any neck discomfort, numbness, or lack of sensation.
- Assisting the athlete to stand or move to the sidelines, if athlete is able to move all extremities and there is no indication of cervical or spinal injury.
- Complete assessment of cognition with SCAT or other assessment tool, including asking the athlete to list the months of the year or count backward.
- Assessment of cranial nerves.
- Romberg test and tandem gait to assess balance.

Low Back Pain

Low back pain is a common ailment of athletes, especially those in sports that involve flexion, extension, and twisting of the spine. Athletes between the ages of 20 and 35 are at greatest risk. Gymnasts, cyclists, weight lifters, and runners are frequently injured. The spine is composed of 24 vertebrae, which protect the spinal cord. Between the vertebrae are gelatinous intervertebral disks that serve as cushions. An injured intervertebral disk may herniate, bulge or even rupture, causing pressure on the nerves. The most common injuries involve L4-L5 and L5-S1. Symptoms vary, but usually include sharp pain radiating down the sciatic nerve in one or both legs and stiffness upon arising. Assessment should include type, intensity, site, and duration of pain, as well as contributing factors (such as position). Range of motion and gait must be assessed. With disk herniation or injury to ligaments, flexion usually increases pain. Complete sensory and motor evaluation should be completed, and the person should be referred for neurological care if there is any indication of serious injury.

Acute Hypoglycemia

Diabetic athletes who take insulin face the danger of **acute hypoglycemia** (hyperinsulinism) as their bodies' demand for energy increases with exercise. Hyperinsulinism can cause damage to the central nervous and cardiopulmonary systems, causing neurological impairment. Causes may include:

- Toxic ingestion of alcohol or drugs, such as salicylates.
- Too much insulin for body needs.
- Too little food or excessive exercise.

Symptoms include:

- Blood glucose <50-60 mg/dL.
- Central nervous system: seizures, altered consciousness, lethargy, and poor feeding with vomiting, myoclonus, respiratory distress, diaphoresis, hypothermia, and cyanosis.
- Adrenergic system: diaphoresis, tremor, tachycardia, palpitation, hunger, and anxiety.

A physician must carefully monitor insulin control. Doses may need to be decreased up to 30% prior to exercise. The athlete must monitor blood glucose levels frequently, and must carry emergency absorbable sugar sources, such as glucose wafers, fruit juice, or sugar water with 2-3 teaspoons of sugar. The trainer must be aware of symptoms and must monitor the athlete carefully.

Common Medical Problems Suffered by Runners

There are a number of **common medical problems** associated with running, including a psychological response ("runner's high," or "running addiction") that may lead runners to ignore pain or injury and continue running. For this reason, the athletic trainer must carefully assess runners for injury. The athlete should be regularly evaluated for the following:

- Heat-related illness, such as hyperthermia, hypothermia, sunburn, or frostbite
- Runner's nipple: fissures and bleeding of the nipple caused by friction of a shirt during running
- Fungal infections of the feet
- Urinary tract abnormalities, such as blood in the urine or myoglobinuria, associated with muscle destruction
- Anemia from lack of adequate iron to meet demands of the body
- Menstrual abnormalities, such as infrequent or light menses or complete amenorrhea
- Dehydration from inadequate fluid intake

Shin Splints

Orthopedic injuries, as for instance shin splints, are very common among runners. Especially common are injuries involving the foot, the leg, and the knee, including:

- **Anterior shin splints:** Runners with high arches have decreased shock absorption, so force is transmitted to the lateral aspect of the foot, radiating to the leg and knee. This can result in anterior shin splints: inflammation of the tibialis anterior muscle and connecting tendons. This condition manifests in pain in the shin area when running. The athlete may need orthotic arch supports to provide better support to the foot, and must reduce stride in order to decrease the pull on the muscle.
- **Posterior shin splints:** This tendinitis involves the tibialis posterior muscle and tendon and is synonymous with posterior tibial tendon dysfunction (PTTD), a non-athletic diagnosis. Runners with low arches are prone to this injury, as excess force is transmitted to the medial aspects of the leg. Stretching the calf muscles as well as using firm arch supports and heel lifts may alleviate symptoms.

Overtraining Syndrome

Overtraining occurs when the athlete does not have adequate rest periods between training. Training must be balanced between exercising to build strength and endurance, and rest periods that allow the body to regenerate. Stress occurs when the athlete trains excessively without adequate rest periods. It may affect those engaged in sprint activities or endurance activities. Over time, symptoms of **overtraining syndrome** appear, and the athlete's performance plateaus and then begins to decline. In some cases, overtraining and over-exercising is related to anorexia as well, adding further stress to the body. Symptoms of overtraining syndrome include:

- Chronic fatigue.
- Increased susceptibility to viral infections, such as the flu and colds.
- Weight loss, poor appetite.
- Increase or decrease in heart rate.
- Muscle aches and cramps.
- Increased injuries.

If evidence of overtraining occurs, the primary intervention is enforced periods of rest. Recovery time varies. Overtraining in one sport for 3-4 weeks requires 3-5 days of rest with a slow return to activity.

Exercise-Associated Muscle Cramps

Exercise-associated muscle cramps, sudden painful spasmodic contractions of the muscle, are common problems for the athlete and may be related to overuse of the muscles and dehydration or muscle strain. They are common in triathletes (67%) and runners (50%). Cramps usually occur during exercise or shortly after stopping, although some athletes have cramps during the night. Athletes should record incidence of cramps to help determine how and if they are related to training. Risk factors include age (cramps are more common in older individuals), high BMI, history of running, family history, and inadequate or irregular stretching before exercise. Proper diet, conditioning, and stretching are essential to avoiding cramps, although some athletes will still experience them. A common preventive treatment is the use of pickle juice (2 ounces consumed 10 minutes before exercise or when cramp occurs) or mustard (1 packet), although no one is sure why these seem to be effective.

Tennis Elbow

Overuse injuries are common among all types of athletes, but sports activities often relate to particular types of injuries. Lateral condylitis is a form of tendinitis of the elbow commonly called **Tennis elbow** because it relates directly to chronic repetitive vibration and force from racquet sports. This overuse injury is caused by injury to the extensor muscles of the wrist, which pull the hand up. This injury is often directly related to poor backhand technique, so steps can be taken to decrease the risk of injury. A poor backhand technique is one in which the person leads with the elbow while stroking, and uses only the upper body muscles to hit the ball. Using a two-handed backhand stroke can relieve pressure on the elbow. Additionally, a change in grip size and shape may help, and dropping the elbow while stroking may prevent injury.

Weight Training Injuries

Athletes who engage in **weight training** are at increased risk of muscle injuries and strains, especially of the lower back, as well as trauma from falling weights. There are a number of risk factors for injury:

- Improper biomechanical technique, resulting in twisting or turning during lifts to compensate
- Using excessive weight, resulting in a lack of control while lowering.
- Inattentive or untrained spotters
- Using inappropriate muscles to complete a lift, such as using back muscles to assist the arm in lifting ("cheat curls")
- Overuse of muscles through overtraining without adequate rest
- Failure to adequately stretch as part of warm-up
- Negative exercises with excessive weight
- General improper training
- Lack of concentration during weightlifting activities

Cycling Injuries

Athletes engaged in **cycling** are at risk for a number of different injuries and health-related conditions, including:

- Heat-related sickness from riding in high heat without adequate shade or fluids. Fluid intake must be monitored carefully.
- Muscle cramping, related to overuse of muscles and dehydration.
- Cold-related injuries from riding without adequate clothing to protect and insulate muscles from cold
- Overuse injuries related to failure to perform adequate warm-up stretching exercises.
- Knee injuries related to falls or overuse, such as racing too fast before proper conditioning, riding too far, riding uphill at low rpms, and incorrect positioning of seat.
- Hypoxia related to failure to acclimate to altitude.
- Injury to ulnar nerves from gripping handlebars.
- Low back pain related to poor posture.
- Erectile dysfunction and pain from nerve damage caused by saddle-related trauma, associated with prolonged sitting on small, hard seats.

Accurately Interpreting Signs and Symptoms of Injuries and Illnesses That Require Referral

It is beneficial for the athletic trainer to accurately interpret signs and symptoms of injuries and illnesses that require referral using the medical history and physical examination because a timely referral to appropriate health care providers will ensure best patient care. Some patients may suffer from life threatening injuries and illnesses and need immediate advanced medical care. The athletic trainer must be able to recognize these situations and refer patients immediately. A good history and physical examination will assist the athletic trainer in identifying these cases.

Other injuries or illnesses will worsen if referral to an appropriate health care provider is delayed. For example, a thorough physical examination of a patient's feet could indicate a referral to a podiatrist is appropriate. If this referral is not made or is delayed, the patient may develop comorbidities such as knee injury secondary to the foot abnormalities. To provide the best patient care, the athletic trainer should recognize when referrals are needed, refer as appropriate, and utilize all the services other health care providers have to offer.

Signs and Symptoms of General Medical Conditions Requiring Referrals

There are many general medical conditions patients may suffer from that require referral to another healthcare professional to provide best patient care. For example, meningitis, an inflammation of the meninges, is a serious, possibly fatal, illness that requires referral. Signs and symptoms of meningitis include a high fever, a very painful headache, stiffness in the neck, photophobia, and sensitivity to sound. Progressive symptoms of the illness include vomiting, convulsions, and coma. Diabetes mellitus is another general medical condition athletic trainers must be cognizant of and be prepared to refer patients suspected of having this syndrome. Type 1 diabetes can have a sudden onset with symptoms to include excessive thirst, hunger, frequent urination, itchy skin, blurry vision, and fatigue.

Performing Off-the-Field Examinations
Performing the Palpation Portion

The athletic trainer should systematically perform palpation of bony and soft tissue structures comparing bilaterally for abnormalities. Palpation should begin with light pressure and then progress to deeper pressure as tolerated by the patient. Palpation should begin away from the injury and gradually move closer to the injury, distal to proximal. The patient should be encouraged to relax and not guard during the palpation process for the athletic trainer to gain the most information possible about the injury.

Possible bony abnormalities that may be palpated include gaping at a joint or a joint that is out of normal alignment. Swelling over a bone can be palpated as well as abnormal protuberances. Possible soft tissue abnormalities that can be detected through palpation include swelling, abnormal tension, temperature variations, deformities, and differences in the texture of the tissues. The athletic trainer can also discover abnormal sensations the patient may be experiencing such as numbness or hypersensitivity.

Performing the Observation Portion

When performing observation during an off-the-field physical examination, the athletic trainer watches the patient looking for wide range of possible abnormalities. Observation can begin as soon as the patient walks into the athletic training clinic and is usually performed simultaneously with the history-taking portion of the examination. Possible abnormalities the athletic trainer may observe include abnormal gait and movement patterns, guarding of the injury, stiffness, and inability to move the injured area. Obvious deformities may be observed, such as protrusions, and the patient may make facial expressions that indicate pain. The athletic trainer should also look for swelling, inflammation, discoloration, crepitus produced when the patient moves the injured body part, and possible atrophy.

Signs and Symptoms a Patient May Display After Suffering a Cerebral Concussion

There is a wide range of signs and symptoms patients may display following a cerebral concussion. The athletic trainer must be acutely aware of the signs and symptoms of a concussion and be able to assess patients using accepted standards for head-injury management. The Sport Concussion Assessment Tool (SCAT3) assists the athletic trainer in identifying various types of concussion signs and symptoms. Clinical symptoms of a concussion include headache, the patient feels as if they are "in a fog," and fatigue. Physical signs include loss of consciousness, amnesia, balance deficits, and decreased coordination. Behavioral changes include irritability, sadness, and emotional extremes. Cognitive impairments include slowed reaction times, difficulty concentrating, and difficulty remembering. Sleep disturbances include drowsiness and difficulty falling asleep.

Assessing Head Injuries Using the Sport Concussion Assessment Tool

The Sport Concussion Assessment Tool (SCAT3) is a standardized assessment tool for use by medical professionals, such as athletic trainers, to evaluate patients for possible concussions. The SCAT3 is designed for patients 13-years-old and older, while the Child SCAT3 is designed for patients 12-years-old and younger. Performing preseason baseline testing with the SCAT3 is beneficial for comparing test results after a patient suffers a head injury. The SCAT3 should be performed when patients are at rest, at least ten minutes after physical activity.

The SCAT3 includes the Glasgow coma scale, Maddocks score to determine patients' situational awareness during a game, and a list of possible concussion symptoms for the athletic trainer to ask the patients if they are experiencing. If patients are experiencing any concussion symptoms, they are asked to rate those symptoms in severity from one to six, six being the most severe. A cognitive assessment is performed in which the patient responds to questions such as what month it is, the date, and approximate time. Memory is tested as well as concentration, balance, and coordination.

Performing and Grading Manual Muscle Testing

Resistive range of motion can be evaluated through manual muscle testing. MMT can give valuable information about the extent of the injury based on the ability of the contractile tissue to move thorough a full range of motion (ROM) against resistance. To perform MMT, the patient must be positioned so that the affected muscle can be isolated and move through a full ROM. The athletic trainer then provides manual resistance as the patient moves the affected body part through its ROM.

A common grading system allots grades of a zero to five for MMT. A five indicates the patient can move the affected body part through its full ROM against gravity and with full resistance applied. A score of a four indicates the patient can move the body part through its full ROM against gravity with partial resistance. A three indicates the patient has full ROM against gravity when no manual resistance is being applied. A two indicates that patient has complete ROM when gravity is omitted. A score of a one indicates slight contractility but no movement and the joint. A zero indicates there is no evidence of the muscle contracting at all.

Assessment of Orthopedic and Non-Orthopedic Injuries

When an **orthopedic injury** occurs, the athletic trainer must assess the injury to determine if the athlete needs referral for more care. Questions related to orthopedic injury include:

- How did the injury occur? What exactly were you doing?
- What sounds did you hear when the injury occurred? Snap, crunch, crack, or pop?
- How was movement or activity limited by the injury? Can you bear weight? Lift? Do you have a complete range of motion?
- How does the injury feel? On a pain scale of 0-10? Numb? Burning? Stabbing?

Non-orthopedic health questions may be more complex because the symptoms and problems are less immediate, but careful observation and questioning must be performed to obtain the following information:

- Description of symptoms, including duration and the specific times of occurrence.
- Medical treatments or consultations.
- Constancy of symptoms and things that affect symptoms.
- Changes of any kind: diet, weight, or medications.

Dental Fractures and Avulsions

Dental fractures, most commonly of the maxillary teeth, may occur in association with other oral injuries. Fractures are classified according to the severity of the fracture:

- Ellis I: chipping of enamel.
    - Rough edges should be smoothed by dentist to prevent mouth injury, but this does not require emergency treatment.
- Ellis II: fracture of enamel and dentin with pain on pressure and air sensitivity.
- Ellis III: fracture of enamel, dentin, and pulp with pain on movement, air and temperature sensitivity. Blood may be evident.
    - For both II and III, refer to dentist promptly so tooth can be saved.
    - Oral analgesics.
    - Alveolar/root fracture: Loose tooth, malocclusion, and sensitivity to percussion. Requires prompt referral to dentist for splinting and/or root canal.

Dental avulsions are complete displacements of a tooth from its socket. Permanent teeth may be reimplanted if within 1-2 hours after displacement. The tooth, left as is, can be transported from accident site to the emergency department in Hank solution, saline, or milk.

CORNEAL ABRASION AND ULTRAVIOLET KERATITIS

Corneal abrasion is direct scratching or scraping trauma to the eye, often related to contact lenses, causing a defect in the epithelium of the cornea. Infection with corneal ulceration can occur along with abrasion. Symptoms include pain, intense photophobia, and tearing. Determining the cause and source of the abrasion is important for treatment, as organic sources pose the danger of fungal infection and soft contact lenses pose the danger of *Pseudomonas* infection.

Ultraviolet keratitis results from injury to the corneal epithelium from exposure to the ultraviolet rays of the sun (as in snow blindness, where the snow reflects UV rays into the eyes) or from artificial light sources, such as tanning beds, halogen lights, or welding torches (flash burn). Symptoms usually occur 6-12 hours after exposure and include pain, tearing, photophobia, diminished visual acuity, and spasm of the eyelids. An accurate history that details exposure to UV rays should be taken. For both corneal abrasion and ultraviolet keratitis, the person should be immediately referred to an ophthalmologist for treatment.

PECTORALIS MAJOR RUPTURE

The pectoralis major is the fan-shaped muscle on the anterior wall of the chest comprising most of the male chest muscle and lying beneath the breast in females. The muscle attaches to the humerus and allows the arm to internally rotate, adduct across the chest, and flex. The muscle is not required for normal function of the shoulder, but is utilized during some athletic activities, such as bench pressing. **Rupture of the pectoralis major** most commonly occurs at the insertion point on the humerus. Symptoms include sudden onset of sharp pain in the anterior shoulder or arm, with edema and weakness. Pain increases on adduction, internal rotation, and flexion against resistance. A bulging or gap in the muscle may be noted on palpation. Rest and the RICE program (rest, ice, compress, elevate) may relieve symptoms, but the injury should be evaluated by a physician.

ANAPHYLAXIS SYNDROME

Anaphylaxis syndrome is a sudden acute systemic immunoglobulin E (IgE) or non-immunoglobulin E (non-IgE) inflammatory response affecting the cardiopulmonary and other systems.

- *IgE-mediated response* (anaphylactic shock) is an antibody-antigen reaction against an allergen, such as milk, peanuts, latex, insect bites, or fish. This is the most common type.
- *Non IgE-mediated response* (anaphylactoid reaction) is a systemic reaction to infection, exercise, radio contrast material or other triggers. While this response is almost identical to anaphylactic shock, it does not involve IgE.

Typically, with IgE-mediated response, an antigen triggers release of substances, such as histamine and prostaglandins, which affect the skin, cardiopulmonary, and GI systems. Histamine causes initial erythema and edema by inducing vasodilation. Each time the person has contact with the antigen, more antibodies form in response, so allergic reactions worsen with each contact. In some cases, initial reactions may be mild, but subsequent contact can cause severe life-threatening response.

Wide range of *symptoms*, can include cardiopulmonary, dermatological, and gastrointestinal responses; may recur after the initial treatment (biphasic anaphylaxis), so careful monitoring is essential. Examples:

- Sudden onset of weakness, dizziness, and confusion.
- Severe generalized edema and angioedema. Lips and tongue may swell. Urticaria.
- Increased permeability of vascular system and loss of vascular tone.
- Severe hypotension leading to shock.
- Laryngospasm/bronchospasm, airway obstruction; dyspnea, wheezing.
- Nausea, vomiting, and diarrhea.
- Seizures, coma and death.

Treatment includes:

- Establishing patent airway (may require intubation).
- Providing oxygen at 100% high flow.
- Monitoring VS.
- Administering epinephrine (Epi-pen® or 1:1000 solution 0.1 mg/kg/wt) if available.
- Transferring to emergency department for treatment, (ex. IV fluids).

SHOCK

There are a number of different types of **shock**, but they all have certain characteristics in common. In all types of shock, there are marked decreases in tissue perfusion related to hypotension, so that there is insufficient oxygen delivered to the tissues and, in turn, inadequate removal of cellular waste products, causing injury to tissue. Other general characteristics of shock include:

- Hypotension (systolic below 90 mm Hg). This may be somewhat higher (110 mm Hg) in those who are initially hypertensive.
- Tachycardia (>90).
- Bradypnea (<7) or tachypnea (>29). This varies depending upon the cause of shock.
- Decreased urinary output (<0.5 mL/kg/hr), especially marked in hypovolemic shock.
- Metabolic acidosis.
- Hypoxemia <90 mm Hg for children and adults birth-50; < 80mm Hg for those 51 to 70 and <70 for those over 70.
- Peripheral/cutaneous vasoconstriction/vasodilation.
- Alterations in mental status with dullness, agitation, anxiety, or lethargy.

HYPOVOLEMIC SHOCK

Hypovolemic shock occurs when there is inadequate intravascular fluid.

- The loss may be absolute because of an internal shifting of fluid or an external loss of fluid, as occurs with massive hemorrhage, thermal injuries, severe vomiting or diarrhea, and injuries (such as ruptured spleen or dissected arteries) that interfere with intravascular integrity.
- Hypovolemia may also be relative: that is, related to the vasodilation and increased capillary membrane permeability from sepsis or injuries or the decreased colloidal osmotic pressure that may occur with loss of sodium and disorders like hypopituitarism and cirrhosis.

Hypovolemic shock is classified according to the degree of fluid loss:

- *Class I:* <750 mL or ≤15% of total circulating volume (TCV)
- *Class II:* 750-1500 mL or 15-30% of TCV
- *Class III:* 1500-2000 mL or 30-40% of TCV
- *Class IV:* >2000 mL or >40% of TCV

Neurogenic Shock

Neurogenic shock is the result of injury to the CNS caused by acute spinal cord injury (both blunt and penetrating injuries), neurological diseases, drugs, or anesthesia. In this form of shock, the autonomic nervous system that controls the cardiovascular system is impaired. Symptoms include hypotension and warm dry skin related to lack of vascular tone, resulting in hypothermia from loss of cutaneous heat. Bradycardia is a common but not universal symptom. The degree of symptoms relates to the level of injury, with injuries above T1 capable of causing disruption of the entire sympathetic nervous system and lower injuries causing various degrees of disruption. Even incomplete spinal cord injury can cause neurogenic shock. *Initial treatment* includes:

- ABCDE (airway, breathing, circulation, disability evaluation, exposure) protocol.
- Transfer to trauma unit or facility.

Revised Trauma Scoring System

The **revised trauma scoring system** is used to rapidly assess persons involved in trauma. It is often used at the scene of an accident by first responders, including athletic trainers. The revised trauma scoring system is composed of 3 elements, with the 3 scores added together:

	Respiratory rate per minute:	**Systolic blood pressure (mm Hg):**	**Glasgow Coma Score (GCS):**
4 points	10-29	>89	GCS 13-15
3 points	>29	76-89	GCS 9-12
2 points	>6-9	40-75	GCS 6-8
1 point	1-5	1-49	GCS 4-5
0 points	Not breathing	No blood pressure found.	GCS 2

Scores range from 12 (best) to 0 (worst). Patients with scores ≤11 require treatment in a trauma center. Scores are often used to predict patient outcomes.

Subarachnoid Hemorrhage

Subarachnoid hemorrhage (SAH) may occur after trauma but is common from rupture of a berry aneurysm or an arteriovenous malformation (AVM). However, there are a number of disorders that may be implicated: neoplasms, sickle cell disease, infection, hemophilia, and leukemia. The first presenting symptom may be complaints of severe headache, nausea and vomiting, nuchal rigidity, palsy related to cranial nerve compression, retinal hemorrhages, and papilledema. Late complications include hyponatremia and hydrocephalus. Symptoms worsen as intracranial pressure rises. SAH from aneurysm is classified as follows: *Grade I:* No symptoms, or slight headache and nuchal rigidity. *Grade II:* Moderate to severe headache with nuchal rigidity and cranial nerve palsy. *Grade III:* Drowsy, progressing to confusion or mild focal deficits. *Grade IV:* Stupor, with hemiparesis (moderate to severe), early decerebrate rigidity, and vegetative disturbances. *Grade V:* Coma state with decerebrate rigidity

Treatment includes: Identifying and treating underlying cause. Observing for re-bleeding. Referral for surgical repair if needed.

Epidural Hemorrhage

Hemorrhage is always a concern after head trauma, because even injuries that appear slight can result in vascular rupture, resulting in hemorrhage between the skull and the brain. **Epidural hemorrhage** is bleeding between the dura and the skull, pushing the brain downward and inward. The hemorrhage is usually caused by arterial tears, so bleeding is often rapid, leading to severe neurological deficits and respiratory arrest. In some cases, there is initial loss of consciousness with apparent recovery for minutes or hours before sudden deterioration. Initially, the body compensates by rapidly absorbing cerebrospinal fluid and decreasing blood flow, but the compensatory measure is soon overwhelmed. This type of injury usually results from skull fractures with middle meningeal artery lacerations or venous bleeding, such as may occur with a blow to the head from contact sports. Referral for immediate surgical repair is imperative.

Subdural Hemorrhage

Subdural hemorrhage is bleeding between the dura and the cerebrum, usually from tears in the cortical veins of the subdural space. It tends to develop more slowly than epidural hemorrhage and can result in a subdural hematoma. If the bleeding is acute and develops within minutes or hours of injury, the prognosis is poor. Subacute hematomas that develop more slowly cause varying degrees of injury. Subdural hemorrhage is a common injury related to trauma to the head, especially with loss of consciousness. Onset of symptoms is earlier in the younger athlete, because some cerebral atrophy is normal with age, giving the older athlete more room for blood to accumulate. Symptoms of acute injury may occur within 24-48 hours, but subacute bleeding may not be evident for up to 2 weeks after injury. Symptoms vary and may include bradycardia, tachycardia, hypertension, and alterations in consciousness. Referral must be made for surgical evacuation of the hematoma.

Diabetes Mellitus

Diabetes mellitus is the most common metabolic disorder in children, affecting about 1.5 million children and adolescents, with 70-85% suffering from Type I and the rest from Type II. The peak age of onset for both types is 10-12 in girls and 12-14 in boys.

Type I: Immune-mediated form with insufficient insulin production because of destruction of pancreatic beta cells. Symptoms include:

- Pronounced polyuria and polydipsia.
- Short onset.
- May be overweight, or recent weight loss.
- Ketoacidosis present on diagnosis.

Treatment: Insulin as needed to control blood sugars, Glucose monitoring 1-4 times daily, and diet control with carbohydrate control and exercise

Type II: Insulin resistant form with defect in insulin secretion. *Symptoms* include:

- Long onset.
- Obese with no weight loss or significant weight loss.
- Mild or absent polyuria and polydipsia.
- May have ketoacidosis or glycosuria without ketonuria.

- Androgen-mediated problems, such as hirsutism and acne.
- Hypertension.

Treatment: Diet and exercise, glucose monitoring, oral medications

> **Review Video: Diabetes Mellitus: Diet, Exercise, & Medications**
> Visit mometrix.com/academy and enter code: 774388

DIABETIC KETOACIDOSIS

Diabetic ketoacidosis (DKA) is a complication of diabetes mellitus. Inadequate production of insulin or administration of insulin results in glucose being unavailable for metabolism, so lipolysis (breakdown of fat) produces free fatty acids (FFAs) as an alternate fuel source. Glycerol in both fat cells and the liver is converted to ketone bodies (β-hydroxybutyric acid, acetoacetic acid, and acetone), which are used for cellular metabolism less efficiently than glucose. Excess ketone bodies are excreted in the urine (ketonuria) or exhalations. The ketone bodies lower serum pH, leading to ketoacidosis. Symptoms include:

- Kussmaul respirations: hyperventilation to eliminate buildup of carbon dioxide, associated with "ketone breath" (fruity odor). General weakness, progressing to stupor. Fluid imbalance, including loss of potassium and other electrolytes from cellular death, resulting in dehydration, excessive urination, and excess thirst.
- Cardiac arrhythmias, related to potassium loss, can lead to cardiac arrest. Hyperglycemia, with glucose levels above normal (i.e., greater than 125). Initial treatment includes referral for Insulin therapy by continuous infusion.

SHARING ASSESSMENT FINDINGS WITH OTHER HEALTHCARE PROFESSIONALS

The Certified Athletic Trainer has a responsibility to refer injured athletes to appropriate medical practitioners for care and **share assessment** findings. The trainer must ensure that the athlete has signed a medical release of information, but must keep in mind that some information may be protected (such as information about sexually-transmitted diseases) and should not be provided to all medical authorities if it is not necessary for care. The trainer should keep detailed and clear medical records about any evaluation and care given. A written report should be sent to any physician to whom an athlete is referred, using correct medical terminology and outlining the results of any testing that was done to determine injury or illness. An injury report should indicate how and when the injury occurred.

EDUCATING PATIENTS AND STAKEHOLDERS ABOUT INJURY FINDINGS, PROGNOSIS, AND THE PLAN OF CARE

Education about findings, prognosis, and the plan of care helps ensure best patient outcomes by increasing compliance because it gets all stakeholders involved and on the same page regarding the patient's injury and the rehabilitative process. By thoroughly communicating the findings, all involved parties can better understand the nature and extent of the injury, trust that a proper diagnosis has been determined, and have confidence that an appropriate course of action has been developed. Clear communication of the prognosis will establish the projected amount of time that will be needed for healing, rehabilitation, and the expected outcome the patient will have at the end of the rehabilitative process. By explaining the plan of care, all involved parties will be able to understand how the rehabilitation will lead to the desired outcome and measure rehabilitative progress towards the end result. When this is all communicated to the patient and involved stakeholders, all can work collaboratively to ensure the patient performs appropriate rehabilitation while not doing anything to inadvertently aggravate the injury. The patient can be encouraged and reminded that they are making progress towards their desired end result.

Health Insurance Portability and Accountability Act

The Health Insurance Portability and Accountability Act (HIPAA) governs how patients' private medical information (PMI) is protected and what steps must be taken for PMI to be shared. HIPAA ensures that patients have access to their own medical information, offers added control over how their medical information is shared, and sets consequences if PMI is not kept private.

There are many occasions in the field of athletic training in which multiple healthcare providers may be caring for the same patient and sharing medical findings would benefit the patient, offering better patient care. For PMI to be shared among these providers, a HIPAA authorization form must be signed. For the HIPAA authorization form to be valid, it must indicate what medical information can be disclosed, who may release the information, who the information can be disclosed to, the purpose for disclosing the information, have an expiration date, be signed and dated by the patient, or if signed by a personal representative their authority to sign for the patient must be identified.

> **Review Video: HIPAA**
> Visit mometrix.com/academy and enter code: 412009

Role and Scope of the Athletic Trainer and the Team Physician

Athletic trainers work primarily under the direction of a team physician, and it is the physician who ultimately is responsible for the medical care of the athletes. However, there are many occasions when the athletic trainer must have the ability to make independent decisions, as they may be the only healthcare provider onsite at the time of an injury. Therefore, the athletic trainer and team physician should share a common philosophy on best practices in patient care to establish a good, working relationship that keeps patients' best interests as a foundation.

Exploring specific duties, the team physician is responsible for compiling complete medical histories, determining medical diagnoses, and determining when patients should be held out of physical activity and when it is safe for them to return. The athletic trainer serves many roles such as injury prevention, emergency care, injury examination, designing and supervising therapeutic rehabilitation programs, developing conditioning programs, and working collaboratively with the team physician to perform pre-participation physical examinations.

Using Goal Setting to Motivate Patient Compliance in Rehabilitation

Athletic trainers can use goal setting as a motivational technique to increase patient compliance to the rehabilitation plan by ensuring goals fit into certain parameters. For example, specific short-term goals should be included that directly lead to the long-term rehabilitative goals of the patient. The patient and the athletic trainer should work collaboratively when developing short-term and long-term goals. The goals should be measurable, challenging, and attainable with satisfactory effort. Goal setting can work as a motivational tool because it decreases the stress of injury, allows the patient to take responsibility over their rehabilitation, provides positive reinforcement, and integrates time management.

Immediate and Emergency Care

EMERGENCY ACTION PLANS

Creating an emergency action plan and keeping it up-to-date benefits the athletic trainer by ensuring proper preparation for any emergency situations that may arise. There are many factors that must be considered to properly respond to emergency situations such as the inclusion of multiple personnel and specialty equipment. During emergencies, time is of the essence, so a well-developed and practiced emergency action plan will help to reduce stress, increase timeliness, and ensure all involved parties know their role in the event of an emergency. A swift and appropriate response could quite possibly be the difference in life or death for the patient. The emergency action plan should account for the proper management of multiple types of emergencies as well as dictate the directions emergency personnel will need to access all venues in which the athletic trainer provides coverage such as the bleachers of a football field or an indoor swimming pool.

NECESSARY COMPONENTS OF AN EMERGENCY ACTION PLAN

There are several components an emergency action plan (EAP) must include and an EAP must be developed for every venue in which athletic trainers provides coverage. EAPs must specify emergency personnel, equipment, and phone lines available. EAPs should establish protocols for the removal of sports equipment such as helmets and shoulder pads. EAPs must plan for easy access to emergencies by establishing which gates, doors, and padlocks must be opened to allow emergency medical personnel access to the site of the emergency.

EAPs assign roles staff members must perform during an emergency. For example, a designated person should call 911 and be ready to communicate all essential information. A person should be designated to meet the emergency medical personnel and direct them to the emergency, another to keep spectators away, and a person should go with the patient to the hospital. All staff should know their role in an emergency. EAPs should not only plan for potential injuries and illnesses to athletes, but also other emergencies that may arise at venues such as a spectator suffering a heart attack. The EAP should be reviewed, updated, practiced, and documented annually.

EMERGENCY MEDICAL EQUIPMENT REQUIRED TO PROPERLY MANAGE EMERGENCY SITUATIONS

There is a variety of emergency medical equipment that needs to be readily available for athletic trainers to properly manage emergency situations that may arise. For example, athletic trainers need a variety of splints for possible fractures, crutches, slings, wound care supplies, and emergency cutting tools for football helmet facemask removal. Additionally, athletic trainers need face shields for CPR, and AEDs readily available at all sites in which athletic training services are provided. Access to cold-water immersion must be available when high heat and humidity makes heat stroke a threat for athletes. When caring for athletes with specific medical conditions, athletic trainers should have access to the patients' emergency medical devices such as EpiPens, insulin injections, and inhalers for asthma. Communication devices must be readily available at all locations to activate emergency medical services as needed.

UNIVERSAL PRECAUTIONS TAKEN WHEN EXPOSED TO BLOOD OR BODILY FLUIDS

The Occupational Safety and Health Administration (OSHA) has established regulations employers must adhere to in order to protect employees and patients from exposure to bloodborne pathogens at the workplace. In the field of athletic training, the employing institution must provide the supplies athletic trainers need to properly follow universal precautions. Athletic trainers must ensure these precautions are followed in the athletic training clinic. Personal protective equipment needed includes disposable non-latex gloves, disposable mouthpieces for resuscitation devices, eye protection, masks, and shields. Also, a container for disposal of biohazardous materials and a container for sharps disposal is needed. For proper cleanliness of the athletic training clinic, disinfectants approved by the Environmental Protection Agency, chlorine bleach, and antiseptics are essential. Finally, any contaminated laundry should be separated from other laundry in biohazard bags and washed separately in hot water with a detergent capable of deactivating bloodborne viruses.

Obtaining Consent to Treat a Minor

Obtaining consent to treat for minors should be achieved prior to the start of the athletic season. To do this, parents or guardians should be asked to sign a consent form allowing medical treatment to be given to their child if necessary. In the event of an emergency, if possible, the parents should be informed of the emergency, what treatment the athletic trainer intends to provide, and should be asked for consent to treat for that specific incident. If the parent cannot be reached, the consent-to-treat form signed at the beginning of the season can be sufficient. If there is no consent form, the patient's implied consent to save their life can be enacted upon. When traveling, the athletic trainer should bring consent-to-treat forms as well as contact information for parents and guardians.

Triage

When managing multiple patients suffering from varying injuries and illnesses, triage is important to determine who needs to receive medical care first. If immediate care is provided to patients suffering from only minor injuries, while other patients with life-threatening conditions do not receive immediate care, their outcome may be detrimental. For example, if two football players hit helmet-to-helmet and both players are injured, the athletic trainer should quickly assess both patients to determine who needs the most immediate care. If one patient reports symptoms consistent with a concussion while the other patient reports symptoms consistent with a spinal injury, the patient with the possible spinal injury should receive immediate care. A responsible adult must monitor the patient with the possible concussion until the patient with the possible spinal injury is transported to an advanced medical care facility. Once this is completed, the athletic trainer can then evaluate and care for the player with the possible concussion.

Compartment Syndrome

Compartment syndrome occurs when muscle perfusion is inadequate because of constriction caused by a cast or tight dressing, or because of an increase in the contents of a muscle compartment because of edema or hemorrhage (often related to fractures or blunt trauma, especially to the anterolateral leg). The result is an increase in soft tissue pressure. It most often affects the forearm and leg muscles. Symptoms include:

- Severe throbbing pain unrelieved by opiates.
- Numbness and tingling as the pressure on nerves increases.
- Cyanosis and decreased or lacking pulse.
- Edema.
- Treatment must be initiated immediately to prevent neurovascular damage and necrosis:
- Elevation of affected limb above the heart.
- Release of constricting cast or dressings.
- Immediate transfer to ED for Doppler ultrasonograph to verify pulses and tissue fasciotomy to relieve constriction if the condition is advanced or does not respond to medical treatment. The wound is left open, allowing the muscle tissue to expand, and covered with moist sterile NS dressing while the limb is elevated.

Skull Fractures

Skull fractures are most common in contact sports, such as football, but may also result from severe blunt trauma, as for instance being hit with a baseball bat. Symptoms will relate to the location and extent of the fracture, but typically include:

- Bruise, swelling, deformity, or laceration at the point of injury.
- Bleeding from nose or ears.
- Clear fluid draining from eyes or ears (cerebrospinal fluid).
- Pain and tenderness at injury site, and more generalized headache.
- Battle's sign—bruising behind the ear—indicates a posterior basilar fracture (delayed sign).
- Raccoon eyes—bruising and discoloration about the eyes—is a sign of a frontal basilar fracture (delayed sign).
- Alterations in consciousness or lack of consciousness.
- Unequal pupils.

Assessment for ABCs should be done first, followed by neurological assessment. The person should be immobilized while awaiting emergency transfer, as skull fractures may be associated with spinal cord injury.

Heat Stress and Heat Exhaustion

Heat-related illnesses include heat stress, heat exhaustion, and heat stroke. Each of these conditions requires different treatment; however, treatment for all types of heat-related illness should begin with immediately removal from the hot environment.

Heat stress may include sunburn, edema, heat syncope, and heat cramps. Immediate treatment includes rehydrating, treating symptomatically, and observing for signs that may indicate impending heat exhaustion or heat stroke.

Heat exhaustion may be related to water depletion if the person is not adequately hydrated, resulting in dry mouth, increased thirst and decreased urinary output. Heat exhaustion may also be related to sodium depletion, even with adequate hydration, if the person is not acclimated to heat, resulting in weakness and headache. With both types of heat exhaustion, flu-like symptoms and pulse and BP changes may occur.

Immediate treatment for heat exhaustion includes:

- Cooling with evaporative techniques (spraying with cool water, fanning) and cold packs to neck, groin, and axillae.
- Monitoring temperature (usually <105 °F and may be normal) and vital signs.
- Slow rehydration with sports drink (0.1% isotonic NaCl), about ½ glass every 15-20 minutes.
- Rest for 2-3 hours.
- If symptoms worsen or do not subside within 2-3 hours, the athlete should be monitored for 24 hours and, in severe cases, transferred to ED for evaluation and intravenous fluids.

Exertion heat stroke (EHS) is the most common type of heat stroke in athletes. Heat builds up in the body faster than it can be dissipated. Typical symptoms include temperature variations, diaphoresis, dizziness, loss of consciousness, and alterations in consciousness, beginning with irritability and progressing to seizure and coma. Heat stroke is life threatening, and the athlete must be transferred immediately to an ED for treatment. Evaporative cooling techniques should be instituted while awaiting transfer.

Heart Attack

Heart attack should be suspected in those with chest pain that lasts more than 10 minutes or who exhibit typical symptoms of heart attack, such as sudden severe chest pain accompanied by nausea, signs of shock, pain radiating to neck and arms (especially left), pallor, and diaphoresis. Females may have less specific symptoms, such as neck pain, epigastric pain, or "severe indigestion." Immediate treatment includes calling 9-1-1 for emergency transfer to ED; giving the person an aspirin if one is available and the person is not allergic; monitoring vital signs; and positioning person in comfortable position (often with head elevated). If the person has nitroglycerine, this should be administered as well. If oxygen is available, that should be administered while awaiting transfer. If the person goes into cardiac arrest, cardiopulmonary resuscitation should be started immediately and should continue until help arrives or the pulse and respirations begin spontaneously.

Cardiac Arrest and CPR

Any person who loses consciousness should immediately be assessed for **cardiac arrest** by observing the chest for respirations and palpating the carotid artery (between the larynx and sternocleidomastoid muscles) for pulse. If there are no pulse or respirations, the trainer should tell someone to call 9-1-1 and begin cardiopulmonary massage immediately, noting the time. If no one else is available to call 9-1-1, the trainer should do that before beginning CPR, unless the victim is a child. In that case, CPR should be done for one minute before stopping to call 9-1-1. The person in cardiac arrest should be placed in supine position on the floor or ground. Compressions are performed on the lower third of the sternum, above the sternal notch, using care to avoid the xiphoid process. Compressions are made with the palm of the hand (fingers raised). The non-dominant hand is placed on the sternum, arms crossed, and the top hand placed on top of the bottom hand.

The top hand does the compression, pushing the bottom hand with the elbow locked and at a 90° angle to the ground. Compressions should depress the chest 1 inch for an infant or young child, and 1.5-2 inches for others. Previous guidelines recommended 15 compressions followed by 2 respirations (for 2-person) and 30 to 2 for one-person, but current guidelines for CPR advise cardiac massage only at the rate of about 100 compressions per minute. Exceptions are children (more likely to suffer respiratory problems) and adults with oxygen deprivation (near drowning). The compressions should continue without stopping until help arrives or until the person begins breathing and develops a pulse spontaneously. If an automatic defibrillator (AED) is available, this should be used as soon as possible, as brain death begins to occur in 4-6 minutes.

Snake Bites

About 45,000 **snakebites** occur in the United States each year, with about 8000 poisonous. In the United States, an estimated 25 species of snakes are venomous. There are two types of snakes that can cause serious injury, classified according to the type of fangs and venom. **Coral snakes** have short fixed permanent fangs in their upper jaw and venom that is primarily neurotoxic, but may also have hemotoxic and cardiotoxic properties:

- Wounds show no fang marks, but there may be scratches or semi-circular markings from teeth.
- There may be little local reaction, but neurological symptoms range from mild to acute respiratory and cardiovascular failure.

Treatment includes:

- Cleansing wound thoroughly of dirt and debris and either leaving it open or covering it with a dry dressing.
- Transporting immediately to ED for administration of antivenin even without symptoms, which may be delayed, and tetanus toxoid or immune globulin.

The second type of snake that can cause serious injury are the **pit vipers.** *Rattlesnakes, copperheads, and cottonmouths* have erectile fangs that fold until they are aroused; their venom is primarily hemotoxic and cytotoxic, but may have neurotoxic properties.

- Wounds usually show 1 or 2 fang marks.
- Edema may begin immediately or may be delayed up to 6 hours.
- Pain may be severe.
- There may be a wide range of symptoms, including hypotension and impairment of blood coagulation that can lead to excessive blood loss, depending upon the type and amount of venom.
- There may be local infection and necrosis.

Treatment includes:

- Cleansing the wound thoroughly and dressing as indicated.
- Circling edema with a permanent marker and recircling every 15 minutes.
- Transporting immediately to an ED for tetanus and antivenin as indicated.
- NSAIDs and aspirin should NOT be given for pain.

Missile/Impalement

Missile/Impalement injuries include arrow, gunshot, paint gun, nail gun, and shrapnel wounds. These injuries are usually circular, oval, or triangular, and may have both an entry (with abrasion at periphery) and exit site. Other residue, such as gunpowder, may be evident at the entry. Puncture wounds are difficult to properly clean and become infected easily, even with treatment, so the athletic trainer should apply compression dressing only to puncture wounds and should not attempt to remove any impaled object. A bulky supportive dressing should be placed about the object to provide compression, decrease bleeding, capture drainage, and prevent the object from becoming dislodged. The person should be transferred to an ED immediately and positioned such that there is no pressure against an impaled object. *Treatment* varies according to the site, type, and degree of injury, and may include tetanus prophylaxis, wound irrigation, removal of any foreign body, and antibiotics as indicated.

Pneumothorax

Pneumothorax is a leak between the lung tissue and the chest wall such that extraneous air is in the pleural space, causing a partial or complete collapse of a lung. Types include:

- *Spontaneous/Simple pneumothorax* is a breach of the parietal or visceral pleura, such as when an air-filled bleb on the lung surface ruptures. *Traumatic pneumothorax* is a lacerating wound of the chest wall, such as a gunshot or knife wound. Open pneumothorax occurs when air passes in and out, causing the lung to collapse; it is indicated by a sucking sound and a paradoxical movement of the chest wall during respiration.

- *Tension pneumothorax* is similar to traumatic open pneumothorax; however, the air can enter the pleural sac but can't be expelled, causing a pronounced mediastinal shift to the unaffected side with severe compromise of cardiac and respiratory function.

Symptoms of pneumothorax vary widely depending on the cause and degree of the pneumothorax, but include:

- Acute sudden pleuritic pain (95%), usually on the affected side.
- Decreased breathing sounds on the affected side, associated with dyspnea and increasing cyanosis.
- Tension pneumothorax: tracheal deviation, distended neck veins, decreased breath sounds, and hemodynamic compromise.

Treatment includes:

- Call for emergency transfer to ED immediately.
- Check airway, breathing, and circulation.
- Administer oxygen if available.
- Bandage all wounds of the neck or chest at once, and cover sucking chest wounds with airtight material, such as plastic wrap or gauze pads coated with petroleum jelly (except for one corner of the gauze, to allow air to escape but not enter).

TRAUMATIC INJURY WITH BLEEDING/HEMORRHAGE

Most sports-related **traumatic injuries with bleeding** are not a life-threatening hemorrhage, although some areas, such as the face, may appear to bleed heavily. The injured person should always be evaluated quickly for signs of shock.

- For minor cuts and lacerations, the immediate care is to apply direct pressure (as with gauze pads) to the bleeding lesion, elevating the area of injury above the level of the heart if possible. Bleeding usually slows almost immediately and stops within minutes, after which a compression dressing can be applied.
- Severe hemorrhage is a medical emergency that requires a 9-1-1 call and immediate transfer to an ED. A tourniquet should not be used, as this may cause more damage, but pressure should be maintained over the wound and the wound should be elevated. The artery feeding the area (such as the femoral artery for the leg and brachial artery for the arms) should be compressed. If signs of shock manifest, the person should be in a supine position with feet elevated while awaiting transfer.

SHOCK

There are a number of different types of **shock**. Hypovolemic shock results from loss of body fluids as with severe diarrhea; cardiogenic shock from heart disorder; hemorrhagic shock from blood loss; neuropathic shock from neurological injury; hypoglycemic shock from hyperinsulinism; and septic shock from infection. Interference with the lungs' ability to receive oxygen or the heart's ability to circulate blood can result in shock. During shock, the cells don't receive enough oxygen to metabolize glucose and, as the cells compensate, lactic acid forms, changing the acid-base balance. This prompts the cells to leak toxins into the blood, at which point cells begin to die. Symptoms include diminished blood pressure, tachycardia dyspnea, pallor, confusion, cool clammy skin, and loss of consciousness. Emergency treatment includes:

- Calling 9-1-1 for emergency transfer to ED.
- Placing the person flat and elevating his or her feet above the level of his or her heart.
- Controlling hemorrhage by compression.
- Administering oxygen if available.

SPINAL CORD INJURIES

(Part I) **Spinal cord injuries** may result from blunt trauma, falls from a height, various types of sports injuries (especially contact sports, gymnastic, diving), or penetrating trauma. Damage results from mechanical injury and secondary responses resulting from hemorrhage, edema, and ischemia. The type of symptoms relate to the area and degree of injury.

- Anterior cord: The posterior column functions remain, so there is sensation of touch, vibration, and position remaining below injury, but with complete paralysis and a loss of sensation of pain and temperature. Prognosis is poor.
- Brown-Séquard: The cord is hemisected, resulting in spastic paresis, loss of sense of position and vibration on the injured side, and loss of pain and temperature on the other side. Prognosis is good.
- Cauda equina: Damage is below L-1 with variable loss of motor ability and sensation, and bowel and bladder dysfunction. Injury is to peripheral nerves, which can regenerate, so prognosis is better than for other lesions of the spinal cord.
- Central cord: Results from hyperextension and ischemia or stenosis of the cervical spine, causing quadriparesis (more severe in upper extremities) with some loss of sensation of pain and temperature). Prognosis is good, but fine motor skills are often impaired in upper extremities.
- Conus medullaris: Injury to lower spine (lower lumbar and sacral nerves).
- Posterior cord: Motor function is preserved but without sensation.
- Spinal shock: Injury at T6 or above, results in flaccid paralysis below lesion, with loss of sensation, loss of rectal tone, bradycardia, and hypotension.

Patients with **spinal cord injuries** should immediately be evaluated for airway control, and their spine kept immobilized. Emergency services must be called to transport the person to an ED. Spinal injury can occur at any point in the spine, with symptoms dependent upon the point of injury. Initial symptoms may be inability or reluctance to move. In severe injuries, there may be decorticate or decerebrate postures. Range of motion and sensory testing can help to determine if there is injury, but these should not be performed if cervical spine injury is suspected. In this case, the head should be immobilized and the helmet left in place unless it interferes with ventilation or fails to hold the head secure. If necessary, the helmet and shoulder pads should be removed simultaneously, so that the cervical area is not hyperextended. One should not attempt to move or roll a person with suspected spinal cord injury unless emergency services are not available.

RUPTURED SPLEEN

Splenic rupture, a concern after mononucleosis, can also occur as a result of blunt trauma to the abdominal area, as from sports where falls or sharp contact are common, such as football, hockey, soccer, snowboarding, mountain biking, and body boarding. Splenic rupture is characterized by initially sharp pain in the left upper quadrant, followed by dull flank pain. If the spleen is leaking more slowly, the person may not exhibit symptoms at first, but then will complain of left shoulder pain (Kehr's sign). In some cases, rupture may occur a month after an injury. Rupture should be suspected in any person who sustains an abdominal injury and has difficulty arising or reports abdominal pain or dyspnea. If the spleen has completely ruptured, the athlete will have signs of shock. This is a medical emergency: 9-1-1 should be called and the athlete transferred to an ED. Any athlete suspected of splenic injury should be removed from play, referred for medical attention, and then barred from play until the spleen has healed.

MONONUCLEOSIS

Infectious **mononucleosis** (caused by the Epstein-Barr virus) is very common among young people and can be caused by exchange of saliva, as from kissing or sharing water bottles. Clothing may also become contaminated, so jerseys and other clothing should not be shared. Incubation periods range from 2-6 weeks and active infection from 3-15 days. Athletes with signs of infection (usually upper respiratory symptoms with enlarged lymph nodes and marked fatigue) should be restricted from play. Of more concern is the fact that the liver and spleen may be affected. The spleen often enlarges, putting the athlete in danger of splenic rupture from blunt trauma. The most dangerous period for rupture is between the 4th and 21st day after the onset of symptoms, so the athlete should be barred from play during this time. After 3 weeks, the athlete may resume light activity if there are no symptoms of liver or spleen disorder and no fever.

BLISTERS

Blisters occur when friction causes fluid to collect in the outer layer of the dermis, especially during hot humid weather. Blisters are common on hands and fingers (gymnasts, pitchers), feet (runners, dancers), and buttocks (bicycle/horse riders). Preventive methods include avoiding socks or wearing light cotton socks; taping vulnerable areas; applying 10% tannic acid to skin 1-2 times daily for 2-3 weeks; and wearing properly-fitted gloves and shoes. Immediate treatment includes:

- Cleaning and leaving small blisters (<1 inch) intact with no other treatment.
- Applying an ice pack for 5 minutes to painful blisters or blisters >1 inch.
- Blisters >1 inch may be washed thoroughly with soap and water and punctured at several points with a sterile needle, while pressure applied to drain blister. Then, a compression dressing should be applied.
- Non-prescription topical antibiotics, such as Neosporin®, may be applied to prevent infection.
- Protective dressings, including foam or moleskin with holes cut above the blister, should be applied over compression dressings for weight-bearing areas, such as the foot.

BAROTRAUMAS

Barotrauma (barotitis media) caused by increased pressure in the air (as for instance when descending in an airplane or diving underwater) is damage to the middle ear. Barotrauma may also occur at high altitudes. Individuals with upper respiratory infections are at greatest risk, so athletes should not attempt to dive with a URI. With barotrauma, the tympanic membrane of the ear is pulled inward, because the middle ear pressure is less than the external pressure. Pain will usually be acute in the affected ear and may be accompanied by tinnitus, decreased hearing, and dizziness. The Valsalva maneuver may reduce pressure: taking a breath, holding the nose, closing the mouth and breathing out while trying to force air into the ears. If symptoms worsen or do not subside, the athlete should be seen by a physician for emergency treatment, as the tympanic membrane may rupture.

Human/Animal Bites

Human "bites" occur when the teeth of one person injure another, not necessarily through intentional biting. This is not uncommon in contact sports. Human bites may also be the result of altercations, and are referred to as "fist-bites." There are three common types:

- Closed fist bite, resulting in a small wound on the metacarpophalangeal joint of the middle finger. Bacteria enter the wound when the person extends the fingers, carrying bacteria to the extensor tendons, which can result in infection.
- Finger bite, in which a finger may be partially or completely severed.
- Puncture bite, usually on the face, from contact with another person's tooth.
- Immediate treatment includes applying pressure to stop bleeding, and then thoroughly flushing the wound with dilute Betadine, dilute peroxide, or normal saline solution. Protective dressings should be applied. Large wounds or those with skin flaps or signs of more serious tissue injury should be referred to a physician.

Exercise-Induced Asthma

Exercise-induced asthma (bronchospasm) is a particular risk for those with pre-existing asthma or allergies, especially with high pollen counts, high levels of smog, and cold dry weather. Athletes usually begin to cough, wheeze, and complain of shortness of breath and chest tightness after about 5 minutes of exercise. The symptoms may increase 5-10 minutes after exercise ceases, but symptoms usually recede by 30 minutes. Athletes should be cautioned to regularly take all prescribed preventive medications and warm up for 5-10 minutes before performing strenuous exercise. Additionally, they should breathe through their noses to warm the air and learn to monitor their own breathing. Immediate care includes stopping activity, positioning the person in an upright position, and having the athlete use his or her inhaled bronchodilator. If the symptoms are severe and do not begin to subside after ceasing activity and using the bronchodilator, the athlete should be transferred to an ED for further treatment.

Conjunctivitis

Conjunctivitis is an inflammation of the conjunctiva, the membrane that lines the eyelid and eye, usually caused by bacteria, virus, or allergen. The inflammation causes small capillaries to rupture, resulting in the "pink eye" appearance. The inflammation is usually accompanied by itching and discomfort in the affected eye. If caused by bacteria or virus, conjunctivitis is contagious while symptomatic, and may be spread by contaminated fingers, towels or washcloths. If inflammation worsens or doesn't begin to clear in 48 hours, the athlete should be referred to a physician. Bacterial conjunctivitis is treated with topical antibiotics, and allergic conjunctivitis with antihistamine eye drops, but there is no effective treatment for viral conjunctivitis. The athlete should be advised to wash his hands often, avoid touching his eye or sharing towels, and avoiding eye makeup. Cool or warm moist compresses to the eye for 10-15 minutes 3-4 times daily may relieve symptoms. The infection usually clears in 1-2 weeks or 1-2 days after antibiotic treatment if bacterial.

Costochondritis

Costochondritis (Tietze's Syndrome), inflammation of the cartilage that attaches the ribs (usually the 2nd and 3rd) to the sternum, can cause sharp pain in the chest wall, sometimes radiating to the arm and accompanied by tightness in the chest. There is usually point tenderness in the affected area. Costochondritis may result from blunt trauma or repetitive trauma from physical activity that causes strain and is of short duration. The athlete should be advised to stop activity and rest. Heating pad or ice may be applied, depending on which provides the most comfort. Non-prescription NSAIDs may relieve discomfort. The person should avoid movements that aggravate the pain, although easy stretching of the chest muscles 4-5 times a day may be useful. Activity should not resume until symptoms subside as they may recur or become chronic.

SYNCOPE

Syncope, fainting, occurs when the blood pressure drops suddenly, and can result from prolonged exertion (especially in hot weather), prolonged straining (as when lifting weights), prolonged squatting followed by standing during which the legs are rapidly perfused (orthostatic), and from holding the breath while weightlifting ("weightlifter's blackout"). It may also result from low blood sugar or use of alcohol or drugs. When an athlete faints, the trainer should immediately check for respiration and check the carotid pulse to make sure that the person has not suffered a cardiac arrest. If there are respirations and a pulse, the athlete should be placed in the supine position with his feet elevated above the level of his heart. This should raise the blood pressure and the person should regain consciousness, but he should remain in this position for 10-15 minutes. Assessment should be made to determine the cause of fainting and further treatment, such as glucose, may be given as indicated. Preventive measures should be taken, such as monitoring the athlete's techniques.

EXERCISE-ASSOCIATED LEG CRAMPS

Exercise-associated leg cramps are painful involuntary muscle contractions, usually in the calf of the leg, occurring during endurance sports, most commonly swimming or running. The cause is not clear. Some theorize it's related to dehydration, changes in electrolyte levels, or abnormal activity of motor neurons. Individuals with diabetes are often subject to cramps. Other risks include old age, family history, increase in BMI, irregular or short stretching exercises, and intensity of training. Immediate treatment includes passively stretching the affected muscle and kneading the cramped area by squeezing and releasing. The athlete can be advised to flex her foot and point her toes upward, and to hold that position until the cramp eases. This is particularly useful for swimming cramps. Ice applied to the area may relieve pain. The athlete should be kept cool and given sports drinks as she rests the limb until cramping eases. If there are multiple or persistent unrelieved cramps, the athlete should be taken to the ED, as muscles may be injured by severe cramping.

PATELLOFEMORAL PAIN SYNDROME

Patellofemoral pain syndrome (runner's knee) occurs more commonly in females and males, usually between 12 and 36 years old, and among those who are physically healthy. The disorder often relates to overstressing the knee while playing sports that require running, such as sprinting, soccer, and basketball. This is a progressive disorder, with pain increasing over time. Usually pain is about and beneath the patella, especially at the inner aspect, and is aggravated by walking or running on a grade, flexing the knee as in squatting, or taking off in running. The knee may have a clicking sound and may feel unstable. Risk factors include flat feet or abnormalities in the femur, such as shortening or turning inward. Immediate treatment includes ice packs for 20 minutes 2 to 4 times daily for 2 to 4 days, followed by applications of heat. NSAIDs may be used for pain. Quadriceps exercises should begin when pain subsides. Assessment should identify the cause, as orthotics or modifications in activities may be needed.

PLANTAR WARTS

Plantar warts are caused by infection with human papillomavirus (HPV), usually on the plantar surface of the feet. They begin as pin-sized lesions, often with dark spots at the center, but a number of them can grow together and cause large lesions called "mosaic warts." Lesions grow as the virus enters cells and causes them to reproduce more quickly. The lesions become increasingly painful as they grow and compress underlying tissue. Plantar warts shed a virus that is contagious to others, so going barefoot in showers or sharing shoes can spread the infection. Cushioning in shoes may be needed for comfort. Medicated pads are available; these can be applied after soaking the foot in soapy water. The pad is left in place for 2 days, and then the white tissue is scraped off and the area is exposed to air for two days. This treatment is repeated for two weeks. Physician referral should be made, as home treatment is time consuming and not always successful.

RICER Therapy

RICE (sometimes extended to RICER) therapy is a frequent emergency treatment after sports injuries, especially for contusions, strains, and sprains. This therapy reduces swelling and discomfort and promotes increased circulation and healing:

- **Rest:** The athlete should immediately cease the activity that caused the problem in order to avoid further damage.
- **Ice:** Ice or cold compresses should be applied for 15-20 minutes for the first 24-48 hours, to reduce swelling.
- **Compression:** An Ace bandage or similar dressing should be used to apply gentle pressure and prevent and/or reduce swelling.
- **Elevation:** The injured area should be elevated above the level of the heart, often by using pillows to elevate the body part.
- **(Referral):** Referral should be made to an appropriate physician for care as needed.

Evaluation of Pain

Pain is subjective and may be influenced by the individual's pain threshold (the smallest stimulus that produces the sensation of pain) and pain tolerance (the maximum degree of pain that a person can tolerate). The most common current pain assessment tool is the 1-10 scale:

$$0 = \text{no pain}$$
$$1 - 2 = \text{mild pain}$$
$$3 - 5 = \text{moderate pain}$$
$$6 - 7 = \text{severe pain}$$
$$8 - 9 = \text{very severe pain}$$
$$10 = \text{excruciating pain}$$

However, there is more to pain assessment than a number on a scale. Assessment also includes information about onset, duration, and intensity. Identifying what triggers pain and what relieves it can be very useful when developing a plan for pain management. Patients may show very different behavior when they are in pain: some may be fearful of disability, some may cry and moan with minor pain, and others may exhibit little difference in behavior when truly suffering; thus, judging pain by behavior can lead to the wrong conclusions.

Constipation and Fecal Impaction

Constipation is a condition in which bowel movements are less frequent than normal for a person, or hard, small stool is evacuated less than 3 times weekly. Constipation results from the colon, where fluid is absorbed. If too much fluid is absorbed, the stool can become too dry. The person may have abdominal distention and cramps and need to strain for defecation.

Fecal impaction occurs when the hard stool moves into the rectum and becomes a large, dense, immovable mass that cannot be evacuated even with straining, usually as a result of chronic constipation. In addition to abdominal cramps and distention, the person may feel intense rectal pressure and pain accompanied by a sense of urgency to defecate. Occasional use of non-prescription laxatives, stool softeners and even enemas (in the case of impaction) can resolve acute constipation, but chronic use only worsens the problem. The athlete should be instructed in dietary modifications (increased fluids and fiber) and referred to a physician if the problem is chronic.

CONTUSIONS OF THE QUADRICEPS MUSCLE

Injuries to the quadriceps muscle in the thigh are common in athletes as the result of direct blunt trauma to the anterior thigh, for instance contact with a helmet in football. **Contusions** are characterized by edema, pain with tenderness in the anterior thigh, and tautness of the muscle on palpation. Ecchymosis begins within hours of injury. Knee flexion may be limited, and the athlete walks with an obvious limp. Immediate treatment includes keeping the knee immobilized in a supported, flexed position (120°) for the first 24 hours, with ice applied for 20 minutes initially and then every 2-3 hours. The limb must be observed carefully, as a severe impact that causes swelling may result in compartment syndrome, which is a medical emergency. Passive stretching or electrical stimulation of the muscle may begin after 24 hours, with icing of the muscle following the stretching/stimulation. Weight bearing should resume gradually as symptoms recede.

SPRAINS AND CONTUSIONS OF THE KNEE

A **sprained knee** is a common sports injury. Usually the athlete will complain of acute pain at the time of injury and may feel the knee snap. Palpation may elicit pain or complaints of numbness. On a physical exam, the athlete may stand unevenly or walk with a limp. Normal range of motion may be impaired such that the knee cannot be straightened. Edema and ecchymosis may develop. The athlete should not bear weight on the knee, although splinting is not necessary. RICE therapy may be used initially to reduce pain and swelling, and the athlete should be referred to medical care.

A **contusion** of the knee is a less serious injury that may include pain and tenderness on palpation, edema, and ecchymosis. Range of motion and ability to walk are not impaired. RICE therapy is usually sufficient treatment.

ACUTE APPENDICITIS

Abdominal pain is not uncommon in athletes. Exercise-related transient abdominal pain (ETAP), a pain in the side, occurs while running in those not properly conditioned. In addition, muscles may be strained or injured by blunt trauma, so the pain associated with **appendicitis** may be overlooked. Appendicitis usually develops over 4 to 48 hours, with some combination of abdominal pain, lack of appetite, nausea, and fever. Pain often begins at the umbilical area and moves to the right lower quadrant, although some people have generalized abdominal pain. Palpation may show point tenderness in the RLQ, especially at McBurney's point (2/3 of the way from the umbilicus to the anterior superior iliac spine), which is the base of the appendix, with rebound tenderness at the point if it is compressed and suddenly released. Athletes with signs of possible appendicitis should be immediately referred to the ED, because an inflamed appendix can burst and cause peritonitis.

NASAL FRACTURES

Nasal fractures are most common in contact sports, such as football, and usually result from direct blunt trauma to the face. Immediate symptoms include intense pain, tenderness and mobility of the bridge of the nose on palpation, and bleeding from the nostrils. Usually deformity is evident. The athlete should be positioned sitting and leaning forward, so that blood doesn't run down the throat. The nostrils should be compressed to control bleeding. If there is clear fluid draining from the nostrils (cerebrospinal fluid), one should not apply pressure. An ice pack may be placed over the injured area to reduce swelling and decrease bleeding. The athlete must be transferred to an ED for further treatment, and should be restricted from sports for about 6 weeks. Upon return, the athlete should wear a protective face guard if engaging in contact sports.

Mandibular Fractures

Mandibular fractures usually result from blunt trauma during contact sports. Initial symptoms include pain; edema and distortion of the jaw; and, on exam, difficulty speaking, swallowing, or opening the mouth. There may be lacerations of the mouth, or loose or knocked out teeth. ABCs should be assessed with attention to airway, and cuts or bleeding lacerations should be treated with pressure to control bleeding. Neurological status should be evaluated. If there is bleeding and no apparent skull or brain injury, the person should be seated upright and leaning forward so that blood doesn't run down the throat. Any dislodged teeth still in the mouth should be removed to prevent aspiration, and the jaw should be immobilized with a wrap around the jaw and top of the head, secured above one ear. Any dislodged teeth should be wrapped as is in moist gauze and transported to the ED with the athlete. When cleared to return to play, the athlete should wear a mouthguard to prevent reinjury.

Injury to the Testes

The **testes** are vulnerable to injury from blunt trauma in a variety of contact sports. The immediate response is severe pain, which may be accompanied by light-headedness, bradycardia, and nausea. The pain may extend from the testicular region to the mid-abdomen. Initial treatment includes:

- Having the athlete lie in the supine position with his knees flexed to the chest until pain subsides.
- Applying ice or cold compress: Ice may increase pain, so the ice pack should not be placed in direct contact with the genitalia. Cold compresses alone often suffice.

Because testes are soft tissue, there may be increasing swelling that can cause compression of testicular tissue. For this reason, the athlete should be monitored for the next hour or more, and if there is increased pain or if pain fails to subside, the athlete should be referred for emergency evaluation, because a surgical operation to decrease pressure must be done within 4 hours of injury.

Corneal Ulcerations

Corneal ulceration is an open lesion on the cornea of the eye. It often occurs during sports played in windy conditions, in which sand or gravel is in the air. It can also be caused small particles becoming embedded in the eye, by irritation from contact lenses, or by infection. Typically, symptoms include tearing, eye pain, photophobia, spasms of the eyelid, blurring of vision, and redness of the eye. Treatment includes the immediate removal of any contact lens, if possible. Because ulceration leaves the eye vulnerable to infection, the athlete should be referred to an ophthalmologist for treatment. The trainer should avoid touching or rubbing the eye, as this may cause further damage. A clean cool moist compress may be placed over the eye for comfort during transit to a physician. Non-prescription drugs, such as NSAIDs, may relieve discomfort.

Otitis Externa

Otitis externa (swimmer's ear), inflammation of the external ear canal, is popularly thought to afflict only athletes in water sports, though it can also afflict other athletes, such as runners, when perspiration runs into the ear and keeps it moist. This warm moist atmosphere leads to the development of bacterial or fungal infections that cause pain, itching, discharge, and sometimes hearing deficit in the affected ear. Upon examination of the ear, discharge or odor may be noted, and pulling on the earlobe usually elicits an increase in pain. The athlete should be referred to a physician for appropriate antibacterial or antifungal medications. The athlete should avoid getting water in the ear for 3 weeks after treatment, and should protect the ear during showering and hair washing. The athlete should be advised to avoid cleaning the ear with objects (such a cotton swabs) or chemical washes. Once treated, the athlete may need to use eardrops recurrently to control flare-ups. Swimmers may need to wear earplugs to protect the ear from chlorine.

SEIZURES

Seizures are sudden involuntary abnormal electrical disturbances in the brain that can manifest as alterations of consciousness, spastic tonic and clonic movements, convulsions, and loss of consciousness.

- *Tonic-clonic (Grand Mal)*: Occurs without warning.
  - Tonic period (10-30 seconds): Eyes roll upward with loss of consciousness, arms flex, and body stiffens in symmetric contractions with cyanosis and salivating.
  - Clonic period (usually 30 seconds or longer): Violent rhythmic jerking with contraction, relaxation, and sometimes incontinence of urine and feces.

Following seizures, there may be confusion; disorientation; impairment of motor activity, speech and vision for several hours; and headache, nausea, and vomiting. During the seizure, the athlete's head and body should be protected from injury, but no attempt should be made to restrain the athlete or insert anything into his mouth. The athlete should be screened from spectators if possible, and turned onto his side if vomiting to prevent aspiration. The athlete should be referred for medical care with prolonged seizures (>5 minutes) or seizures without prior history of epilepsy.

ETHANOL OVERDOSE

Ethanol overdose affects the central nervous system, as well as other organs in the body. Typical *symptoms* of ethanol overdose include:

- Altered mental status with slurred speech and stupor.
- Nausea and vomiting.
- Hypotension.
- Bradycardia with arrhythmias.
- Respiratory depression and hypoxia.
- Cold and clammy skin or flushed skin (from vasodilation).
- Acute pancreatitis with abdominal pain.
- Loss of consciousness.
- Circulatory collapse leading to death.

If people are easily aroused, they can usually safely sleep off the effects of ingesting too much alcohol, but if the person is semi-conscious or unconscious, emergency medical treatment should be initiated. One should not give the person coffee to "awaken" them or encourage them to "walk off" the overdose but should, instead, transfer the person to a physician for care. A warming blanket may be applied to maintain body temperature.

SMALL CUTS AND LACERATIONS

When an athlete gets a **cut or laceration** from blunt or sharp trauma, he or she may react to the trauma by becoming faint; additionally, if there is excessive blood loss the person may develop shock as the blood pressure falls, so the overall condition and amount of blood loss should be assessed. (Hemorrhage requires immediate emergency transfer to an ED). Pressure should be applied to a bleeding lesion to stop bleeding, at which point the area should be thoroughly flushed with soap and water or saline, especially if the wound is contaminated. For small cuts, skin edges should be aligned, Steri-strips® placed over the wound, and a protective dressing should be placed over the cut/laceration. Antibiotic ointment, such as Neosporin®, may be applied to reduce the chance of infection. The person should be referred to a physician for suturing and a tetanus injection as indicated.

Fracture of the Wrist

A **wrist fracture** can occur in the distal radius (thumb side), ulna, or the wrist joint. The radius is the most commonly fractured, but both the radius and ulna may be fractured. Fracture usually occurs when a weight falling on an outstretched hand, resulting in hyperextension, or during direct blunt trauma. It is most common in sports like football, soccer, hockey, skiing, and ice-skating. Pain is usually severe, and deformity may be obvious. Mobility is often markedly decreased, and the athlete has an inability to bear any weight on his wrist. Edema often begins immediately, and there may be tingling or numbness as nerves are compressed. Any bleeding should be controlled with compression; dressings applied to open wounds; splinting of the wrist; and the athlete transported to an ED for treatment and casting. If both bones are broken, internal fixation may be required.

Fracture of the Knee Joint

A **fracture of the knee joint** can occur as the result of blunt trauma or a fall. Fractures can occur in the distal femur, proximal fibula, or patella, and they may be difficult to diagnose. Typical symptoms include edema, deformity of the joint, and pain or tenderness to palpation. If the knee straightens easily, there is no obvious deformity, and a posterior tibial pulse is present, the knee should be splinted above and below the injury, with all joints splinted as well as the associated side of the trunk. If there is considerable deformity but a posterior tibial pulse/dorsal pedal is still evident, then no attempt should be made to straighten the leg, but it should be splinted in the position in which it is found to prevent further injury. If the posterior tibial pulse is absent and the area below the injury is pale or frankly cyanotic, this is a medical emergency requiring immediate transfer. In all cases, the person should be transferred to an ED for treatment.

Knee or Patellar Dislocation

Dislocation of the knee or patella can occur as the result of a sharp blow to the knee joint. Symptoms include immediate acute severe pain and obvious deformity of the joint. The posterior tibial/dorsal pedal pulse is often absent, so immediate medical care is critical. The knee should be splinted in the present position during transfer to an ED. Patellar dislocations are a less severe injury than knee dislocation, and may result from twisting injuries or blunt trauma. There is less pronounced deformity than with a knee dislocation, although patellar dislocation may be obvious on comparison with the other knee. Edema and pain may be present. Immediate treatment includes RICE therapy and splinting the knee in the position found without attempting to realign the kneecap. The athlete should be referred for medical treatment.

Fracture of the Finger

Fracture of a finger may occur as the result of fall or other blunt trauma during sports activity. The athlete may still be able to move the injured finger, but will complain of acute pain. There may be deformity (if the bone is misplaced) and edema at the site of injury. On palpation, the athlete may complain of point tenderness or some lack of sensation. Testing includes placing the hand flat on a hard surface with the injured finger straight, if possible. Then, the trainer gently taps the end of the injured finger in the direction of the wrist. Fracture elicits pain in the finger, sometimes radiating into the hand. The fracture should not be aligned but splinted by buddy-taping the finger to an adjoining finger or cupping the fingers about padding held in the palm of the hand and securing the arm and hand to a rigid splint. A thumb may be splinted with figure 8 taping about the thumb. Ice may be applied during transfer for medical care.

FINGER DISLOCATIONS AND SPRAINS

Finger dislocation is a common sports injury. The athlete complains of immediate acute pain on injury and examination shows an obvious deformity with edema. The injured finger appears shortened, and mobility is markedly impaired. Treatment is similar to that of a fracture. The trainer should make no attempt at realigning the finger. The finger may be splinted as for fracture and an ice pack applied during transfer for medical care.

Sprain of a finger may result from compression, twisting, or being stepped on. The pain is less severe than with a dislocation and there is no deformity, but pain and edema may occur over the joint and palpation elicits tenderness on both lateral aspects of the joint. The athlete usually has limited mobility, cannot make a fist, and exhibits weak grip with pain. Buddy taping (or figure 8 for thumb) and ice (for twenty minutes) can be applied. If symptoms have not subsided, then further medical care should be sought.

HAND OR FOOT NAIL EVULSIONS

Nail avulsion occurs when injury partially or completely tears a nail away from the nail bed. The athlete complains of acute pain, and the nail bed may bleed. Immediate care includes flushing the area with soap and water if dirty, gently applying pressure to control the bleeding, and applying antibiotic ointment (such as Neosporin®) to the nail bed. If the nail remains partially adhered, it should be secured intact (not trimmed) over the nail bed with adhesive bandaging. If the nail has been completely torn away, a dressing should be applied over the nail bed to protect it from further injury. The athlete should be referred to a physician for further treatment as necessary. The nail bed must be protected while the nail grows back, so protective bandaging or cushioning may be necessary during sports activities.

REFERRALS FOR PSYCHOLOGICAL PROBLEMS

The Certified Athletic Trainer is in a unique position to observe athletes for **psychological problems**. If the trainer and the athlete have a relationship of mutual trust and respect, the trainer should be able to discuss concerns about the athlete's psychological status. It is important, however, that the trainer remain supportive but refrain from trying to provide psychological counseling unless qualified to do so. In some cases, conflicts may arise among team members or between the trainer and an athlete, and these problems should be dealt with directly rather than avoided, as avoidance will only worsen the problem. It is normal that athletes express anxiety and fears, especially after an injury or loss: psychological problems are those that are chronic and impair functioning. Athletes with psychological problems should be referred to mental health practitioners.

CHEMICAL EYE BURNS

Chemical eye burns are caused by the splashing of chemicals (solid, liquid, or fumes) into any part of the eye, often related to facial burns. Chemical burns may damage the cornea and conjunctiva, although other layers of the eye may also be damaged, depending upon the chemical and degree of saturation. Many injuries are work-related and involve alkali (> 7 pH), acid (< 7 pH) (muriatic acid or sulfuric acid), or other irritants (neutral pH) such as pepper spray. Alkali chemicals (such as ammonia, lime, and lye) usually cause the most serious injuries. *Symptoms* include:

- Pain.
- Blurring of vision.
- Tearing.
- Edema of eyelids.

Immediate treatment includes irrigating the eye and other contacted areas with copious amounts of water or normal saline. A history should be obtained to determine the cause of the injury, and the person immediately should be referred for further emergency care and eye exam.

HYPHEMA

Hyphema is bleeding in the fluid-filled anterior chamber lying between the cornea and the iris. This injury occurs from direct impact of the eye, as by a hand or ball. Initially, the blood in the chamber impairs vision, and the athlete may report dramatic vision loss. If there is a large amount of bleeding, the entire eye may appear red, but smaller bleeds may not be evident. As the blood settles, vision begins to clear. Often, this problem resolves and the blood is reabsorbed, but a hyphema is a medical emergency requiring referral to an ophthalmologist or ED so that the extent of injury can be assessed. The eye should be left uncovered. Initial treatment includes bed rest for 48-72 hours to reduce stress on the eye and prevent further bleeding, as sometimes an initial small bleed is followed by more severe bleeding in 3 to 5 days. The athlete must not return to sports activities until participation is cleared by an ophthalmologist.

ORBITAL BLOWOUT FRACTURE

Orbital blowout fracture damages the bones that comprise the eye socket, most often those of the orbital floor. In sports, it is most often caused by severe blunt trauma, as from a baseball bat or elbow, directly to the eye socket. Symptoms include severe pain about the eye and socket; edema; bruising about the eye; diplopia; and, in some cases, proptosis (protrusion of the damaged eye from the socket). On palpation, crepitus from air in the subcutaneous tissue may be noted, and the person may complain of numbness in the cheek on the affected side, caused by pressure on the infraorbital nerve. Sometimes nosebleeds occur as well, and pain in the eye may increase with nose blowing. There may be reduced eye movement and pain on eye movement, especially vertical. Immediate treatment includes applying soft dressing to cover the eye and ice pack (15-20 minutes) to reduce swelling. This is a medical emergency and the athlete should be transferred immediately to an ED for evaluation by ophthalmologist.

ELBOW DISLOCATION/FRACTURE

Dislocation or fracture of an elbow may present with similar symptoms and radiograph may be needed for diagnosis. The injury usually results from a fall or blunt trauma to the elbow. The athlete complains of severe pain, and muscle spasms may occur. Mobility is limited and there may be obvious deformity. Usually edema begins immediately after injury. There may be pallor and coolness of the arm and hand distal to the injury. The person may exhibit signs of shock. Immediate care includes treating for shock, monitoring pulses, and splinting the elbow. No attempt should be made to change the position of the elbow, as it may increase damage to nerves and vessels. It should be splinted as found and ice should be applied while in transit to the ED for further medical treatment.

FRACTURE OF THE FEMUR

Although **femur fractures** are not common in sports, they can occur, especially in sports such as skiing where the athlete falls with force. Stress fractures may occur as well. The athlete will have acute pain and often reports hearing or feeling the bone snap. There may be considerable blood loss and edema at the site of injury, depending upon the amount of displacement of the bone. Immediate treatment includes treating the person for shock as indicated by symptoms. The person should be flat with the uninjured leg raised above the level of the heart. Any hemorrhage of an open wound should be controlled by compression. An open wound should be covered with a dressing, and the injured leg should be splinted to prevent movement. The posterior tibial/dorsal pedal pulse should be monitored to ensure that circulation is not impaired. The athlete should be transferred to the ED immediately for further treatment.

FRACTURE OF TIBIA/FIBULA

Fracture of the tibia or fibula, or both bones, may occur as a result of a twisting injury at any point from the proximal to the distal ends. The fibula is more protected by tissue, and fracture of this bone alone may be more difficult to detect, as the tibia provides a natural splint. There may be little obvious deformity, and the person may be able to walk. Tibia fractures are more likely to result in an open fracture because of proximity to the skin surface. If both bones are fractured, there is usually pronounced deformity and edema at the site of the fractures, with severe pain and marked tenderness on palpation. Immediate treatment includes stopping blood flow with compression, monitoring pulses, applying dressing to an open wound, and splinting the leg with rigid splints on each side of the leg to prevent the legs from rotating. (The legs can be tied together if splints are unavailable.) Ice should be applied and the athlete should be transferred to an ED.

SHIN SPLINTS

Shin splints most often result from repetitive stress and inadequate warm-up exercises. This injury is common among runners. Symptoms include aching pain in the shin area that recedes after stopping activity. Treatment includes both preventive measures before activity and treatment after activity, as well as modifying activities to prevent further injury.

- Pre-exercise interventions include applying ice pack for 15-20 minutes before beginning exercise and applying compression dressing with 3-inch elastic stretch bandage in a spiral wrap from distal to proximal end of the shin.
- Post-exercise intervention includes RICE therapy.
- NSAIDs (such as aspirin and ibuprofen) may relieve discomfort for adults.
- The athlete should be advised regarding restriction of activity until he or she is pain-free and has made modifications in training to prevent recurrence.

FOOT AND ANKLE INJURIES

Foot and ankle injuries are very common in athletes. Sprains and fractures may be differentiated by palpation: Pain over the back edge of the malleolus, the fifth metatarsal or the navicular bone may indicate fracture. Usually, the athlete will be able to take at least 4 steps on a sprained ankle but will be unable to walk if there is a fracture. While some advocate leaving the shoe in place to provide compression, this is not a safe practice, as the foot should be examined for circulatory impairment.

If there is NO apparent fracture, immediate treatment includes:

- RICE therapy to decrease edema for 24-48 hours.
- If edema persists for three to seven days, contrast baths of cold water (45-60° F for 1 minute) and warm water (100-105° F) for 4 minutes twice daily for 1-2 weeks. The baths should be followed by passive flexion and extension of the foot.
- Weight bearing should wait until swelling and pain subsides.

HERNIA

A **hernia** occurs when the abdominal wall separates, allowing the protrusion of abdominal tissue. The most common hernia for males is the inguinal hernia, and for females, the femoral hernia. Hernias may be caused by inherent weakness in the muscles, straining (as for heaving, lifting, or bowel movements), or stress on the muscles from obesity. Hernias are often not associated with pain but present as a soft bulge in the abdomen, groin, or scrotal area. The bulge enlarges on standing and often reduces when lying flat. There may be sharp or dull aching pain associated with the hernia, usually increasing with straining. Hernias are only medical emergencies if they become incarcerated (a loop of bowel protrudes and twists, cutting off circulation). With incarceration, there is acute severe pain, sometimes with nausea and vomiting. Hernias must be examined by a physician, and the athlete should be restricted from activities until cleared by the physician. Surgical repair is usually performed.

TREATMENT OF DEBRIS IN THE EYE

It is not uncommon for athletes to get small **debris in their eyes**. The immediate symptom is photophobia, tearing, and discomfort. The person may feel something gritty within the eye. Debris in the eye can cause corneal abrasion, so protective eyewear should be worn when possible. The athletic trainer should wash his or her hands before examining the eye under a good light. The lower lid is pulled downward while the athlete looks up, and then the upper lid is pulled upward while the athlete looks down. If debris is imbedded or there is obvious corneal irritation, the eye should be covered with a clean pad and the athlete should be transferred for treatment immediately. If a small speck of debris is noted in the sclera (white part of eye), it may be removed gently with a cotton swab. If no debris is seen or it cannot be easily removed, the eye should be flushed with clean water; if symptoms persist, the person must be seen by an ophthalmologist.

SHOULDER DISLOCATION

Shoulder dislocations are common injuries resulting from blunt trauma or hyperextension. Usual symptoms include the injured athlete holding the arm away from his body (fractured humerus usually causes the person to hold his arm against his body with his arm across his chest. There is usually acute severe pain in the shoulder, obvious squaring deformity, and functional loss. There may be numbness or partial paralysis of the arm from compression on nerves or blood vessels. The trainer should not attempt to reduce the dislocation, as this could cause further damage. The arm should be supported by placing a pillow or other roll (such as a blanket) between the chest wall and the arm. Then, an arm sling with swathing may be applied to prevent pressure on the joint. Pulses and circulation must be monitored. The person should be transferred for medical care.

EMERGENCY CARE PROCEDURES REDUCING THE RISK OF MORBIDITY AND MORTALITY

Using appropriate emergency care procedures can reduce the risk of morbidity and mortality because when patients are given the advanced medical care they need in a timely fashion they have better outcomes. Planning for various emergency situations that may arise in the multiple venues in which an athletic trainer provides coverage increases the timeliness and effectiveness of care during emergency situations. For example, having an AED readily available will increase the likelihood of a patient surviving a sudden cardiac arrest with ventricular fibrillation. Having appropriate splints readily available and properly splinting a fractured bone before moving a patient limits secondary damage to the surrounding tissues, prevents the fracture from being further displaced, and lessens the extent of the injury and recovery time. There are many other emergency scenarios, that when given appropriate emergency care, decrease patients' risks of morbidity and mortality.

MECHANISMS OF INJURY
CERVICAL FRACTURES

Possible mechanisms of injury for cervical fractures include an axial load to the top of the head combined with neck flexion and forceful hyperextension of the head. Signs and symptoms of a possible cervical fracture include pain in the cervical region of the neck, pain in the chest, point tenderness on the neck, restricted movement, spasm in the cervical musculature, loss of sensation in the limbs or trunk, loss of strength in the limbs or trunk, inability to move the limbs or trunk, and loss of control over the bowels and/or bladder. Proper management includes immediate immobilization of the cervical spine, activation of advanced emergency medical services, and spine boarding by emergency medical personnel prior to transportation for advanced medical care.

SKULL FRACTURES

The mechanism of injury for a skull fracture is usually a forceful blow such as a baseball or a shot put hitting the head. Signs and symptoms of a skull fracture include unconsciousness or severe headache and nausea. Blood may be observed in the middle ear, the ear canal, and the nose. Ecchymosis behind the ear (Battle's sign) and around the eyes (raccoon eyes) may develop. Cerebral spinal fluid, which is straw-colored, may appear in the ear and nose. A skull fracture is a medical emergency and the patient must be immediately referred for advanced medical and be seen by a neurosurgeon. With a skull fracture it is not the actual fracture itself that makes the injury such an emergency, it is the complications from intracranial bleeding, bone fragments on the brain, and possible infection.

SECOND-IMPACT SYNDROME

Second-impact syndrome occurs when a patient suffers from a second injury to the head before they have fully recovered from their first head injury. The second injury to the head results in quick swelling and herniation of the brain creating a life-threatening emergency condition. The second impact does not even have to be severe or a blow to the head to result in second-impact syndrome. For example, if a patient is hit in the chest, causing the head to move around quickly, this can create enough force to cause a second injury to the already damaged tissue in the brain.

Initially, a patient suffering from second-impact syndrome may seem normal but within a few seconds to several minutes their condition rapidly deteriorates. They may display dilated pupils, lose the ability to move their eyes properly, and collapse. Patients suffering from second-impact syndrome need immediate advanced medical care. This is a life-threatening condition, and about half of patients who suffer from second-impact syndrome die from it. Preventing second-impact syndrome from occurring is the athletic trainer's primary defense. Making wise, cautious decisions about return-to-play following a head injury, and following nationally accepted practices for head injury management is key to preventing this life-threatening condition from occurring.

SUBDURAL HEMATOMA

A subdural hematoma is a life-threatening medical condition resulting from acceleration and deceleration forces that cause injury to the brain. These forces result in torn vessels between the dura mater and the brain causing bleeding and increased intracranial pressure. Acute subdural hematomas are the most common cause of death for athletes. These acceleration and deceleration forces can be produced by a blow to the head, such as a player being hit in the head by another player, an object, or hitting their head on the ground. Signs and symptoms of a subdural hematoma vary but can include a headache that gets worse, one pupil dilated, nausea, dizziness, lethargy, and unconsciousness. Patients suffering from an acute subdural hematoma need immediate advanced medical care for best possible results.

MANDIBULAR FRACTURES

The mechanism of injury for a mandibular fracture is direct blow to the lower jaw. In the athletic environment, this injury usually occurs in contact sports. Mandibular fractures are the second most common facial fracture, second to nasal fractures. As with all injuries to the face, the athletic trainer should also suspect and evaluate the patient for a possible head injury as well. Signs and symptoms of a mandibular fracture include a mandible deformity, malocclusion of teeth with possible bleeding, numbness in the lower lip, pain with biting, and trismus, which is a reduced ability to open the jaw. Proper management requires immediate immobilization with an elastic wrap and referral for advanced medical care. A physician must reduce and fixate the patient's mandible. Full return-to-play following this injury typically takes two to three months.

MAXILLARY FRACTURES

Maxillary fractures typically occur from a powerful blow to the upper jaw such as being hit by a hockey puck or ball traveling at a high speed. The front of the maxilla is thin and, therefore, is usually where fractures occur. However, a severe fracture of the maxilla, called a Le Fort fracture, occurs when the maxilla becomes detached from the skull. This is uncommon in sports and is more likely to occur in a motor vehicle accident. Fractures of the maxilla are the fourth most common fractures to the face.

Signs and symptoms of a maxillary fracture include swelling over and around the maxilla and possible numbness in the area if there is involvement of the infraorbital foramen and nerve. Occasionally, there is associated bleeding of the nose (epistaxis). With a Le Fort fracture, there will be significant malocclusion of the teeth and epistaxis. Proper care depends on the severity of the fracture. A Le Fort fracture must be referred immediately for advanced medical care. For a less severe fracture that does not contain malocclusion or excessive epistaxis, ice, ibuprofen, and a referral to a physician within 24 hours is appropriate. If numbness is present, the patient should be referred for a CT scan right away to determine proper care.

ZYGOMATIC COMPLEX FRACTURES

A fracture to the zygomatic complex (cheekbone) usually occurs from a forceful blow to the area. There are three different attachment sites for the zygoma to the surrounding facial bones. The zygoma attaches to the frontal bone, the maxilla, and the temporal bone. Since the zygoma is such a thick bone, fractures usually occur along the suture lines where it attaches to the surrounding bones. Signs and symptoms of a fracture to the zygomatic complex include pain, swelling, possible trismus (reduced opening of the jaw), and possible numbness. There will not be an obvious deformity unless all three of the attachments to the facial bones are fractured. In that case, the zygoma usually rotates downward causing in a decreased prominence of the cheekbone when compared bilaterally. Proper management depends on the severity of the fracture. If an obvious deformity is present, an immediate referral for advanced medical care is warranted. If the fracture is not displaced, ice, ibuprofen, and a referral to a physician within 24 hours is sufficient.

TOOTH SUBLUXATION, LUXATION, AND AVULSION

The mechanism of injury for tooth subluxation, luxation, and avulsion is a blow to the mouth. Signs and symptoms for a tooth subluxation is slight looseness of the affected tooth without any misalignment. The patient may report that the tooth does not feel right and may be sensitive to touch and biting. With a tooth luxation, the affected tooth is very loose and out of place, either shifted forwards or backwards. An avulsed tooth is completely knocked out.

Proper management differs on the extent of the tooth injury. For subluxation, the patient should be referred for a dental examination within 48 hours of the injury. With luxation, the athletic trainer should attempt to realign the affected tooth if it moves easily and the patient should be referred for immediate dental care. With a tooth avulsion, the tooth should be rinsed clean but not scrubbed or scraped. The athletic trainer should then try to reimplant the tooth as the sooner the tooth is reimplanted, the better the outcome. If the tooth cannot be reimplanted, the tooth should be stored in a tooth-saving kit, in the patient's saliva in a plastic bag, milk, saline, or inside the patient's mouth between their cheek and gum. Regardless of if the tooth can be successfully reimplanted or not, the patient should be referred for immediate dental care.

ORBITAL FRACTURES

The mechanism of injury for an orbital fracture is a blow to the eye in which the eye is pushed backwards into the socket. This creates compressive forces that can result in a fracture to the bony structure surrounding the eye. Signs and symptoms of an orbital fracture include limited eye mobility, double vision, edema, the affected eye may appear downwardly displaced, and the patient may experience pain or numbness to the area. The athletic trainer should immediately refer a patient suffering from a potential orbital fracture for immediate advanced medical care. Most orbital fractures require surgical repair along with antibiotics.

PROCEDURES FOR WOUND CLEANSING, DEBRIDEMENT, AND DRESSING

To properly cleanse an open wound, the athletic trainer should irrigate the wound with a nontoxic solution such as simple saline or tap water as soon as possible to remove any debris, exudate, and bacteria from the wound. However, if bone or tendon is visible, tap water should not be used. Antiseptics such as iodine and hydrogen peroxide may harm patients' tissues causing a delay the healing process and therefore should be used with caution.

If needed, debridement should be performed to remove any necrotic tissue and foreign bodies from the wound to promote healing. Wounds should be covered with a proper dressing that is selected based on the type of wound and the needs of the patient. Occlusive dressings have been shown to increase healing and decrease the risk of infection. The athletic trainer should inspect the wound daily and check for possible signs of infection. If signs of infection are present, the athletic trainer should refer the patient to a physician.

REMOVING A PATIENT WITH A SUSPECTED CERVICAL SPINE FRACTURE FROM A POOL

When a patient in a swimming pool has a suspected cervical fracture, the proper procedure for removing the patient from the pool must be followed for best patient outcomes. The athletic trainer must call for emergency services, get into the water with the patient, and immobilize the patient's head and neck while waiting for additional help to arrive. The patient's neck can be effectively immobilized by positioning the patient face up in the water, extending the patient's arms overhead, extending their elbows, and squeezing their arms together against their head, stabilizing the cervical spine.

Once a spine board and a second rescuer are available, extraction from the pool can be performed. The primary rescuer continues to immobilize the head and neck while the second rescuer places the spine board under the patient. The second rescuer then stabilizes the patient's head and neck while the primary rescuer securely straps the patient to the spine board at the levels of the head, chest, hips, and thighs. Once the patient is secured to the spine board, one rescuer will get out of the pool while the other stays in and both rescuers work together to slide the patient out of the pool while keeping them securely fastened to the spine board. Finally, the patient can be transported to an emergency medical treatment facility.

SHOCK

Shock can occur during all types of injuries but is more likely to develop when serious injuries are present such as with fractures, internal injuries, and severe bleeding. Shock occurs due to a dilation of blood vessels that allows the liquid portion of the blood to leave the blood vessels and enter tissue spaces of the body. This leaves the blood cells in the vessels with limited plasma, resulting in lowered blood flow and not enough oxygen being transported throughout the body, especially the nervous system. This causes tissue death and will lead to death of the patient unless advanced medical care is given.

There are steps the athletic trainer should take to prevent a patient from suffering from shock. The athletic trainer should remain calm, reassure the patient, keep bystanders away, and not let the patient look at their injury if it is serious. Clothing should be loosened, the patient's body temperature should be maintained, and elevation that is appropriate to the injury should be provided.

Different types of shock:

- Hypovolemic shock occurs from trauma that results in a large amount of blood loss. The lowered blood volume makes the body incapable of effectively transporting oxygen to the body organs.
- Respiratory shock occurs when the body cannot deliver enough oxygen throughout the body due to an injury to the lungs or the breathing control center.
- Neurogenic shock occurs as a result of general dilation of the blood vessels, which results in inadequate oxygen delivery throughout the body.
- Psychogenic shock is caused by a temporary dilation of the blood vessels, resulting in a lowered amount of blood flow to the brain. Fainting is the common term for psychogenic shock.
- Cardiogenic shock occurs when the heart is unable to pump blood throughout the body.
- Septic shock occurs as a result of a severe infection, usually bacterial in nature.
- Anaphylactic shock occurs as a result of a patient being exposed to something they are extremely allergic to such as a food or insect stings.
- Metabolic shock occurs when a severe medical condition goes untreated over time.

CONTROLLING BLEEDING

There are actions athletic trainer can take to control external bleeding and with all these actions, universal precautions must be used. Direct pressure can be applied by pressing a sterile gauze pad onto the injured tissue firmly. Elevation of the injured body part should also be performed if necessary. If direct pressure and elevation do not control bleeding, applying pressure to the appropriate pressure point should be employed. There are 11 pressure points on each side of the body. The two most common pressure points used to control hemorrhaging are the brachial and femoral arteries.

Internal hemorrhaging can be a life-threatening condition. If a patient is suspected to have internal hemorrhaging within the abdomen, thorax, or skull they should not be moved and the athletic trainer must call for immediate advanced medical care. To prevent shock, the patient should be kept calm and their body temperature should be sustained.

SIGNS EXHIBITED BY UNCONSCIOUS PATIENTS

There are many potential conditions that may cause a patient to lose consciousness. The physical signs of the patient may help the athletic trainer to determine the cause of unconsciousness. When a patient suffers heat syncope, signs they may display include a pulse that is fast and weak, breathing that is shallow and fast, dilated pupils, and their skin may be cold and clammy. When a patient suffers a concussion that causes unconsciousness, signs they may display include a pulse that is irregular and weak, shallow and irregular breathing, and their skin may appear pale and feel cool to the touch. A patient suffering from Grand Mal Epilepsy may display a fast pulse, noisy breathing that turns deep and slow as time progresses, and dilated pupils.

When a patient suffers from a brain compression and injury their decent to unconsciousness is usually gradual. Their pulse will gradually get slower, breathing may be noisy and slow, skin hot to the touch and flushed, and pupils may be unequal. When a patient suffers a heatstroke, they may have difficulty breathing, have a fast pulse, and their skin may be hot to the touch. When a patient becomes unconscious from a diabetic coma, signs they may display include a weak but fast pulse, deep breathing with sighing, and an acetone smell to their breath. An unconscious patient suffering from shock may display a weak but fast pulse, breathing that is rapid and shallow, clammy skin that is cold to the touch, and dilated pupils.

Primary Injury Survey vs. Secondary Injury Survey

The primary and secondary surveys are both parts of the on-the-field injury assessment. During the primary survey, the athletic trainer assesses the patient for life-threatening conditions such as unconsciousness, lack of respiration, no circulation, severe bleeding, and shock. The primary survey is performed first and if any threat-to-life is determined, the athletic trainer must call for advanced medical care and provide appropriate immediate care. If the patient is conscious and stable, a primary survey is not needed and the athletic trainer can proceed directly to the secondary survey. During the secondary survey the athletic trainer determines specifics about the injury. Pertinent information about the injury from the patient is gathered, vital signs are observed, and the athletic trainer determines the appropriate steps to be taken to properly care for the patient's injury.

Seizure Disorders

There are various causes for seizure disorders. For example, some patients suffer from seizure disorders as a result of genetic predisposition, others from alterations in brain metabolism, and others suffer seizure disorders as a result of previous injuries. When determining activity restrictions for patients who suffer from seizure disorders, the needs of the individual must be considered. If a patient's seizures are properly controlled, then limited or no activity limitations are needed. However, patients with seizure disorders should not swim by themselves, scuba dive, or participate in activities at high heights. If a patient's seizures disorders are not properly controlled and they experience severe daily or weekly seizures, the patient should not participate in collision sports. To care for a patient suffering from a seizure, the athletic trainer should not restrain the patient, assist them to the ground if possible, keep them away from anything that may cause them injury during the seizure, loosen any tight clothing, and remain calm.

Suspected Drug Overdose

When a patient suffers from a suspected drug overdose the athletic trainer should immediately activate emergency medical services and contact their local poison control center. While waiting on emergency services to arrive, the poison control center can give directions on how to immediately care for the patient. The poison control center will need specific information to provide the best care. They will need to know the name and age of the patient, the name of the drug that was taken along with the amount taken and the time it was taken if known, signs and symptoms the patient displays, vital signs, and the name and location of the person calling.

Removing the Facemasks of Football Helmets

There are several tools used to remove the facemasks of football helmets. These tools cut, unscrew, or release the fasteners that attach the facemask to the helmet. Athletic trainers must be familiar with the fasteners used on the helmets their athletes wear and have the needed tools to remove those fasteners, detaching the facemask within 30 seconds. Before removing a facemask, a trained rescuer should immobilize the patient's head to limit any movement.

There are usually four fasteners that attach the facemask to the helmet. The two side fasteners should be removed first and then the two fasteners on the top should be removed. The tools used should be equipment-specific, based on the type of fasteners used on the helmets. For quick-release fasteners, a quick release tool is required. The use of an electric screwdriver can be faster and produces less movement than cutting tools such as the FM Extractor and Anvil Pruner. However, these cutting tools must always be available in case a screw fails and cannot be removed with a screwdriver.

DIABETIC COMA AND INSULIN SHOCK

A diabetic coma is a life-threatening condition that may develop when a patient's diabetes is not properly managed. Prevention of a diabetic coma is the best course of action. This can be achieved through monitoring blood glucose levels, ensuring a proper diet, and urine dipstick testing. Signs and symptoms of a diabetic coma include difficulty breathing, extreme thirst, a fruit-smell to the breath, flushed skin, mental confusion, and nausea. Emergency medical care is required and an insulin injection may be advisable.

Insulin shock occurs when the diabetic patient has too much insulin and suffers low blood sugar. Signs and symptoms of insulin shock include a tingling sensation, weakness, headache, irritability, shallow breathing, and a rapid heartbeat. If the hypoglycemia is mild, the patient may respond well to glucose tablets, orange juice, or candy. However, if the reaction is severe, or the patient has a loss of consciousness, emergency medical care is required.

POLICE

The acronym POLICE stands for protection, optimal loading, ice, compression, and elevation which are appropriate treatments following common acute musculoskeletal injuries. Protection is implemented to keep the damaged tissue from suffering from additional damage and bleeding. Depending on the injury, this may require the use of crutches, braces, or slings. Optimal loading is achieved by introducing appropriate mechanical loading to the tissue after a brief period of protection. This will optimize healing by improving the physical qualities of collagen.

Ice application serves many functions. It works as an analgesic, which can reduce muscle guarding secondary to pain. It promotes vasoconstriction, which limits excessive edema and decreases intravascular pressure. It also lowers the tissue's metabolism and its need for oxygen, which reduces cell death due to hypoxia (lack of oxygen.) Compression decreases bleeding and swelling by placing pressure on the injured area and increases lymphatic drainage. Elevation assists in preventing excessive edema accumulation by allowing gravity to aid in lymphatic drainage. The higher the elevation of the involved area, the more effective it is. Both compression and elevation should be performed as often as possible for 72 hours following the injury.

MAKING PATIENT-CARE DECISIONS DURING AN EMERGENCY SITUATION

The athletic trainer, emergency medical technicians, and team physician should all work collaboratively to ensure the proper management of emergency situations that may arise. Prior to an emergency situation, all involved parties should discuss their roles in patient care so any emergencies can be handled efficiently to provide best patient care. Generally, the athletic trainer has more emergency management training than the team physician so the athletic trainer should be able to determine appropriate management for emergency situations. If it is determined that emergency medical services will be needed, they will be called to the site of the emergency. Once on scene, the emergency medical technicians will determine proper management of the injury as they have the most training in emergency management. Throughout the emergency situation the athletic trainer should remain readily available to assist the emergency medical personnel, pass on pertinent information, and assist with athletic equipment such as football facemask removal.

TAPING AND BANDAGING

There are a number of different types of tape used for **taping and bandaging:**

- Zinc oxide tape is non-elastic and is used to strap joints or prevent blisters, but it shouldn't be used to enclose muscles or areas that may swell with exercise, as it may interfere with circulation.
- Self-adhering tape sticks to itself but not to the skin and is elastic. It can be used to strap joints, provide compression, and finish (top layer) bandaging.
- Elastic adhesive bandages are elastic with zinc oxide and are used around muscles that may expand during exercise.
- Foam tape may be used to provide a cushion beneath other types of tape.

There are a number of purposes for taping and bandaging:

- Provide support for muscles and joints and protect unstable joints.
- Limit mobility of injured joints or prevent abnormal movement.
- Protect skin from infection and blistering.
- Secure protective equipment.
- Provide compression to control hemorrhage.

CRUTCHES

Crutches should be properly fitted before the athlete attempts ambulation. Correct height is one hand-width below axillae. The handgrips should be adjusted so that the athlete can support his body weight comfortably with his elbows slightly flexed rather than locked in place. The athlete should be cautioned not to bear weight under the axillae, as this can cause nerve damage, but to hold the crutches tightly against the side of the chest wall. The type of gait that the athlete uses depends on the type of injury. Typical gaits include:

- Two-point, in which both crutches are placed forward and the healthy leg advances first to the crutches.
- Three-point, in which the injured extremity and both crutches are advanced together, at which point the healthy leg advances to the crutches.

The athlete should be advised whether there is partial or no weight bearing, and demonstration should be provided. Stair climbing should be practiced:

- Ascending: Healthy foot goes first, followed by crutches and injured extremity.
- Descending: Crutches go first, followed by the healthy foot.

WOUND HEALING AFTER A SOFT TISSUE INJURY

There are 4 primary phases to wound healing:

- **Hemostasis** takes place within the first few minutes after injury and bleeding, when the platelets begin to seal off the vessels and secrete substances that cause vasoconstriction. Thrombin is produced to stimulate the clotting mechanism, forming a fibrin mesh.

- **Inflammation (lag or exudative) phase** occurs over the first four days after the injury. During this phase, there is erythema and edema along with pain, as the blood vessels release plasma and neutrophils or polymorphonucleocytes to begin phagocytosis, which removes debris and prevents infection.
- **Proliferative/granulation (fibroblastic) phase** occurs over days 5 to 20 after injury. During this phase, fibroblasts produce collagen to provide support and granulation tissue starts to form. Epithelization and contracture of the wound occur.
- **Maturation (differentiation, remodeling or plateau) phase** occurs after day 21, and lasts for an indeterminate duration. The fibroblasts leave the wound and the collagen tightens to reduce scarring. The tissue gains tensile strength. This stage can last up to 2 years, and the wound can break down easily again during this phase.

REMOVAL OF TICKS

Ticks can spread a number of different diseases, including Babesiosis, ehrlichiosis, Lyme disease, and Rocky Mountain spotted fever. Those in tick-infested areas should be cautioned to avoid tall grass and shrubby areas, use repellants (DEET), and wear light-colored clothing with their arms and legs covered and their pants tucked into their socks. Athletes should shower and examine their skin immediately after returning indoors, as ticks often wander about the body for 30 minutes before biting and feed 12-24 hours before spreading infection. The groin, axillae, and neck are common sites for ticks. The CDC recommends removing ticks with tweezers, and NOT using petroleum jelly, nail polish, alcohol or other methods, as these may cause the tick to regurgitate and spread infection. The tick should be grasped near the skin and pulled upward without twisting. Then, the skin should be washed with soap and water. The tick should be saved in a plastic bag in case testing is needed. Burrowed ticks must be removed by a physician.

SPLINTING A FRACTURE

PROPERLY SPLINTING A FRACTURE

When a fracture is suspected, the injured patient should not be moved until the fracture is immobilized. The fracture must be splinted in the position it is found. Do not attempt to realign displaced bones. In the event of an open fracture, the wound must be dressed to prevent infection and blood loss.

A splint must be selected that can immobilize the joint above and the joint below the fracture. If there is a suspected lower-leg fracture, both the knee and foot must be immobilized. A rapid form vacuum immobilizer is commonly used for this type of injury. Possible wrist fractures require the fingers and elbow to be immobilized which can be accomplished with a SAM splint. The injured arm should also be placed in a sling. For suspected fractures around the shoulder a sling is applied and the injured arm is secured to the upper body. For possible femur fractures a special splint is made that properly immobilizes this injury, the half-ring splint.

Once the appropriate splint is applied, the distal pulse and the color of the patient's fingers or toes should be monitored to insure proper circulation. The patient must be referred to receive immediate medical care.

Application of Splints

Splinting is used in the case of suspected or obvious dislocations and fractures before the person is moved to prevent further injury. Before applying a splint:

- Control bleeding through compression and apply dressing to cover open wounds.
- Monitor circulation, sensation, and mobility (CSM). If circulation is impaired and pulse is absent, gently partially realign the limb while assessing circulation until pulse is felt or cyanosis subsides.
- Rule of thirds: For injury to the proximal third of a bone, splint both below the injury and the joint above the injury. For injury to the middle third, splint joints above and below the injury. For injury to distal third, splint above the injury and the joint below the injury.
- If possible, one person should stabilize the limb while splinting is done.
- Provide splints on both sides of the injury to prevent rotation.

Splinting Related to Specific Injuries

The type of splinting required depends upon the site of injury:

- **Shoulder:** The arm should be placed in a sling, with the wrist/hand above the level of the elbow.
- **Humerus:** A rigid splint should be applied on the lateral humerus, and the arm secured in a sling across the chest with a swath binder.
- **Elbow:** Splint in position found. If straight, splint from axilla to wrist along medial aspect with splint tied in place. If bent, place rigid splints from upper arm to wrist and support in sling.
- **Forearm:** Place rigid splint, or SAM splint, on both sides of arm with thumb upward from palm and extending past elbow. Then, support in sling with swath binder about body.
- **Pelvis and hip:** Provide firm backboard and avoid lifting legs.
- **Femur:** Rigid splints on both sides of leg can be used, or buddy splinting can be used if necessary. Traction splints are preferred, but usually only available with EMS.

Types of Splints Used for Immobilization

There are a number of different types of **splints** that may be used for immobilization. There are many commercial splints available, but in an emergency, rolled-up newspapers or other material may be used:

- *Anatomic or "buddy" splints* involve using adjacent body parts to provide immobilization, such as taping fingers together, tying legs together, or securing an arm across the chest.
- *Rigid splints* are not flexible and may be plastic boards or wooden boards, padded or unpadded, or heavy cardboard. Molded SMA splints fit around the limb. Rigid splints must be of sufficient length to extend well above and below the point of injury.
- *Soft splints*, such as pillows, may be used if no other splints are available for support of fractures of the lower arm or leg. Inflatable splints are also available and can provide very good immobilization.

Hyperventilation

Hyperventilation can occur in response to emotional stress, diabetic ketoacidosis, shock, and high-altitude sickness. Symptoms include feelings of lightheadedness, dizziness, anxiety, and agitation. If prolonged, calcium levels may drop and paresthesia with numbness and tingling or muscle twitching may occur. Dyspnea is >40/min. If related to altitude sickness, the person should not climb further but, once stabilized, should descend until dyspnea subsides. Contrary to common practice, the person hyperventilating should not be asked to rebreathe using a paper bag, as this does little to alter blood gas and can stress the cardiopulmonary system. Instead, the trainer should provide reassurance and calmly coach the person to breathe more slowly, inhale through the nose, hold the breath for a short period, and then exhale slowly until breathing slows.

EMERGENCY ACTION PLANS FOR SPORTS-RELATED ACTIVITIES

The Certified Athletic Trainer and others in a sports program should establish **emergency action plans** that include the following:

- Map of facility with specific designations for first-aid equipment and plans for entry and exit routes for EMS personnel, as well as the location of any necessary keys.
- Immediate telephone access (usually cell phone).
- Fully-stocked first-aid kits, fire extinguishers, and flashlights with easy access.
- Medical release, physical examination, incident, and transfer forms.
- CPR and other first-aid training for support staff.
- Identification of all support staff on site and external support (EMS, fire department, etc.).
- Posting of telephone numbers for EMS, physicians, medical facilities, Hazmat team, etc.
- Chain of command for managing emergencies, calling 9-1-1, contacting family/guardians, and reporting to media.
- Medical supervision.
- Medical supplies: splints, dressings, tape, etc.
- Budget.

ESTABLISHED REFERRAL STRATEGIES TO INCREASE THE TIMELINESS OF CARE

Having established referral strategies increases the timeliness of care because it simplifies the referral process and ensures that appropriate healthcare professionals are readily available to provide specialized care as needed. There are a multitude of injuries and illnesses the physically active population experiences and many times the athletic trainer will be the first member of the healthcare team to see these patients. It is important for the athletic trainer to recognize those injuries and illnesses that require referral and have a specialist in that field of healthcare available for referral. For example, athletic trainers may see patients who suffer from injuries and illnesses that require referral to a dentist, a podiatrist, an orthopedic surgeon, a psychiatrist, a neurologist, and a cardiologist, just to name a few. Having healthcare professionals in these fields available to evaluate and treat these patients will ease the stress and uncertainty patients and their families may experience and can make setting up appointments more efficient.

COOPERATING WITH OTHER MEMBERS OF THE HEALTH CARE TEAM

The Certified Athletic Trainer is just one of a group of **healthcare providers** working together to reduce morbidity in athletes. Other members of the healthcare team may include:

- *Physician:* The team physician or family physicians provide medical support and assessment, evaluating the criteria for safe participation and return to play.
- *Physician's assistant (PA):* The PA assists with diagnosis and treatment.
- *Physical therapist (PT):* The PT devises and supervises exercises and activities for strengthening and recovery.
- *Chiropractor:* Treatments may reduce pain, especially related to pulled muscles or nerve compression.
- *Acupuncturist:* Similar to chiropractor.
- *Massage therapist:* Treatment increases circulation, stimulates muscles, and reduces pain.

- **Personal trainer:** This person helps the athlete to devise a personal plan for strengthening or exercise, and assists in the implementation of the plan.
- **Sports nutritionist:** The nutritionist helps the athlete maintain an adequate intake of nutrition and fluids, appropriate to the sport.
- **Psychologist:** Mental health care helps the athlete deal with stress.

Therapeutic Intervention

PATIENTS' PLANS OF CARE

Creating, evaluating for effectiveness, and revising patients' plan of care results in enhanced patient outcomes because it allows for the plan of care to adapt to the changing needs of patients. Initially, creating a plan of care helps to inform patients and stakeholders about the estimated amount of time the patient will need to recover, the goals of rehabilitations, and steps to be taken to achieve those goals. Frequently evaluating the effectiveness of the plan will ensure that the desired results are being obtained from the rehabilitative plan. If the results are not being obtained, the athletic trainer will be able to recognize areas of the plan of care that will need to be modified to meet the desired rehabilitative results. Appropriately revising the plan ensures that it fits the actual needs of the individual patient as they progress towards their rehabilitative goals.

DEVELOPING PATIENTS' PLAN OF CARE

PHASES OF THE HEALING PROCESS

Athletic trainers must be cognizant of the healing process, be able to determine what stage of the healing process patients are in, and design plans of rehabilitation that optimize the conditions for healing. The three phases of the healing process can overlap but progress from the inflammatory phase, to the fibroblastic repair phase, and finally the maturation-remodeling phase. During the inflammatory phase, patients may experience swelling, loss of function, increased pain, redness, and an increase in the skin temperature surrounding the injury. For proper healing, the inflammatory phase must occur, however the athletic trainer can take steps to prevent excessive swelling and pain through ice, compression, elevation, and anti-inflammatory medications if necessary. The inflammatory phase generally lasts up to 4 days following the initial injury.

During the fibroblastic repair phase, regeneration occurs leading to scar formation. This phase generally lasts from around 4 days after the injury to around 6 weeks post-injury. Cardiorespiratory endurance, muscular strength, and flexibility should all be maintained throughout healing. During the maturation-remodeling phase of healing, scar tissues can be restructured to eliminate functional limitations using functional strengthening techniques. This phase can take 2 to 3 years to fully complete.

PROPOSED THEORIES OF PAIN CONTROL

The three models of pain control are theories. Research is still underway to fully understand how pain modulation occurs. However, these theories can be utilized to help decrease patients' levels of pain.

- The gate control theory of pain modulation proposes that an increase in neural activity triggers a release of encephalin from the dorsal horn, which inhibits the transmission of pain information by "closing the gate" through which the neural information is transmitted. Athletic trainers can utilize electrical stimulation to provide an increase in neural activity and "close the gate," therefore preventing the transmission of pain information.
- The descending pathway pain control theory proposes that pain impulses can be inhibited and are influenced by previous experiences, emotions, and sensory information, which affect the perception of pain. High intensity electrical stimulation near a noxious level can stimulate the descending neurons and prevent transmission of pain information.

- The release of ß-endorphin theory proposes that painful stimulus triggers the release of an analgesic chemical, similar to an opiate called ß-endorphin. Point stimulation with electrical currents near the site of injury or along trigger points can trigger the release of ß-endorphin.

Age-Related Changes

The athletic trainer should be aware of physiological changes that occur throughout the aging process and be able to apply this information for best patient outcomes. For example, degenerative diseases and preexisting injuries are more prevalent in older-adult patients. Being aware of this can help the athletic trainer screen for these conditions and provide appropriate care. The athletic trainer may find that a patient suffers from osteoarthritis and compensatory biomechanics from a previous injury. The athletic trainer can then address and correct these concerns with therapeutic exercises.

Older adults also have a higher incidence of diabetes and arteriosclerosis, which may affect wound healing. To ensure optimal wound healing, nutritional advice should be given to ensure patients are consuming their recommended daily allowances of Vitamin C, K, A, zinc, and amino acids. Safe exercise should also be promoted to the older adult population as many studies show that regular physical activity can delay and prevent many degenerative changes that occur with aging.

Pharmacological Protocols

Athletic trainers must follow the regulations regarding pharmacological practices within their state for the patient population they serve. If athletic trainers are allowed to administer over-the-counter drugs, the following guidelines for adult patients can be followed if no contraindications exist.

Fever: If a patient has a fever ranging from 99.5 to 102 degrees Fahrenheit, the patient may be administered 325 mg of acetaminophen every 4 hours as needed. If the patient's fever is 102 or greater, a physician should be consulted.

Watery nasal discharge: If a patient has watery discharge from the nose, 30 mg of pseudoephedrine (Sudafed) can be administered every 6 hours if needed. Pseudoephedrine should not be administered 4 hours prior to activity or if the patient is in postseason play.

Cough: If a patient has a cough with no mucus or clear mucus, 10 mL of Robitussin DM can be administered every 6 hours if needed. Robitussin DM may cause drowsiness and should not be administered 4 hours prior to activity. The patient should be encouraged to drink fluids. If the patient coughs up green or rusty colored mucus or has a continuous severe cough, a physician should be consulted.

Healing Processes of Acute and Chronic Injuries

Acute injuries originate from one event, such when a patient changes directions quickly and suffers an ACL sprain. Chronic injuries occur over time from cumulative micro-traumas. For example, iliotibial band syndrome develops over time from overuse and excessive stress on the involved structures that may originate from biomechanical abnormalities. While acute injuries are generally only in the inflammatory response phase for around 4 days following the initial injury, chronic injuries generally are in the inflammatory phase longer and are more resistant to physical and pharmacological treatments. Therefore, chronic injuries may take an extended amount of time to resolve the inflammatory process. Correcting the causes that led to the chronic injuries must be addressed, or it is highly likely that they will reoccur.

Scope of Practice for Various Health Care Providers and Reasons for Referral

Dentist: A team dentist oversees the dental needs of patients and should be available for emergency dental care such as a tooth luxation or avulsion.

Neurologist: A specialist treating neurological conditions that can be referred to in order to help patients with head or nervous system injuries.

Ophthalmologist: An eye specialist who can be referred to treat eye injuries and provide vision-correcting services.

Podiatrist: A foot specialist that should be referred to for surgical procedures, the correction of foot biomechanics, and the construction of specialty orthotics.

Sport psychologist: A specialist in psychology as it pertains specifically to sports. They can be referred to in order to help patients cope with the injury and rehabilitation process.

Rehabilitation When a Surgical Procedure is Involved

The phases of rehabilitation when a surgical procedure is involved are the preoperative phase, the acute inflammatory response phase, the fibroblastic repair phase, and the maturation-remodeling phase. These phases align with the phases of the healing process.

- Preoperative phase: This phase is used to improve patient outcomes by allowing the initial inflammation following the injury to resolve prior to surgery while maintaining strength, flexibility, and cardiorespiratory endurance.
- Acute inflammatory response phase: During this phase, the body works to clean up the injured area to create an environment conducive to healing. The athletic trainer can assist this process by protecting the injured tissues, encouraging optimal loading, application of ice, compression, and elevation. While immobility of the injured body part may be required, the patient should still perform appropriate exercises to maintain strength, flexibility, and cardiorespiratory endurance that do not exasperate the injury.
- Fibroblastic repair phase: During this phase scar tissue is being developed to repair the damaged tissue. Appropriate exercises should be performed to maintain fitness, while regaining full range of motion and neuromuscular control.
- Maturation-remodeling phase: During this phase, the scar tissue can be realigned through dynamic, functional sport-specific exercises to regain functional strength.

Rehabilitation Following the Surgical Repair of an ACL Sprain

During the preoperative phase, goals for a patient who suffers from an ACL sprain include resolution of the initial inflammatory response, regaining full range of motion, maintaining strength as tolerated, and psychological preparation for the surgery. During the acute injury phase, goals are to reduce pain, swelling, and hemorrhaging from the surgery. Full knee extension should be established by the end of the first week after surgery. Knee flexion should be worked towards, as well as quadriceps control, and neuromuscular control. During the fibroblastic repair phase, goals should be to maintain full extension, increase flexion, achieve a normal gait, strengthen the surrounding musculature, maintain cardiorespiratory endurance, increase neuromuscular control, and begin gentle functional exercises. During the maturation-remodeling phase, goals include functional progression that leads to readiness for full return to activity.

Nonfeasance, Malfeasance, Misfeasance

There are legal actions patients may pursue if they are harmed. The athletic trainer must act within their scope of practice and provide the best available care to prevent possible litigation. Nonfeasance is failing to act when an action should have been taken. For example, if an athletic trainer did not follow proper lightning-safety protocols and a patient suffered from a lightning-strike injury, the athletic trainer could be sued based on nonfeasance. Malfeasance is providing a service that a person is not permitted to perform that results in further injury to the patient. For example, if athletic trainer attempted to realign a fractured bone, which resulted in the patient suffering further injury, the patient could sue based on malfeasance. Misfeasance occurs when a person performs a service they are allowed to perform, however it is done improperly, which results in further injury to the patient. For example, if an athletic trainer performed an ultrasound treatment using improper parameters that resulted in further injury to the patient, the patient could sue based on misfeasance.

Factors Affecting Normal Range of Motion

Normal **range of motion** is the maximum possible movement of a joint. There are a number of factors that can affect flexibility and the normal range of motion:

- **Immobilization**: If a joint has been immobilized because of injury, it may lose muscle flexibility and range of motion until the muscle is stretched through exercise. The same can occur after surgery, such as rotator cuff repair, in which range is limited because of damage to the muscles. Lack of flexibility in a joint most often relates to muscle limitations.
- *Scar tissue or injury/disease* of the joint capsule and/or ligaments: If the joint itself is damaged or scarred, this can impact the range of motion. This type of injury may be more difficult to repair.
- *Loss of strength*: Injuries or diseases that decrease muscle strength can have a profound effect on range of motion, because the muscles may not support the full range and, over time, this has the same effect as immobilization, compounding the problem.

Range of Motion

One of the first focuses in a rehabilitative sports exercise program should be on retaining and improving flexibility and **range of motion** because, without adequate range, the athlete's performance is limited. Exercises to increase flexibility should be performed early so that other exercises, which depend upon the flexibility of the joint, can be performed subsequently. Without flexibility, the athlete increases the chance of re-injuring the joint during rehabilitation and after, when sports activities are resumed. Additionally, during the healing process, scar tissue begins to form. Over time, this scar tissue normally contracts, but in a joint, excessive contraction can result in a limited range of motion. During the remodeling phase of healing, stretching exercises can reduce the chance of contracture; therefore, the program of exercises should be based upon the phase of healing to ensure maximum benefit.

Rehabilitation Issues Related to Strength and Endurance

Once range of motion is achieved, the focus of rehabilitation shifts to **strength and endurance**. Strength of the muscle is the maximal force it can exert, and endurance is the ability to maintain strength while engaged in prolonged or repetitive activities. Both strength and endurance must be considered during rehabilitation, because both are necessary for normal function in sports. There must be a balance between strength and endurance exercises, because improving one parameter improves the other. Therefore, it may be beneficial to focus on strength and, when that plateaus, to shift focus to endurance until the muscle strength increases enough the rehabilitation can again shift to strength exercises. Determining where to focus the energy in a rehabilitation program requires careful observation and monitoring of the individual response to exercise.

Principles of Rehabilitation

With all types of rehabilitation and reconditioning, sound **principles** should be followed in order to prevent further deconditioning. An athletic trainer needs to ensure that all muscles and circulation are exercised while the injury is being rehabilitated:

- Begin with a thorough evaluation and assessment.
- Establish short-term and long-term goals.
- Initiate treatment early after injury, usually within the first 24-48 hours, because people can lose 3-4% of muscle strength per day.
- Provide ongoing reevaluation and assessment, and modify the program as needed, especially during the first week.
- Promote compliance with the rehabilitation program by keeping the athlete informed and intervening if the athlete fails to attend sessions or perform exercises.
- Plan an appropriate rehabilitation for both the type of injury and the individual needs of the athlete.
- Increase the intensity of the rehabilitation program as indicated, without increasing injury to the affected body part or injuring other muscles.
- Remember that the injury is a part of the whole and not the sole focus of rehabilitation.

Establishing Goals

Establishing both **long- and short-term goals** is a necessary component of rehabilitation, in part because it motivates the athlete. Long-term goals are often easier to define, as they generally involve returning the athlete to full strength. Short-term goals that identify outcomes need to be established throughout rehabilitation and continually reassessed. Goals should be measurable by objective means as much as possible, although some assessment, such as the determination of pain, is by nature subjective. However, using a 0-10 pain scale can help to increase objectivity. Measurable goals should be stated clearly: "In one week, the athlete will have 3/5 strength in the X muscle." Depending upon the goals, measurements, such as muscle girth, should be taken on a regular basis so that progress can be plotted. Goals should be realistic and made with the individual in mind. A highly motivated individual may achieve goals more readily than someone who is depressed or less motivated.

Improving Treatment and Rehabilitation Outcomes by Educating Patients

Educating patients using appropriate information improves treatment and rehabilitation outcomes because it allows the patient to fully understand their injury, how the rehabilitative process will help them to obtain an optimal recovery, and therefore can increase compliance to the rehabilitative plan. Also, when the athletic trainer can thoroughly answer all the patients' questions, this may increase their trust in the athletic trainer's ability to evaluate, provide treatment, and develop an effective plan of care that will help them to achieve their desired results.

For example, if a patient suffers from a MCL sprain they will need to be compliant during several stages of a rehabilitative plan of care to have an optimal recovery. If the athletic trainer explains the injury, the steps of the rehabilitative plan, and the physiological reasoning why each step is included, then the patient can see the whole picture and understand the importance of compliance throughout the plan of care. When the patient understands the importance, they will be more likely to follow-through with the rehabilitative plan and, therefore, achieve optimal results.

Educating Patients About Surgery and Rehabilitation

There are many steps an athletic trainer should take when educating a patient about surgery and the rehabilitative process. The patient's injury should be explained thoroughly in a way the patient can understand using anatomical charts or models. The patient should feel comfortable asking questions and receive clear answers. It is important that the athletic trainer ensures the patient understands the extent of the injury as well as consequences for not following the plan of rehabilitation to improve patient compliance. The prognosis should be realistic and not give false hope. The healing process should be explained as well as the estimated amount of time the patient can expect the process to take. The overall plan of rehabilitation should be explained, giving the patient reasons why the exercises and modalities are selected. Finally, the patient should be encouraged to keep a positive outlook on their rehabilitation, as their attitude greatly affects their outcome.

Evidence-Based Practice

Incorporating evidence-based practice allows the athletic trainer to make informed decisions about patient care while taking into account evidence from research. The five steps of evidence-based practice are to develop a clinical question, look through related available research, determine the research's strength of evidence, implement the best practices found in the research review, and evaluate patient outcomes for effectiveness.

When developing a clinical question, the athletic trainer should use the PICO format to ensure they are addressing the patient outcomes, interventions available, comparing alternatives, and the desired outcomes. Next, the athletic trainer searches the literature available through databases that that include evidence-based practices using keywords from the clinical question. The strength of the evidence of research found should be considered. The NATA uses the SORT scale to rate the strength of evidence. After reviewing the literature, the athletic trainer chooses the best options for treatment while taking into account the individual patient's values and preferences. Finally, after treatments have been offered, the athletic trainer should evaluate the effectiveness of the treatment plan and make any adjustments as necessary.

Increased Incidence of Noncontact ACL Injuries in Females vs. Males

There are many factors that have been researched to explain the increased incidence of noncontact ACL injuries in females versus males. The most important contributing factors are neuromuscular, such as latencies in muscular activation, improper muscle recruitment patterns, and stiffness of joints. Also, a strong contraction of the quadriceps muscle group during eccentric contraction is a big contributor. Other possible reasons include an increased Q-angle, lower-leg malalignments such as excessive genu valgum, knee recurvatum, pronation, and external tibial torsion. Currently, there is no consensus that sex-specific hormones play a role in the increased incidence of ACL sprains for females, so no restrictions during the menstrual cycle of female athletes is warranted.

Increasing Patients' Adherence to Rehabilitation Programs

Patients' noncompliance to plans of rehabilitation can be the biggest deterrent to successful return to play. Therefore, athletic trainers must do all they can to increase patient compliance. Steps to increase patient compliance include offering encouragement, providing positive reinforcement, keeping an upbeat attitude, being creative when designing the plan of rehabilitation, including variation in exercises, and ensuring rehabilitation is as pain-free as possible. The athletic trainer can also ask for support from patients' peers and families asking them to encourage patients in their rehabilitation and ensure patients make time for rehabilitation in their schedule. The athletic trainer can also ask for support from the coaching staff to reinforce the importance of rehabilitation and offer discipline if patients do not follow their plan of care. Finally, thoroughly explaining the plan of rehabilitation and writing it down for patients will help to increase compliance.

VISUALIZATION

Visualization (therapeutic imagery) is used by athletes for a variety of purposes:

- Relaxation and reduction of stress
- Performance improvement
- Rehabilitation

The principles behind all of these are the same, although the focus of concentration is different. Visualization is the process of creating a visual image of a desired outcome and imagining or "feeling" oneself in that place or situation. For example, if the focus is on healing and recovery of an injured leg with limited range of motion, then the athlete imagines how it "feels" to extend and flex the limb in normal range of motion, and imagines walking and using the limb, with his mind focused on the goal of therapy. All of the senses may be used to imagine a scene—what it looks like, smells like, feels like, and sounds like.

There are a number of methods used for **visualization**. Some include audiotapes with guided imagery (e.g., self-hypnosis tapes), but the athlete can be taught basic techniques, including the following:

- Sit or lie comfortably in a quiet place, away from distractions.
- Concentrate on breathing while taking long, slow breaths.
- Close the eyes to shut out distractions and create an image in the mind of the desired place or situation.
- Concentrate on that image, engage as many senses as possible, and visualize details.
- If the mind wanders, breathe deeply and bring consciousness back to the image, or concentrate on breathing for a few moments and then return to the imagery.
- End with positive imagery.

Sometimes, athletes are resistive at first, or have a hard time maintaining focus, so guiding them through visualization the first few times can be helpful.

COMMUNICATION DURING TREATMENT AND REHABILITATION

Communication is an important component of a rehabilitative program. One must exercise judgment when deciding how to communicate with an injured athlete. If an athlete is in pain or under stress, retention decreases: this is the time to provide support and compassion rather than a detailed explanation of treatment. However, at some point the athlete should be provided information about the injury and the plans for rehabilitation in terms that he or she can understand, avoiding unnecessary use of medical jargon. The trainer should cultivate the following habits of communication:

- Reflecting back what the athlete says: "I hear you say that you don't believe you will regain strength."
- Making observations: "I see that you are doing only half of your exercises."
- Keeping at eye level with the athlete to avoid "looking down" while speaking.

It's important that the athlete feel a part of decision-making and be allowed input. The trainer should always take time to answer questions.

KÜBLER-ROSS STAGES OF GRIEF

Kübler-Ross described 5 **stages of grief** that people go through when dying or suffering other severe loss. Many sports psychologists have applied these stages to injured athletes. Understanding these stages can help the athletic trainer provide better support to the athlete:

- *Denial:* The athlete may feel that rehabilitation is not necessary because the injury is less severe than reported and may be optimistic and cheerful. At this stage, the athlete may be resistive to exercises because he/she feels they are not necessary. The athlete may be unrealistic about goals.
- *Anger:* As the athlete recognizes that the injury will not go away, he/she may feel that others are to blame for the injury, or that life is unfair. The athlete may lash out at his or her trainer, family, and team members in frustration. The trainer should be supportive without telling the athlete everything will be all right, because the athlete is not receptive at this point.
- *Bargaining*: This involves if-then thinking: "If I work twice as hard, then I'll get better twice as fast." The athlete must be cautioned not to overstress an injury, because he or she may exercise more than is safe in order to hold up his or her end of the "bargain."
- *Depression*: As the athlete begins to accept the injury, he or she may become depressed, feeling no one understands. Providing support and reassurance by showing progress from objective measurements can help to reduce anxiety. If this stage is prolonged, or the athlete becomes profoundly depressed, it may affect efforts at rehabilitation because the athlete may feel that exercise is futile. In that case, the athlete may need to be referred for psychological counseling.
- *Acceptance*: This final stage represents a better understanding on the part of the athlete that realistic long- and short-term goals can be achieved. The athlete is often more cooperative and less stressed, which facilitates the rehabilitation process.

IMPLEMENTING APPROPRIATE THERAPEUTIC EXERCISES

Implementing appropriate therapeutic exercises assists patients' recovery and function because they offer many benefits such as maintaining or regaining full range of motion, preventing atrophy, and stopping proprioceptive losses. Maintaining or regaining patients' full range of motion allows for proper function of the affected body part. This also prevents new injuries from developing throughout the kinetic chain due to limitation in motion. By preventing atrophy, patients will not lose significant muscular mass and will therefore make the rehabilitative plan can become more effective. Implementing exercises that train patients' proprioception limits proprioceptive losses, allowing patients to maintain more effective movement patterns that make return-to-activity a smoother process.

THERAPEUTIC EXERCISE PROGRAM AFTER ACUTE INJURY

It is important to avoid stress to an **acute injury** initially while clotting is taking place and during the first 3-5 days when the inflammatory process is occurring, as there is a great deal of cellular activity in the wound. However, a **therapeutic exercise** program considers not only the injured part but also the cardiovascular status and other parts of the body. If one has an injured right leg, then exercises can be done for the left leg and upper limbs. Usually, by the beginning of the second week, remodeling occurs, with collagen type III replaced by collage type I. At this point, some range of motion and beginning strength exercises may be initiated, except for in the case of tendon injuries, which are restricted from strengthening exercises for at least 3 weeks. Range of motion is especially important during weeks 3-5, because after 2 months collagen hardens and becomes less flexible.

Cardiovascular Conditioning

Cardiovascular conditioning is especially important after injury or illness, because cardiovascular/respiratory fitness can decrease rapidly with inactivity. The type of cardiovascular exercises will depend upon the site of injury and the phase of healing. For example:

- If there is an injury of a lower extremity, then non-weight-bearing exercises, such as swimming, weightlifting, or upper body cycling may be indicated.
- If there is an injury to an upper extremity, then weight-bearing exercises, such as climbing stairs, running, aerobics, or use of elliptical machine is more appropriate.

In all cases, the type of cardiovascular conditioning should be tailored to the individual and his or her habits. Cardiovascular endurance requires training at least 3 days per week, with both continuous and interval training.

Aquatic Therapy
Increasing Range of Motion and Balance

Aquatic therapy may be used effectively to increase range of motion for both upper and lower extremities, as well as to improve balance by strengthening the trunk and abdomen. The number of repetitions and the duration of the exercises will vary depending on the condition and purpose. Exercises are often done 3 times weekly, but may be done 5-6 times weekly in some cases:

- *Shoulder* (internal rotation and extension): This exercise is done while standing in water to the level of the waist and using a buoyant barbell to increase resistance. The barbell is held with both hands behind the back, with the barbell floating. The person squats slightly, forcing his arms to rise, and holds the squat for about 30 seconds before returning to standing. This is repeated to tolerance.
- *Shoulder* (flexion, bilateral). This exercise increases both strength and endurance of shoulder muscles and is performed while standing in water to the shoulder level. Feet are in a striding position, and the arms are at the side of the body with the palms facing anteriorly. Both arms are raised simultaneously to shoulder level, the palms are rotated until they face posteriorly, and then the arms push downward past the vertical line of the body. This exercise may be varied by the addition of buoyancy equipment or gloves to increase resistance or changes in stance. For instance, the exercises can be performed while standing on one leg.
- *Lower extremity* (hips, knees, and ankles, with focus on knee flexion): In water to the shoulders and with the trunk upright, the knees flexed (60-80°), and the tibia vertical, the person does lunge walking to the point of fatigue. This exercise is usually done about 3 times weekly.
- *Trunk stability & abdominal, arm, and shoulder strength:* This exercise is done standing in water to the upper chest level (shoulders above the water). The arms are extended in front of the body with both hands holding onto a Styrofoam barbell. The muscles of the abdomen are tightened, and the arms are pulled down with the elbows straight until the barbell rests against the thighs. Then, the barbell is raised again to the beginning position in a controlled manner, with resistance against buoyancy. This exercise may be varied by standing in water to above the shoulder, or by increasing the size of the barbells to increase resistance.

- **Hip & knee mobility and balance:** Standing vertically on one leg in water to chest level, the person tightens the muscles of his abdomen and kicks the other leg forward and then backward behind the vertical line of his body, keeping his knee straight. Note: this exercise is usually performed near the edge of the pool so that the person can hold on for support if necessary; if the emphasis is on balance, the person should avoid holding onto the edge.
- **Balance:** This exercise is performed while submerged in water to the upper chest level, and begins with the arms extended out to the sides floating at the top of the water and one foot raised, with the knee flexed and the thigh at a 90° angle to the vertical line of the body. The purpose is only to maintain balance. Once stabilized in this position, the arms should be pulled into the body and crossed in front of the chest.

BUOYANCY AND HYDROSTATIC PRESSURE

There are a number of issues to consider when **aquatic therapy** is part of rehabilitation and reconditioning:

- **Buoyancy** provides support to weakened muscles and allows exercise with less discomfort. In some cases, flotation devices may be required to assist with buoyancy, depending upon the type of injury. Buoyancy is force in opposition to gravity, so exercises (such as raising a limb) which outside of water would have gravity as a resistive force, are assisted by buoyancy in the water. The opposite is true also for lowering a limb, as buoyancy increases resistance. Thus, adding buoyancy devices (such as cuffs) while lowering a limb increases resistance even more.
- **Hydrostatic pressure** varies according to depth and provides pressure that may reduce edema, reduce elevations in blood pressure, and reduce spasticity. Resistance increases with depth and is proportional to the speed of movement in the water, with rapid movement increasing resistance.

PHYSIOLOGICAL EFFECTS

Immersing an athlete in water produces a number of **physiological effects** unrelated to the exercises. Cardiovascular changes include increased cardiac and intrapulmonary blood volume, with increased pressure in the right atrium, increased volume at the left ventricular diastole, increased stroke volume, and overall increased cardiac output. At the same time, there is a reduction in peripheral circulation and lung expansion, decreasing vital capacity. Often, the heart rate remains unchanged or significantly lower than when the individual is performing similar exercises outside of the water, depending upon the depth of the water and speed of exercise. Resistance in water increases with immersion up to about the middle of the body, at which point buoyancy counterbalances resistance. Exercises with water up to the waist result in similar heart rate and consumption of oxygen as exercise out of the water.

REHABILITATION OF LOW BACK INJURIES

Low back pain is a common complaint of athletes, and is most often related to the overuse of muscles. Injuries are most often soft-tissue, especially in the younger athlete, although persistent or severe pain should be evaluated for lumbar disk pathology, spondylolysis, or spondylolisthesis. There is no real consensus treatment of low back pain, but recent studies indicate that the traditional program of bed rest and immobilization is no more effective than remaining active within tolerance. While there is little evidence that massage decreases low back pain, it is often used along with specific exercises and may provide some measure of comfort. There is some evidence that specific exercises decrease low back pain, although exercise may be ineffective if pain is acute, and studies are inconclusive on the value of exercise for chronic pain. Acupuncture or vertebral manipulation may reduce pain in some instances. Traction is also used to relieve acute pain, although studies are inconclusive as to the value of this therapy.

WILLIAMS' FLEXION EXERCISES

Both Williams' flexion exercises and McKenzie extension exercises have been used for low back pain, but studies indicate that McKenzie extension exercises are more effective in relieving pain than Williams' flexion exercises. For this reason, Williams' exercises are not routinely used, although trainers should be familiar with them. **Williams' flexion exercises:** This exercise program aims to flex the lumbar area (correcting lordosis) in order to open the vertebral foramen and more evenly distribute weight across the intravertebral disks. Williams' flexion exercises include:

- *Sit-ups*, which have been modified to the use of the crunch, as sit-ups tend to strain the lower back.
- Posterior pelvic tilt.
- *Trunk flexion*, which involves lying in the supine position and drawing both knees to the chest.
- *Long sit and reach*, which is no longer used, as it worsens sciatica.
- *Iliotibial band stretch*, otherwise known as the front lunge.

STAND TO SQUAT/STAND TO SIT.

MCKENZIE EXTENSION EXERCISES

McKenzie extension exercises are used to decompress nerves in cases of lumbar herniated disks. These exercises push the disk anteriorly away from the root of the nerve, although the exercise program actually includes both flexion and extension. Studies show that these exercises are more effective than Williams' flexion exercises. McKenzie exercises are done about every 2 hours, and usually require intensive work with a therapist. The exercises performed are specific to the type of pain; they aim to "centralize" the pain, or relieve the pain in the leg and move it to the back where it can be more easily tolerated. Extension or flexion exercises are prescribed depending upon which one moves pain to the center of the back. Extension exercises, for example, may focus on standing and sitting correctly, or may focus on the prone position, from which the trunk to can be gradually raised to extend the back. The sequencing of exercises is individualized.

STRENGTHENING THE MUSCLES OF THE BUTTOCKS AND HIPS

One of the exercises that **strengthen** the muscles of the **buttocks and hips** (gluteus maximus and hip lateral rotators) is *prone hip extension*. This is a non-functional exercise that helps the athlete to develop kinesthetic muscle awareness before beginning functional exercises. While strengthening the gluteus maximus, this exercise also stretches the muscles of the anterior thigh.

- The athlete lies prone on a firm surface, with a pillow under his abdomen.
- Squeezing and tightening the muscles of his buttocks, the person, holding his leg straight, barely lifts his leg off of the surface and holds it there for a few seconds before lowering his leg back to the surface.
- The exercise is repeated using the other leg.

A set of exercise is usually about 10 lifts per leg, but the number of sets may vary according to the individual plan of therapy.

Improving Body Alignment for Standing Activities

Therapeutic exercise to improve **body alignment** for standing activities includes exercises that strengthen the hip and lower extremities and maintain proper balance, such as the ***walk in stance (position I)***, which helps to train the athlete to move her body over the hip correctly.

- The athlete stands upright with pelvis, hips, knees, and feet pointing forward in a staggered stance, with the affected leg in the forward position.
- The athlete slowly bends the forward hip and knee, and leans slightly forward toward the leg, being careful not to bend the knee beyond the foot. The athlete then stops and holds for 10 seconds.

Squeezing the gluteal muscles and holding the abdominal muscles taut, the athlete tightens the quadriceps muscle to straighten the leg while holding the arch up and keeping the toes on the surface.

Walk in stance with single limb (position II) begins with the end of position I:

- As the front leg straightens, the athlete lifts the heel of the back leg, maintaining forward facing alignment of pelvis, hips, knees, and feet. This position is held for 3 seconds.
- The knee is bent and the leg swung forward as if to take a step, but then this position with the foot elevated off of the surface is held for 30 seconds.

Walk in stance with split squat (position III) begins with the same beginning stance as for position I:

- The athlete slowly bends downward, flexing his knee and hip but being careful not to bend the knee past the foot and keep weight on the front leg, until the hip moves out of body alignment.
- The athlete then slowly rises and repeats the up-and-down exercise while maintaining position over the front foot.

Improving Balance with Strengthening Exercises

Strengthening exercises to improve **balance** include stepping exercises that increase muscle strength in the back, hip, knee, ankle, and foot. These exercises are done with the pelvis level:

- ***Stepping up:*** The athlete stands in front of the step and steps up with one foot with the toes down but the arch elevated, leaning forward over the foot but keeping the pelvis level, and then returning to the starting point.
- ***Stepping down:*** The athlete stands on a step and lifts and flexes the knee on the side that will step down, while flexing the hip and knee on the other leg (being careful not to bend past the foot). The athlete positions the foot as though to step down but does not touch the ground and holds the foot above the surface for 10 seconds, finally returning to the start position.

Increasing Flexibility by Stretching the Quadriceps Muscles

There are a number of different exercises that can be done to stretch and increase the **flexibility** of the **quadriceps** muscles. Extension of the lumbosacral area should be avoided during these exercises:

- *Prone:* With a strap attached around her ankle, the athlete lies in a prone position with a pillow under her abdomen. She then grasps the strap over her shoulder and pulls the foot of her affected side forward toward her buttocks until a pull is felt in the anterior thigh, holding the stretch position for 15-30 seconds before returning the leg to the start position.
- *Lateral:* The athlete lies on the opposite side of the affected leg and flexes the knee of the affected leg, reaching back with her hand to grasp the foot and pulling the leg toward her buttocks until a pull is felt in the anterior thigh, holding for 15-30 seconds.
- *Standing:* Similar to lateral position, but done while standing and holding onto a bar for support.

Increasing Range of Motion with Extension and Flexion Exercises for the Knee

Extension and flexion knee exercises that increase range of motion include both sitting and prone lying exercises:

- *Sitting:* This exercise is used to improve both flexion and extension, and can be done throughout the day. The athlete sits in a chair that allows her leg to swing back under her body. The athlete extends her knee and her leg as far as possible, holds briefly, and then flexes it back as far as possible. If necessary, the stronger leg can be used to increase extension by looping the foot behind the ankle of the affected leg and providing some passive extension.
- *Prone:* This exercise focuses on extension to stretch taut muscles. The athlete lies prone on a table with her knee extending over the edge and a folded towel under her anterior thigh. The knee is extended and held as straight as possible for 1-2 minutes. Ankle weights may be used.

Stretching Exercises for Hamstrings

A **hamstring stretch** may be performed in either the standing or supine lying position. The number of repetitions and duration of exercises varies according to tolerance and condition:

- *Standing:* This exercise is done with the athlete standing, facing a table that is about hip height. The athlete places the foot of his affected leg on the table, keeping both the knee on the affected leg and the supporting leg straight and extended. Then, the athlete, bending forward at the hips, reaches out with the contralateral hand to the foot, until a stretch is felt in the hamstrings.
- *Supine:* The athlete lies flat on a table with the affected leg extended straight upward and held at 90°, and with the hands clasped about the distal thigh. The knee is extended fully until a stretch is felt in the hamstrings; it is held in that position for a moment, and then relaxed.

STRETCHING EXERCISES FOR HIP MUSCLES

There are a number of **stretching** exercises that can be done for the **hip muscles:**

- *Flexor:* The athlete places his hands on the floor with the affected hip and leg extended, supporting his weight on his toes with his heel elevated. The contralateral foot is flat on the floor, with the knee flexed and the torso leaning parallel to the thigh, so the person is in a position similar to take-off for running. The person pushes his hips forward until stretching and tightness occurs in the extended hip.
- *Adductor:* This exercise is done with the athlete sitting on the floor. The knees are flexed and separated, and the soles of the feet brought together and held by the hands. The athlete uses his forearms to exert downward pressure on the legs until an adductor stretch is felt.
- *Iliotibial band:* This exercise is done with the athlete lying stretched out on his side on a table, with his top leg hanging over the side of the table for about 5 minutes. The trainer may hold the hip to stabilize the pelvis and apply downward pressure to the leg to increase the stretch.
- *Internal rotator:* The athlete sits on the side of a table with his legs hanging over and knees flexed, while the trainer grasps one leg above the ankle and places the other hand on the anterior thigh, applying external rotation to the hip and pushing the foot past the other leg until stretching is felt in the internal rotators.
- *External rotator:* This is done the same as for internal rotator stretch, except that the hip is rotated internally while the trainer stabilizes the distal femur and pulls the foot laterally.
- *Piriformis supine:* The athlete begins in the supine position on the floor with his knees flexed and his feet flat on the floor. The affected leg is crossed over the contralateral leg, and the athlete grasps his contralateral leg below the knee (with arms under the affected leg) and pulls the legs toward his chest, forcing the affected leg to point toward his contralateral shoulder.
- *Piriformis prone:* In the prone position with the affected knee flexed fully and under his body in line with the contralateral shoulder, and with the foot in front of the contralateral knee, the athlete presses downward, applying pressure on the affected hip and forcing the knee on the affected leg closer to the contralateral shoulder until stretch is felt in the buttocks.

USUAL PROGRESSION OF STRENGTHENING EXERCISES

Strengthening exercise progression:

- *Isometric exercises* are performed with the muscle and limb in static position, with no movement of the joint or lengthening of the muscle. The muscle is contracted against resistance.
- *Isotonic exercises* include movement of the joint during exercise (such as running and weightlifting) and both shortening and lengthening of the muscles through eccentric or concentric contractions. Isotonic refers to tension, indicating that the tension is constant during shortening and lengthening of the muscle.
- *Isokinetic exercises* utilize machines (such as stationary bicycles that can be set with various parameters) to control the rate and extent of contraction as well as the range of motion. Both speed and resistance can be set so that the athlete is limited by the settings of the machine.
- *Plyometrics* is a particular type of exercise program that uses activities to allow a muscle to achieve maximal force as quickly as possible; the sequence is a fast eccentric movement (to stretch) followed quickly by a strong concentric movement (to contract).

Isotonic Strengthening Exercises

Strengthening Exercises for the Femoral Muscles

Isotonic **strengthening** exercises for the **femoral muscles** include two standing exercises:

- *Hamstring curl:* This exercise may be done with the athlete lying prone in a hamstring curl machine and curling the weighted bar to a 90° angle by pulling his heel toward his buttocks while holding his abdominal muscles taut. The hamstring curl can also be done with the athlete standing against a table with his quadriceps muscle flush against the table. In this position, the athlete flexes his knee completely, lifting his heel toward his buttocks and holding this position briefly before extending his knee back to beginning position. This exercise is usually done 10 times for two or three sets. Ankle weights are often added to increase resistance and enhance strengthening, usually in increments of five pounds.
- *Hip extension:* This exercise may be done with or without an elastic ankle strap.
  - With the strap attached to the affected ankle and fastened to the front of a chair (by extending the strap beneath the chair), the athlete faces the back of the chair and holds onto the back while pulling his leg with the strap backward against the strap's resistance.
  - Without the strap, the athlete leans forward over a table to support his upper body while extending the knee on the affected leg and raising the leg upward as far as possible without external rotation. Ankle weights are often added to increase resistance, usually in increments of 5 pounds.

Strengthening Exercises for the Leg

Isometric exercises for **strengthening** the **leg** are usually done in 2-3 sets of 10 and include:

- *Quadriceps:* The athlete may perform isometric quadriceps exercises in a variety of positions: standing, sitting, or supine. In each case, the knee of the affected leg is fully extended, and the athlete attempts to maximally contract the quadriceps muscle, holding it for 10 seconds before relaxing the muscle and repeating. The muscle should be palpated during contraction, and if contraction is insufficient or the wrong muscles (such as the hamstrings or gluteals) are contracting, electrical stimulation or biofeedback may help the athlete isolate and contract the correct muscle. Sometimes, it is sufficient for the trainer to provide feedback and instruction to help the athlete recognize when the contraction is correct, both by how the muscle feels and by palpating to feel the contraction.

Positions are usually held for 10 seconds and performed in sets of 10:

- *Reverse quadriceps:* This exercise is done with the athlete lying in the prone position on a table, with the heel of the affected leg elevated and the toes on the table. The knee is extended fully to straighten the leg until the femur lifts away from the table. The position is held for 10 seconds before relaxing.
- *Hamstrings:* The athlete sits with his foot flat on the floor or lies supine with his knee flexed and his foot flat on the table or floor, pressing downward with his heel to tighten the hamstrings. The leg should be palpated by the trainer to ensure that the correct muscle is tightening.
- *Quadriceps & Hamstrings:* In the same positions as for hamstring exercises, the athlete first tightens his quadriceps and then presses downward with his heel to tighten the hamstrings.

STRENGTHENING EXERCISES FOR THE HIP

There are a series of isometric **strengthening** exercises for the **hip** that are an important part of rehabilitation after injury. Usually, each position is held for 10 seconds after the muscles tighten, and the exercises are done in sets of 10.

- *Abduction*: The athlete sits with his knee flexed and foot on the floor, and places his contralateral hand against the lateral thigh (distally, above the knee) and uses his hand to pull inward while his hip tightens with abduction force to resist movement.
- *Adduction*: The athlete sits with his knees flexed and feet on the floor, and places both fists beside each other between the distal thighs, maintaining this position while the thighs press against the fists and attempt to adduct.
- *Extension*: This exercise is done with the athlete in a standing position with his back about 6 inches away from a wall and holding onto a chair or other support for balance. The athlete places the heel of his foot against the wall and pushes against the wall until muscles tighten.
- *Internal rotation:* The athlete sits on a chair with his knees flexed, his ankles crossed, and his affected leg on the bottom. The trainer tries to pull the bottom foot away from the top while the athlete resists.
- *External rotation:* The athlete sit on a chair with his knees flexed and parallel and his feet flat on the floor, touching along the medial aspects, and tries to push the affected foot against the other foot in an attempt to force the contralateral leg to externally rotate.

STRENGTHENING EXERCISES FOR THE TRICEPS SURAE AND THE SQUAT

General **strengthening** exercises for the **lower extremities** include:

- *Triceps surae:* This exercise strengthens the triceps surae, which includes both the gastrocnemius and soleus muscles. The athlete sits in a chair with his affected knee either flexed or extended and his foot balanced on the edge of a stool. The athlete holds a hand weight or other resistance aid over the distal thigh above the knee while plantar flexing his ankle against the resistance. This exercise is done in two positions to exercise both sets of muscles. With the knee extended, the gastrocnemius is exercised; with the knee flexed, the soleus is exercised.
- *Squat:* Holding free weights or other devices, the athlete squats, holds, and repeats. This can be done with a single leg or both legs, and with various ranges of motion, depending upon the degree of limitation.

PROPRIOCEPTIVE NEUROMUSCULAR FACILITATION

Proprioceptive neuromuscular facilitation (PNF) is specific exercise to increase flexibility (usually of the arm or leg), strength, and range of motion, targeting particular muscle groups with both stretching and contracting. Proprioception is movement and sensory awareness, and this is incorporated into exercises that include spiral and diagonal movements with 3 components: flexing/extending, adducting/abducting, and rotating. Conditioning exercises should always precede PNF, to avoid damage to soft tissues. A typical exercise includes extending the muscle as completely as possible until the stretch is felt, and then contracting maximally (to tolerance) for 5 seconds against resistance (such as provided by trainer) to prevent movement. Then, the muscle is relaxed, and the trainer carefully pushes the muscle group (such as in the hip or shoulder) slightly beyond the normal range of motion and holds for 30 seconds. This is followed by 30 seconds of relaxation before repeating the procedure (the entire sequence is usually repeated 4 times).

Stretching During Warm-Up and Cool-Down

Stretching is done for a variety of reasons: increasing fitness, relaxing, preventing injury and soreness, and increasing flexibility. Stretching is important in both warm-up and cool-down activities:

- *Warm-up:* Stretching alone is not an adequate warm-up routine but is an important part. Warm-up exercises should be performed before stretching, in order to increase circulation and warmth in the muscles and allow them to stretch more easily. Neither isometric nor active stretching is appropriate for a warm-up routine, as these may tire the muscles prior to exercise. Rather, warm-up stretching should include static stretching followed by dynamic stretching.
- *Cool-down*: Following vigorous exercise, cool-down exercises should take place. As with the warm-up, stretching exercises should be only a part of the cool down, which should include about 5 minutes of slowing activity related to the sport, followed by dynamic stretching and finally static stretching (the opposite of warm-up stretching).

Types of Stretching Used in Rehabilitation and Reconditioning

Stretching must be done properly to be effective. Muscles should be stretched in isolation, because isolated stretching reduces muscle resistance from agonistic muscles. Stretches should be done using good leverage and avoiding the risk of injury, especially with stretches that involve rotation (which increases the danger of ligament and tendon strains) or pressure on the vertebrae (which can cause low back injury). There are a number of different types of stretching exercises:

- *Active (static-active):* This type of stretching involves stretching, holding, and using the agonist (contracting) muscles only to hold the position. An example of an active stretch is standing and extending the leg with no support to hold the leg up. The contraction and tension of the agonist muscles help the stretched (antagonist) muscles to relax through a process known as reciprocal inhibition.
- *Ballistic stretching:* This type of stretching can be counterproductive because it extends the muscle beyond the normal range of motion in a forceful, bouncing, jarring manner, such as by repeatedly changing from extension to flexion by rapidly bending to touch the toes. No time is allowed for the muscle to recover, so muscles may begin to tighten.
- *Dynamic stretching:* This type of stretching is always done in a controlled manner, slowly increasing the stretch and movement speed to the limit of the range of motion but not forcing it beyond (as with ballistic). Exercises are stopped when muscles become tired and/or when maximal range of motion is achieved.
- *Isometric*: This type of stretching uses isometric contractions of muscles without motion to increase flexibility and strength.
- *Passive (relaxed):* This type of stretching requires assistance in the form of a partner, equipment, or the floor/wall in order to maintain the stretch. For example, if the leg is extended, the trainer may hold the leg in the extended position. The person is passive in the sense that he or she does not actively stretch to increase range of motion. Passive stretching is particularly useful in the cooling down period after exercise, as it can relieve soreness.
- *PNF (proprioceptive neuromuscular facilitation):* PNF combines passive and isometric stretching techniques with awareness of movement and position to increase flexibility. A common technique is called slow-reversal-hold-relax, although there are a number of variations, such as hold-relax-swing.

- ***Static stretching:*** This type of stretching is similar to passive (indeed the terms are used interchangeably sometimes) except that there is more active stretching to maximal range of motion, after which the stretch is held. This type of stretching does not include repeated motions.

STRENGTHENING THE ABDOMINAL AND BACK MUSCLES OF THE TRUNK

The **trunk** muscles are those of the back, and lower and upper abdomen. These muscles are involved in almost all activities:

- ***Sit-ups:*** This exercise uses primarily the upper abdominal muscles and hip flexors of the trunk when done properly. The athlete should lie on the floor with his arms folded across his chest or "boxed" about his head. The knees should be flexed and feet flat on the floor, spaced in line with the shoulders. The trainer holds the feet, and the athlete tightens his abdominal muscles and curls his body upward, touching his knees with his elbows. This position is held to a count of 6, at which point the athlete slowly uncurls and lowers his trunk back to the starting point, keeping his abdominal muscles taut until his shoulders contact the floor.

Unfortunately, sit-ups increase the risk of strain of the back muscles, especially if done improperly, and much of the "lift" relates to contractions of the hip flexors rather than the abdominal muscles.

- ***Crunch (partial sit-up or curl-up):*** This exercise uses primarily the upper abdominal muscles and erector spinae musculature to strengthen and stabilize the lower back. The athlete lies on the floor in the same leg, foot, and back position as for sit-ups, with the chin tucked. The athlete inhales and tightens his abdominal muscles, then slowly raises only his head and shoulders off of the floor while exhaling, curling toward the knees, and then holds the position for a count of 6 before slowly lowering his body back to the floor. It is important that the neck remain in the extended position and that the arms and hands are not used to pull the neck forward, as this will strain the muscles. Folding the arms across the chest mitigates this problem. Placing weights on the chest or performing the exercise with the head in a slightly declined position increases resistance.
- **Leg curls:** This exercise focuses on strengthening the lower abdominal muscles and trunk flexion. The athlete sits on the edge of a bench or table so that his buttocks are supported, but his legs are over the edge. Holding onto the bench or table for support, the athlete extends his legs in front, brings them together, and then raises both legs simultaneously about 4 inches above the level of the bench or table. Then, the knees are flexed as the legs are drawn up as close as possible to the athlete's chest. Keeping the abdominal muscles tight, the athlete extends his knees while lowering his legs until they return to the previous point of extension 4 inches above level of the bench or table.

CIRCUIT TRAINING

Circuit training is used both for routine training and for rehabilitation and reconditioning, as it increases the range of motion, strength, and endurance of the whole body. During circuit training, athletes perform a series of exercises for short periods of time, with rest periods in between. Typically, an athlete might perform 5 exercises in a circuit, such as 30 seconds of as many pushups as possible followed by 30 seconds of rest, and then 30 seconds of as many squats as possible followed by 30 seconds of rest, and so on, repeating the series of exercises for a set number of times or set period of time. A timer signal is used to pace the exercises. The choice of exercises depends upon the needs of the individual athlete and may include flexibility exercises, calisthenics, aerobic exercise, and weight training. It's important to start circuit training slowly to prevent injury, and to do warm-up and stretching exercises beforehand.

Exercises After Rotator Cuff Repair
Using the Pendulum

After repair of a **rotator cuff** injury, a sling that partially immobilizes the arm is used for 2-3 days and continued for 6 weeks at night. During the months after surgery, a progression of exercises is introduced and usually performed three times a day in sets of ten. Flexion exercises are usually performed prior to abduction, and the athlete should take care not to lean on the arm or carry more than 5 pounds of weight during the early stages after surgery:

- **Pendulum exercises**: This simple exercise may be introduced within 48 hours of surgery. The athlete bends to 90° at the waist, supporting his body with a hand on a stool or chair and, with the affected arm hanging down, rotates his trunk in a circular motion to move the arm first in a clockwise and then counterclockwise direction. Usually 10 rotations are performed in each position.

Assisted Exercises

These exercises for mobility usually begin about a week after surgery for rotator cuff repair, although they may be used for injuries as well. The series of exercises includes:

- **Shoulder rotation with support:** With the athlete sitting, the forearm of the affected arm is placed flat against a table or other surface and the forearm slid back and forth to tolerance in an arc to the side, forcing the shoulder to rotate.
- **Assisted flexion**: The athlete uses his contralateral hand to clasp the hand on the affected side and lifts both arms upright, flexing the shoulder as much as possible, with the elbow extended and the uninjured side supporting and lifting the affected side. This exercise can be done in the supine or sitting position.

Active Exercises

Active exercises after **rotator cuff** repair:

- **Active finger walk-up:** The athlete stands arm-length in front of a wall or door frame and extends his elbow so the arm is straight, and then "walks" up the wall with the fingers as far as possible, marking progress.
- **Active internal rotation:** The athlete stands and reaches the hand of his affected arm behind his back at about the level of the lumbosacral area, and then moves his hand and forearm up his back as far as possible, forcing his shoulder to rotate internally.
- **Active flexion:** The athlete stands with arms at sides and, with his elbow extended, raises his arm as far as possible toward the ceiling in a forward arc, holding the position for 10 seconds before lowering the arm.
- **Active abduction:** With the athlete in sitting position and the elbow extended, the arm is raised laterally to shoulder level in an arc to the side of the body, and held in this position before the arm is lowered.

Isometric Exercises

Isometric exercises after **rotator cuff** repair (Part IV):

- ***Isometric extension:*** The athlete stands with his back flush against a wall, arms to the side, elbow extended and the palmar surface facing the wall. The athlete then pushes the affected arm against the wall and holds it there for 5 seconds before relaxing.
- ***Isometric external rotation:*** The athlete stands with his side and affected arm flush against a wall; with his elbow flexed to 90°, he pushes the arm against the wall, holding for 5 seconds before relaxing the arm.
- ***Isometric internal rotation:*** The athlete stands facing the corner of the wall with trunk pressed against the wall and affected arm wrapped around the corner, elbow flexed to 90°, and pushes the arm against the wall, holding for 5 seconds before relaxing.
- ***Isometric adduction:*** The athlete sits in a chair with a small pillow between the affected arm and his body; with the elbow flexed comfortably, he pushes the pillow against the side of his body, holds for 5 seconds, and then relaxes the arm.

Isometric Exercises and Rotation Exercises with Weights

Isometric and rotation exercises with weights after **rotator cuff** repair (Part V):

- ***Isometric abduction:*** The athlete sits perpendicular to the back of a chair or wall with his elbow flexed and his arm against the surface of the chair or wall and pushes against it, holds for 5 seconds and then relaxes his arm.
- ***Internal rotation with weights:*** The athlete lies on his affected side with his head supported and holds a light weight in his hand with his elbow flexed to 90°. The hand with the weight is raised toward the abdomen and then lowered slowly.
- ***External rotation with weights:*** The athlete lies on the contralateral side with a small rolled-up towel between his upper arm (distally) and the side of his body. Holding a light weight with his arm flexed to 90°, the weight is lifted toward the ceiling and slowly returned to starting position.

Open Kinetic Chain Exercises vs. Closed Kinetic Chain Exercises

Open kinetic chain exercises and closed kinetic chain exercises have to do with both movement and weight bearing of the extremities:

- **Open kinetic chain exercises (OKCE):** These exercises include movement of the foot and hand through motion at the elbow and hip or knee, but do not involve weight bearing. Single joints, and often single muscles, are involved in activities, such as biceps curls or knee extensions. Shearing force is created.
- **Closed kinetic chain exercises (CKCE):** In these exercises the hand or foot stays stationary against a surface (floor or machine). CKCE do involve weight bearing. Multiple joints, and often multiple muscles, are involved in these activities, examples of which include push-ups and back squats. Compressive force is created.

Short Arc Quadriceps Exercise

Strengthening exercises usually begin early in rehabilitation, while athletes are still non- or partial-weight bearing. Isotonic open kinetic chain exercises include:

- ***Short arc quadriceps:*** This exercise strengthens the quadriceps muscles in knee extension but applies pressure to the anterior cruciate ligament, so it should not be used early after an injury or after reconstruction of the ligament. The athlete does this exercise either in the supine position or while sitting (which increases the difficulty). Lying down, a folded towel is placed under the affected posterior thigh above the knee to slightly flex the knee. The uninjured knee is kept flexed. The injured knee is straightened, the leg is fully extended, and the leg is lifted about 6 inches from the floor. The leg is held in that position for 5 second, and then slowly lowered as the knee is flexed to relax the muscles. The exercise is usually repeated 10 times.

DAPRE Technique

The **Daily Adjustable Progressive Resistance Exercise (DAPRE)** technique is based on the principle that redeveloping strength after injury occurs more rapidly after initial development. The athlete performs progressive resistance exercises on a regular schedule to increase strength. Exercises are performed independently on each side of the body, so that the injured part does not depend on its uninjured counterpart, using the performance of the uninjured side as a baseline. A set of 10 repetitions is done with ½ working weight, followed by another set with ¾ working weight. The 3rd set is performed to maximal ability with full working weight, and the results of this third set are used to adjust the number of repetitions and working weight of the 4th set and the set for the following day. When the strength of the injured side is about 90-95% of the strength of the uninjured side, the focus of the exercise program changes from building strength to maintaining strength and increasing endurance.

Specific Adaptation to Imposed Demands Principle

The **Specific Adaptation to Imposed Demands (SAID)** principle suggests that when a person is injured or stressed, the person will attempt to overcome the problem by adapting to the demands of the situation. This principle is based on Wolff's law (systems adapt to demands). So, if one hand is not usable, the person adapts and uses the other hand. Unfortunately, this adaptation can lead to increasing disability, so when the SAID principle is applied to rehabilitation, it means that the person must do exercises that specifically aim to correct the problem. Thus, the functional needs of the person should always be considered when designing a specific exercise program for that individual (such as treadmill running for soccer players). The exercise activities should mirror the functional activities as closely as possible. For example, if the goal is increased strength rather than endurance, the exercise program should rely more heavily on strengthening exercises.

Plyometrics

Plyometrics is a particular type of exercise program that allows a muscle to achieve maximal force as quickly as possible. Plyometrics considers both concentric and eccentric contractions. Concentric contractions shorten a muscle to cause movement, while eccentric contractions lengthen the muscle just before contraction to increase the force. So, the sequence for a plyometric exercise is a fast eccentric movement (to stretch), followed quickly by a strong concentric (to contract) movement. It is important that the sequence be fast, because otherwise energy will dissipate. This sequence is called the "stretch shortening cycle." The exercises aim to strengthen the muscles and train the nerves to stimulate a specific type of muscle contraction. Plyometric training may reduce the overall time needed to train in order to achieve maximal output. However, plyometric training may lead to increased injuries if the athlete is not physically fit.

Weight Bearing

Before beginning **weight-bearing exercises**, the athlete should be advised as to how much weight to bear (e.g., 50%, 75%) and should be carefully monitored and assisted, as he may not be able to judge his own capacity for weight bearing. Studies have indicated that target weight bearing is rarely achieved by simply telling people what to do. Demonstrations and monitoring must accompany instructions. While exercising, the person should be careful to keep his leg straight (knee in line with feet), avoiding rotation, and should not hyperextend his knee (this is sometimes done unconsciously to increase stability). While walking, the muscles of the thigh and buttocks should contract together. At present, some trainers use machines that harness and support the athlete and control the amount of weight bearing on an injured limb. Equipment includes the Zuni® Incremental Weight-bearing System and the Pneu-Weight® Unweighting system. This equipment is increasingly used for non-injured athletes as well, with results are similar to aquatic exercises.

Gait/Running Cycle

An athletic trainer must have complete understanding of the **gait/running cycle** in order to evaluate runners for technique to prevent injury. The gait/running cycle begins when one foot contacts the ground and completes when the same foot again contacts the ground. The phases include:

- *Stance/Contact:* This phase has 3 parts:
    - *Contact:* The heel makes contact with the ground and cushions the impact, with the foot pronating until it flattens.
    - *Mid-stance:* The foot is still pronating while supporting the body weight with maximum pressure on the arch, as the other foot is in the swing phase.
    - *Take-off/propulsion:* The great toe dorsiflexes, the plantar fascia tightens, and the heel rises from the ground, the foot supinating and providing a lever for propulsion.
- *Swing:* This phase occurs when the foot is not touching the ground.
    - *Follow through:* The toe lifts from the ground.
    - *Forward swing:* The foot swings forward.
    - *Descent:* The heel descends. This phase ends just before contact.

Improving Recovery by Utilizing Appropriate Therapeutic Devices

Recovery from injuries is improved when athletic trainers utilize appropriate therapeutic devices because these devices can limit excessive damage to already injured tissues as well as prevent recurrences of injuries, which provides for best patient care. For example, if a patient is unable to bear weight on an acute ankle sprain, crutches can allow for ambulation without excessive loading of the damaged tissue. Throughout the healing process, the patient may progress to weight bearing while wearing a walking cast. Once the patient has completed rehabilitation, the previously sprained ankle may still have excessive motion in the joint due to laxity of the ligaments, predisposing them to recurrent ankle sprains. In this case, an ankle brace can be used to provide support, prevent reoccurring ankle sprains, and therefore offering best patient care.

Selecting Therapeutic Modalities Based on Evidence from Research

Athletic trainers should incorporate evidence-based practices when selecting therapeutic modalities for patients' treatment plans. This goes beyond analysis of information provided by manufacturers about their therapeutic equipment. The athletic trainer should look for evidence of modality effectiveness in scientific research data. To do this, professional literature should be searched to determine the effectiveness of a selected modality for a specific injury. For example, an athletic trainer could search a research database such as Articles Plus with the clinical question, "Is laser therapy effective for wound healing?" The research can then be reviewed for the strength of the evidence as well as the strength of the research itself. After selecting a modality for treatment using research as a guide, the athletic trainer can analyze their specific patient's outcomes and use that as guide for further decision making through the rehabilitative process.

Acute and Chronic Injuries and the Selection of Therapeutic Modalities

Acute injuries originate from a specific event and it is important to create an optimum environment for healing during the inflammatory process, which occurs immediately after the injury. This can be achieved by providing protection, optimal loading, ice, compression, and elevation. Heat should not be applied to an acute injury, so moist heat packs and thermal ultrasound would be contraindicated. However, electrical stimulation could be used to reduce the patient's pain if needed.

Chronic injuries develop little by little and accumulate over time. These injuries can be more difficult to treat as they may be in the inflammatory phase for a longer period. The athletic trainer must look for signs of the inflammatory process such as redness, heat, swelling, and ecchymosis. If there are signs of active inflammation, the injury can be treated with ice and electrical stimulation if appropriate. However, if no signs of the inflammatory process are displayed, then modalities selected may change. For example, moist heat packs can be used to reduce muscle tension and ultrasound can be administered to optimize the conditions for healing.

Cryotherapy and the Inflammatory Process

When cryotherapy is used intermittently after an acute injury, it reduces negative effects of the inflammatory process. For example, ice application causes vasoconstriction to the arterioles and venules, which helps to limit excessive edema. Also, following a trauma, less oxygen can be delivered to cells around the injury. Ice application lowers the metabolic rate of the cells, decreasing their need for oxygen, which results in less cell death due to ischemia. Cryotherapy also effectively reduces muscle guarding, which decreases cellular waste products that irritate the muscles and cause spasm. Cold application also lowers the excitability of the nerves resulting in the reduction of pain.

Electrical Stimulation to Reduce Patients' Perceptions of Pain

Gate control: Electrical stimulation can be used to lower the patient's perception of pain by "closing the gate" through which sensation is experienced. This can be achieved by applying electrical stimulation at an intensity that feels tingly to the patient, does not cause muscular contraction, with a high frequency.

Descending pathway: Electrical stimulation can elicit the descending pathway for pain modulation by use of a high intensity electrical current along trigger or acupuncture points for a short period. The intensity should be set high, near a noxious level, the pulse duration should be set at 10 microseconds, and the frequency should be set at 80 pulses per second.

Opiate pain control: Electrical stimulation can be used to trigger the opiate pain control mechanism by producing an electrical current of high intensity, as much as the patient can tolerate, near the site of pain or along acupuncture or trigger points for the injury. The pulse duration should be as high as the machine allows, and the frequency should be between 1 and 5 pulses per second.

Paraffin Bath and Ice Massage

Paraffin bath treatments are effective at providing heat to chronic conditions affecting angulated body parts such as the fingers, wrist, ankles, feet, and elbows. Paraffin bath should not be used over open wounds or in areas with a decrease in circulation. It is very important that the patient's body part that will receive paraffin bath treatment is thoroughly cleaned before the treatment, otherwise the paraffin wax may become contaminated. Ice massage is used to reduce pain and inflammation of a small area of the body such as a tendon or bursae. Ice massage should not be performed if a patient has an adverse reaction to cryotherapy. The patient's level of comfort during the treatment should be continuously monitored and the treatment adjusted accordingly.

USING THERAPEUTIC MODALITIES

SAFETY PRECAUTIONS TO FOLLOW

There are many safety precautions athletic trainers must take when using therapeutic modalities. Manufacturers' guidelines for care and maintenance of the equipment must be followed. Regular checks for equipment functionality must be performed. Patients must always be supervised when receiving therapeutic modality treatments so that the athletic trainer can quickly address any possible adverse reactions. The comfort of the patient must be maintained and the treatment stopped if the patient experiences an adverse reaction. Before performing any therapeutic modality treatment, the athletic trainer must ensure the treatment is not contraindicated and is appropriate for the injury and the patient's phase of the healing process.

PHARMACOLOGICAL CONCERNS

Iontophoresis and phonophoresis both are used to push medicines into patients' affected body tissues. Iontophoresis uses direct electrical current through an iontophoresis generator to push the charged ions of medications though the skin and into target tissues. The most commonly used medications for iontophoresis are dexamethasone and hydrocortisone. The athletic trainer must ensure they are following the laws within their state when considering the use of iontophoresis. Chemical burns from the direct current used are a common problem with iontophoresis.

Phonophoresis uses the acoustic energy from the ultrasound machine to push medications through patients' skin and into target tissues. The most commonly used medication with phonophoresis is hydrocortisone. Many clinicians choose ointments with a 10% concentration of hydrocortisone and occasionally lidocaine is added for its analgesic effects. Once again, athletic trainers must ensure they are practicing within their scope of practice in their state before performing this procedure.

LEGAL CONCERNS

Each state governs the use of therapeutic modalities in the field of athletic training. Therefore, the athletic trainer must be knowledgeable about their state's laws regarding the use of therapeutic modalities and follow them precisely. When therapeutic modalities are used, they must be checked for safety, properly maintained, and be used only for their intended purposes to ensure patient safety.

When selecting a therapeutic modality for use, the athletic trainer should select the best modality available to treat the target tissues while keeping in mind the patient's stage of healing. The athletic trainer must know the indications, contraindications, and any special precautions for all therapeutic modalities they use. Additionally, many manufacturers provide recommended protocols for their equipment, and while the athletic trainer may follow these protocols, they can also adapt them as necessary to meet the needs of the patient. However, decisions to alter the protocol must be based on sound evidence.

ENSURING THE SAFETY OF ALL ELECTRICAL THERAPEUTIC MODALITIES

There are many steps the athletic trainer must take to ensure the safety of all electrical therapeutic modalities in the athletic training clinic. First, the athletic training clinic must be assessed for safety.

Three-pronged outlets must be checked to ensure they are properly grounded. Ground-fault interrupters should be used with all electrical modalities. Extension cords and multiple adaptors create safety hazards and therefore should not be used with electrical modalities. Once the clinic is checked for electrical safety, the athletic trainer should ensure manufacturers' guidelines for care and maintenance of electrical modalities are followed. Electrical modalities must be calibrated yearly and must comply with National Electrical Code guidelines. Finally, common safety sense should be followed to ensure patient protection.

ELECTRICAL STIMULATION FOR MUSCLE REEDUCATION

Surgical procedures can result in difficulties for patients to contract their muscles surrounding the surgical site. Electrical stimulation can be used for muscular reeducation, assisting patients in achieving a contraction of the affected muscle while helping them relearn how to contract the muscle on their own. This is achieved by setting the electrical stimulation intensity high enough to achieve a muscular contraction at 30 to 50 pulses per second with either an interrupted or surged current. As the electrical stimulation of the muscle begins, the patient should be instructed to feel the initiation of the involuntary contraction and try to voluntarily contract the muscle along with the electrical stimulation. This treatment should last 15 to 20 minutes and can be performed several times a day. Not only can this technique assist patients in relearning how to fire the muscles, it can also help prevent atrophy following immobilization.

USING KNOWLEDGE OF THE INFLAMMATORY PROCESS TO ASSIST IN SELECTION AND USE OF APPROPRIATE THEAPEUTIC DEVICES

Athletic trainers use knowledge of the inflammatory process to assist in selecting appropriate therapeutic modalities. For example, the goals of rehabilitation during the initial inflammatory process are to control swelling, decrease pain, and protect the injury from further damage. This can be assisted with specific therapeutic modalities such as the *Game Ready Accelerated Recovery System* that will apply compression as well as cryotherapy to reduce swelling and pain. Interferential currents can be used to decrease patients' pain along with ice. Cold whirlpool can also be selected to decrease pain and swelling. Finally, non-thermal ultrasound can be used during the inflammatory process to reduce pain and swelling.

NEUROLOGICAL RESPONSES PRODUCED BY THERAPEUTIC MODALITIES

Certain therapeutic modalities can create beneficial neurological responses for patients. For example, electrical stimulation units can be used to reduce a patient's perception of pain as well as create involuntary muscular contractions. Pain reduction can be achieved multiple ways such as using the gate control theory of pain modulation to offer neurological stimulus with electrical currents that effectively block the patient's perception of pain. Involuntary muscular contractions can be used to reduce swelling using the muscle-pumping action from muscular contractions to assist lymphatic-system drainage. Muscular strengthening can also be achieved with the use of electrical stimulation. A more powerful muscular contraction can be achieved with electrical stimulation than the patient could produce without the electrical stimulation post-injury. Finally, involuntary muscular contractions can also be used to help a patient relearn how to contract a muscle after a serious injury or surgery.

PHYSIOLOGICAL RESPONSES TO THERMOTHERAPY

When heat is applied to the body, numerous physiological responses occur. The responses vary based on the type of heat that is used, the duration of the treatment, the temperature of the thermotherapy, and the type of body tissue being heated. For example, superficial tissues are heated more easily while deeper tissues can be more difficult to effectively heat. Possible responses to heat application are decreased pain, muscle spasm, joint stiffness, and inflammation. Also, heat application increases blood flow to the area and tissue extensibility. However, for an increased extensibility of tissues to occur, stretching activities must be combined with thermotherapy.

Various types of thermotherapies transmit thermal energy into the body in different ways. For example, conduction occurs when heat is directly applied to the skin such as with moist heat packs and paraffin baths. To avoid tissue damage, the heat applied should not exceed 116.6 degrees Fahrenheit (47 degrees Celsius). Convection occurs when heat is transferred through gasses or fluids such as with warm whirlpools. Radiation occurs when heat is transferred between objects such as with short wave diathermy. Finally, conversion occurs when one type of heat is transferred to another energy form such as with ultrasound as it uses sound waves to produce heat in body tissues.

Physiological Responses to Cryotherapy

The physiological responses to cryotherapy vary based on the type of cold therapy being applied, the duration of the treatment, and the type of tissue being cooled. For example, muscle tissues have a high water content and therefore are more easily cooled. Fat tissue works as an insulator in the body and can be a barrier to cooling. Studies have shown that individuals with less than 0.5 inch of subcutaneous fat have significant cooling in muscular tissue after 10 minutes of cryotherapy while individuals with greater than 0.8-inch subcutaneous fat have minimal muscular cooling with the same treatment time. Typically, the longer the cooling time, the greater the decrease in tissue temperature. However, cryotherapy should not be applied for more than 45 minutes to an hour at a time.

The effects of cryotherapy include decreased pain, decreased muscle guarding, and a lowered metabolic rate, which reduces cell death and therefore decreases rehabilitation time. Wet ice has been shown to be a more effective cooling therapy than chemical cold packs due to the energy needed to melt the ice and the greater amount of surface area contact.

Therapeutic Ultrasound Treatment

Ultrasound treatment uses acoustic vibrations from inaudible, high-frequency sound waves for therapeutic effects. Ultrasound can be used for thermal effects as well as non-thermal therapeutic effects that facilitate the healing process. A coupling agent must be used to effectively transmit the sound waves into the desired body tissues. When determining the settings to use for ultrasound treatment, the athletic trainer must consider the phase of the inflammatory process the patient is in, the tissue that is affected, and the desired results.

For thermal effects, the ultrasound should be set on continuous waves. The frequency settings control the depth of the treatment. The 1 MHz setting is used for heating deeper tissues while the 3 MHz setting is used to heat more superficial tissues. The intensity setting controls the amount of sound energy delivered and ranges from 0.1 to 3.0 W/cm2. To utilize the non-thermal effects of ultrasound, pulsed ultrasound should be used or continuous, low-intensity ultrasound. Contraindications for ultrasound treatment are pregnancy and treatments over areas of the body that are highly fluid such as the eyes and heart. Acute injures should not be treated with thermal ultrasound, and only limited ultrasound should be performed on the epiphyseal areas of children.

Hydrocollator Pack Treatment

Hydrocollator packs are used for pain reduction, relief of muscular spasms, and general relaxation. They mainly heat superficial tissues as deeper tissues cannot be significantly heated with hydrocollator packs. They are made of a silicate gel contained within a cotton pad and are kept immersed within a hydrocollator machine that maintains hot water at a temperature of 160-170 degrees Fahrenheit. To use for treatment, the hydrocollator pack must be carefully removed from the machine, drained for a few seconds, and covered with a commercial cover or several layers of towels. The patient should be positioned in such a way that the affected area can be heated without the patient laying on the heat pack. The hydrocollator pack should be placed on the patient's affected area for 15 to 20 minutes. A contraindication for the use of moist-heat packs is acute injuries.

CRYOKINETIC TREATMENT

Cryokinetic treatment is a combination of cold therapy and exercise. The cold can be applied through various ways such as cold whirlpool, ice packs, or ice massage. Once the patient's affected area is numb, after approximately 12-20 minutes of cold application, the patient will perform exercises while affected body area is numb, approximately 3-5 minutes. Exercises should work to achieve full range-of-motion using progressive resistance exercises. Once the area is no longer numb, ice is reapplied for 3-5 additional minutes, until numbness is reestablished. This procedure is repeated five times and exercises should increase in intensity within the physiological limitations of the patient's current phase in the healing process.

INTERFERENTIAL TREATMENT

Interferential treatment is an electrical modality that can be used for pain management, reduction of swelling, and restricted mobility. To properly administer interferential treatment, the athletic trainer must determine the area to be treated, for example, the exact area the patient is experiencing pain. Then four electrodes with adhesive backs are placed in a square pattern surrounding the treatment area. To do this, the first pair of electrodes run by the same generator are placed directly across from each other. Then the second pair of electrodes run by the same generator are placed directly across from each other. The four electrodes will effectively box in the patient's area of pain. The frequency selected for the electrical currents depends on the patient's needs. For pain modulation, currents of 50 to 100 pps is acceptable, while for muscular contraction, 20 to 25 pps is required.

LOW-LEVEL LASER THERAPY

Low-level laser therapy is used to facilitate wound and soft tissue healing as well as pain reduction. Helium neon (HeNe) and gallium arsenide (GaAs) are two types of low-level lasers used. HeNe lasers emit a red light and offer more superficial treatments with direct penetration of 0.07 to 0.5 inches. GaAs lasers are invisible and offer deeper treatments with direct penetration of 0.4 to 0.8 inches. To perform low-level laser therapy, the athletic trainer sets the desired pulse frequency and treatment time. Then, gentle contact with treatment area is performed in a perpendicular manner over 1-cm squares of the treatment area at a time. Contraindications include treatment over cancerous tissue, during the first trimester of pregnancy, and directly into the eyes.

HELPING PATIENTS MAKE FULL RECOVERIES BY ADMINISTERING APPROPRIATE MANUAL TECHNIQUES

Administering appropriate manual techniques can help patients make full recoveries because manual therapy is a beneficial tool that athletic trainer can use to aid in the recovery of many various injuries. For example, manual therapy is beneficial in breaking up muscular adhesions that limit proper motion of the affected muscle. Muscular adhesions can also be quite painful and cause secondary injuries to develop because other areas of the body must compensate for the limited function of the affected muscle. The athletic trainer can use various manual techniques to break down the muscular adhesions and restore full function to the affected muscle. Examples of manual techniques athletic trainers use include myofascial release, soft tissue mobilization, the Graston technique, joint mobilization, traction, massage, and the strain/counterstrain technique.

Healing Process Guides Decisions for Selection of Appropriate Manual Techniques

The patient's current stage in the healing process guides all decisions regarding the plan of rehabilitation, including the selection of appropriate manual therapy techniques. For example, massage should not be performed for an acute injury that is in the inflammatory phase of healing. During the maturation-remodeling phase, manual therapy such as massage and mobilization techniques can be employed to assist in realigning scar tissues to a more functional pattern. Additionally, some manual therapy techniques can cause a small amount of trauma to tissues to initiate the healing process and break down abnormal adhesions. Examples are the Graston technique and deep transverse friction massage. It is important to be cognizant of the effects of all manual therapy techniques and select the best ones to meet patient outcome goals at the appropriate time in the healing process.

Mobilization Techniques, Deep Transverse Friction Massage, and Dry Needling

Mobilization techniques are performed to restore full range of motion to a joint. To perform this technique, the athletic trainer stabilizes part of the affected joint while gliding another part of the joint. For example, the knee can be mobilized by stabilizing the femur while the tibia is glided posteriorly to increase knee flexion. Mobilization should not be used on lax joints, as this will increase laxity. Manipulations, which are forceful joint glides that result in a pop in the joint, should only be done by professionals specifically trained in this technique.

Deep transverse friction massage is used to restore normal motion to soft tissues just as mobilization techniques are used to restore normal motion to a joint. Using this technique, a massage is done across the grain of the affected tissue to release adhesions. This technique should not be performed on acute injuries or areas with swelling.

Dry needling is a technique used to relieve muscular conditions by inserting a needle into active muscular trigger points and relieving tension in the muscles. The legality of athletic trainers using dry needling varies from state to state so athletic trainers must ensure they practice only within the scope of athletic training allowed by their state. Dry needling requires specialized training to perform safely.

Traction and the Graston Technique

When performing traction, the traction force should be applied gradually and the patient should be monitored for comfort. When selecting the amount of weight for traction, a good guideline to follow would be around half of the patient's body weight for lumbar traction and 20 to 50 pounds for cervical traction, starting with a lighter weight and working up to a heavier weight, as tolerated by the patient.

The Graston technique is an advanced soft tissue immobilization technique that requires special training to perform. It utilizes tools to break up scar tissue and muscular adhesions that cause pain and loss of mobility. A specialized lubricant must be used when performing this technique to prevent skin irritation. Patient discomfort and bruising can occur with this treatment, which the patient should be educated about prior to the treatment.

Ensuring Patient Privacy and Athletic Trainer Integrity with Massage Treatments

There are several steps that should be taken to ensure patient privacy and the integrity of the athletic trainer while performing massage treatments. As massage requires direct physical contact, the athletic trainer should take every precaution to ensure the massage treatment can in no way be misinterpreted as being inappropriate. This is especially important when providing massage treatments to minors and patients of the opposite sex. When performing a massage, only the treatment area should be exposed and the patient should be covered with clothing, sheets, and/or towels. It can be advisable to perform the massage with another person in the room or to perform the massage in an area visible in the athletic training clinic so that there are witnesses to treatment in case any issue may arise.

HARD-SHELL PAD

A hard-shell pad is used to protect a patient's injured area from further injury. Steps for constructing a hard-shell pad:

- Select appropriate material
    - Thermo-moldable plastic
    - Felt
    - Scissors
    - Elastic wrap
- Determine the size and shape the pad will need to be by palpating the patient and marking areas of point-tenderness
- Cut felt to fit the area of point-tenderness
- Heat thermos-moldable plastic until pliable
- Put the plastic on the felt and wrap both onto the patient's area of point-tenderness with an elastic wrap to shape the plastic
- After the plastic has cooled, remove and trim to the needed shape
- If a soft, inner-layer is needed to properly protect the area, create one
    - Select soft foam and cut a doughnut hole the size of the injured area
    - Cut foam identical to plastic
    - Attach both pieces of foam to the plastic with either tape or adhesive

THERMO-MOLDABLE PLASTICS

Thermo-moldable plastics can be used for a variety of purposes such as protecting a deep contusion from further injury, providing support to an injured joint, and correcting abnormalities of the feet. Two categories of thermo-moldable plastics are heat-forming plastics and heat-plastic foams. Heat-forming plastics are the most commonly used in sports medicine and the most popular types are Orthoplast and X-Lite. Heat-forming plastics become pliable at a lower temperature, from 140-180 degrees Fahrenheit. Once heated, they can be formed into the exact shape desired around the patient's affected body part.

Heat-plastic foams have a different density due to the addition of crystals, liquid, or gas within the foam. They are commonly used for orthotics and padding of body parts. The most commonly used are Plastazote and Aliplast. When using thermo-moldable plastics, the athletic trainer must be aware of the rules of the sport to ensure the device will be allowed during competition.

ANKLE BRACES

There are many different types of commercial ankle braces available that are used to prevent ankle sprains. There are lace-up ankle braces, lace-up braces with added straps for support, rigid support braces, and rigid support braces with added straps. Many studies have been done to test the effectiveness of ankle braces, and while results vary, most studies find that ankle braces are effective in preventing ankle injuries. Bracing has little-to-no effect on performance and does not loosen much during exercise, like ankle taping does. Several studies have found a beneficial effect with semi-rigid ankle braces and several studies have shown lace-up braces to be superior to ankle taping in preventing ankle sprains.

Closed Basket Weave Ankle Taping Technique

- Apply two anchors
    - One anchor strip 5-6 inches above lateral malleolus and below the belly of the gastrocnemius (1)
    - One anchor strip around the instep of the foot over the styloid process of the fifth metatarsal (2)
- Apply a stirrup strip posterior to the malleolus and attach to the anchor (3)
    - For an inversion sprain, pull the ankle into eversion
    - For an eversion sprain, pull the ankle into a neutral position
- Apply horseshoe strip under malleolus and attach to the instep anchor (4)
- Repeat alternating stirrup and horseshoe strips overlapping by at least half of the previous strip for a total of 3 each of stirrup and horseshoe strips (5-8)
- Apply 2-3 heel locks (9-10)
- Close the tape job by applying Gibney strips up the ankle. (11-17)
- Add arch support by applying 2-3 circular strips around the arch. (18-19)

Achilles Tendon Taping Technique

- Position the patient
    - Patient lies prone on taping table
    - Affected foot hangs off edge of table in a relaxed position
- Apply two anchors
    - Apply first anchor loosely 7-9 inches above the malleoli using 1.5-inch adhesive tape (1)
    - Apply second anchor around ball of foot using 1.5-inch adhesive tape (2)
- Attach 3-inch elastic tape about 8-10 inches in length to both anchors (3)
- Apply another 3-inch elastic tape that is cut on both ends to the anchor strips (4)
- Secure the elastic tape by closing the tape job using 1.5-inch adhesive tape loosely around the arch (5-7) and around the lower leg (8-13)

X Teardrop arch Taping Technique

The X Teardrop arch taping technique is used to support the longitudinal arch and the forefoot. Athletic tape 1-inch in width is used along with tape adherent. The patient should be positioned prone on a taping table with the affected foot hanging off the edge of the table. Tape adherent is sprayed on the foot and an anchor strip is applied around the ball of the foot. Then, a teardrop shape is applied starting at the base of the first toe, going around the back of the heel, over the arch, and back to the starting point on the great toe. Next, another teardrop shape is applied that starts at the base of the fifth toe, goes around the back of the heel, and ends at the starting point at the base of the fifth toe. These two teardrop shapes are repeated another two to three times and then another piece of tape is applied around the ball of the foot to lock the tape strips in place.

Kinesio Taping Technique

Kinesio taping is a taping technique that has become popular in the United States and is used for many purposes such as reduction of pain and swelling, and facilitating motor activity. However, there is currently no evidence-based research that supports the effectiveness of Kinesio taping for achieving these results. It is proposed that Kinesio taping works by improving the circulation of the circulatory and lymph systems, assisting in strengthening weaker muscles, suppressing the neurological system which results in pain reduction, and reducing muscle tension which improves the biomechanical positioning of joints. Since athletic trainers are effective in multiple taping techniques, they can learn and perform many Kinesio taping techniques as needed for patients.

KINESIO TAPING TECHNIQUE FOR PATELLOFEMORAL PAIN

To apply Kinesio taping for a patient with patellofemoral pain, the athletic trainer will need 2-inch width Kinesio tape. The patient should be seated on a taping table with the knee extended. The athletic trainer will cut a piece of Kinesio tape 10-inches long, make a cut in the middle of one end of the tape the long way, split that end of the Kinesio tape until the split end is 5-inches long, leaving the other 5-inches of the tape un-split. The athletic trainer then places the un-split end of the tape on the front of the patient's thigh so that the beginning of the Y-shaped split is positioned against the superior patella. Then, the split ends of the tape are wrapped around the sides of the patella with little-to-no stretch being applied to the Kinesio tape. The athletic trainer then cuts a piece of Kinesio tape 6-inches long, and splits one end of tape again until half of the tape is split, while half remains un-split. The Kinesio tape is then applied so that the Y-shape at the split is positioned at the inferior patella, and the split ends wrap around the patella with little-to-no stretch being applied to the Kinesio tape.

HIP SPICA WRAP

The **hip spica wrap** is used to support the hip and limit abduction after hip flexor or groin injury when the athlete returns to sports activity or competition. Commercial adjustable elastic wraps are available and are easily applied, but usually the spica wrap is applied with 6-inch elastic bandage (e.g., an Ace® bandage). The athlete stands with the foot of his affected side turned slightly inward to relax the muscles. The wrap begins by anchoring the bandage twice about the proximal thigh, with the end at the lateral aspect, and wrapping toward the medial aspect, spiraling upward. With the second wrap around the thigh, the bandage is brought over the trochanter on the affected side and around the waist. Then, it is brought back around the inner thigh (figure 8), around the hip, and back around the waist, continuing to spiral upward until the hip is secure. The wrap should end on the thigh, and the bandage should be secured thoroughly with elastic tape.

A hip spica can be applied to alleviate discomfort and provide support to patients who suffer from leg injuries such as a strain to the hip adductors. To apply a hip spica for a hip adductor strain, a 6-inch, double-width, elastic wrap is needed as well as 1.5-inch athletic tape. The patient should stand on a taping table, be instructed to place their weight on their uninjured leg, and relax and internally rotate their injured leg. The athletic trainer should start the wrap on the internal upper affected thigh, continuing posteriorly around the back of the thigh, back around the thigh, up over the patient's lower abdomen, around the iliac crest of the unaffected leg, around the patent's back, and then back to the affected leg repeating this pattern until all the elastic wrap is used. The wrap should then be secured with the athletic tape, making sure the athletic tape is not applied too tightly where it will cut off circulation but tight enough to keep the wrap secure during activity.

TRACTION

Traction is used to treat several conditions including spinal nerve root impingement that is caused by disk herniation, prolapse, or spondylolisthesis. It is also used to treat muscular guarding, strain of the spinal muscles, or sprain of the spinal ligaments.

- Manual traction: The athletic trainer provides a manual stretching force, relieving pressure from the spinal disks. This is highly adaptable as the athletic trainer can change the force and the direction of the pull easily.

- Mechanical traction: The patient is secured in a harness that attaches to a machine, which applies a mechanical stretching force either through intermittent or continuous traction.
- Positional traction: The patient is placed in a position that produces traction such as laying supine with hips and knees supported at 90 degrees, relieving pressure on the lumbar disks.
- Wall-mounted traction: Cervical traction can be achieved with an inexpensive wall-mounted unit that uses weights and a harness that goes around the patient's head to relieve pressure on the cervical disks.
- Inverted traction: A special piece of equipment is used to invert the patient and use the force of gravity to relieve pressure from the patient's intervertebral disks, as they lay inverted, secured to the equipment.

INTERMITTENT COMPRESSION

Intermittent compression is used to prevent and reduce swelling by applying an appropriate amount of pressure to the affected area. Intermittent compression pushes excessive fluid accumulated out of the injured area, which facilitates lymphatic drainage, and removes byproducts of the injury process. The injured extremity should be elevated during intermittent compression to achieve best results.

The parameters the athletic trainer must set for intermittent compression treatment are the amount of pressure applied, total treatment time, and the on/off time. The on/off time dictates how much of the total treatment time the compression is applied and can vary from 1 minute on, 2 minutes off to 4 minutes on, 1 minute off. On/off times should be determined based on the comfort of the patient. Treatment times generally last 30 minutes and pressure settings vary based on the body part being treated. For upper extremities, suggested pressures are between 30 to 50 mm Hg and for lower extremities 30 to 60 mm Hg pressure is recommended.

MCCONNELL PATELLAR TAPING TECHNIQUE

McConnell taping is a taping technique used to correct many patellofemoral alignment abnormalities. The tape applies tension to realign the patella into a more biomechanically correct position. This technique also increases proprioception of the patient's knee joint. McConnell taping can be used to correct a lateral gliding patella, a patella with a lateral tilt, rotation of the patella, and anteroposterior alignment abnormalities.

All McConnell taping techniques require two types of very sticky tape. Fixomull and Leuko Sports Tape are commonly used. The area to be taped must be prepared by cleaning, shaving, and applying tape adherent. Two strips of Fixomull are applied over the front of the knee from the lateral femoral condyle. The application of the Leuko Sports Tape varies based on the alignment abnormality of the patient's patella but it will serve to apply tension effectively pulling the patella into the biomechanically correct position.

MASSAGE TECHNIQUES

There are several different massage techniques the athletic trainer can employ to relieve patients' muscular tightness, adhesions, and pain.

- Effleurage: Stroking movements performed during the beginning and ending of a massage to increase relaxation.
- Petrissage: Kneading motion to loosen muscle adhesions. Kneading can be performed by rolling muscular tissue between the thumb and index finger.

- Friction: Deep pressure applied in a circular motion to stretch the tissue and increase circulation to the area. Friction massage is commonly performed to break up scar tissue and relieve muscular tension.
- Tapotement: Percussion techniques used during massage that includes cupping, pinching, and hacking.
- Vibration: A quick back-and-forth motion used for relaxation. Commonly a vibration machine is used for this technique.

Using Sports Massage for Rehabilitation and Reconditioning

Massage therapy is commonly used in sports, and may be employed before activities, at breaks during activities, and after the activity is completed. Many types of massage are used in sports, and some massage therapists specialize in sports massage, but all trainers should know the basic techniques of sports massage as it is used to both treat and prevent injuries. Sports massage is based primarily on Swedish massage, although the massage may be deeper and targeted toward a particular injury. Also, other types of massage may be incorporated into a sports massage program. Massage of an injured area is delayed for the first 48-72 hours to prevent further injury to tissues.

Different techniques include:

- *Compression:* Deep rhythmical compressions of the muscles increase circulation and temperature and make muscles more pliable. Compression may be performed prior to deeper massage techniques.
- *Effleurage:* This is usually the beginning massage. It begins softly and increases in intensity, with the hands gliding over the tissue (with some type of oil or emollient). Massage is performed in broad, rhythmical strokes with the palms of the hands. This massage helps to relax the athlete and identify areas of tightness or pain that may require additional attention.
- *Friction:* These are massages either in line with muscle fibers or across the muscle fibers to create stretching and to reduce adhesions and scarring during healing. The tissue is pressed firmly against the underlying tissue, and then pressure moves the underlying tissue until resistance is felt. Friction massage may be quite deep and can be uncomfortable. Usually the thumb or fingers are used for this type of massage.
- *Pétrissage:* This is a kneading massage, and is usually performed on large muscle areas, such as the calf or thigh. It increases circulation, so it is useful for relaxation and improves circulation and drainage. The full hand is used for this massage, with the heel and thumb stabilizing the tissue while the fingers squeeze the tissue.
- *Tapotement:* This type of massage features quick, rhythmic tapping, usually with the edge of the palm and little finger or the heel of the hand with the fingers elevated. It is performed to increase circulation or relieve cramped muscles.
- **Vibration:** Vibratory massage is used for deep muscle relaxation and reduction of pain. Usually the entire hand is placed against the skin, compressing the muscle and then vibrating the hand to cause movement.
- **Trigger point:** Pressure is applied with a finger or thumb to areas of point tenderness to reduce spasticity and pain.

Thigh Wraps

Thigh wraps support the muscles of the thigh after hamstring and quadriceps sprains and strains and iliotibial band syndrome. Commercial adjustable wraps are available in different sizes and styles. Some are seamless stretch elastic and slide over the foot and up the leg. Others are secured by Velcro® or straps. An elastic stretch wrap (such as a 6-inch Ace® bandage) is also commonly used. It is applied while the athlete is in standing position. The wrap begins at the distal thigh, with the bandage applied around the thigh, spiraling upward and overlapping each time around by about half a bandage width. Pressure should be even and the trainer should avoid increasing pressure at the proximal end, because this could impair circulation. The wrap ends at the proximal thigh and the bandage is thoroughly secured with elastic tape.

SPLINTS AND CASTS

Splints and casts immobilize joints and protect injured bones. They may be applied after surgery. Casts are custom fit and made of plaster or fiberglass with padding underneath the cast, which is solid and cannot be adjusted. Splints, on the other hand, may be custom fit, but standard-sized splints are also available. Splints, also made of plaster or fiberglass, provide partial support and may cover only half or part of a limb but can be adjusted in the event of swelling or infection. Fiberglass is more difficult to mold than plaster, but it is lighter and sturdier. In some cases, a splint may be applied for the first 48-72 hours until edema subsides, at which point a cast is applied. The same rules apply for both:

- Keep the limb elevated above the level of the heart for 48-72 hours.
- Move fingers or toes often.
- Apply ice to the outside of the cast/splint over the injured area.
- Immediately report burning, numbness, or inability to move fingers and toes.

USING TRACTION FOR REHABILITATION OF LOW BACK PAIN

Lumbar traction is used to stretch the muscles and tissue around joints when changes in posture or stretching exercises don't relieve compression that is causing acute pain. Traction should not be used as an exclusive therapy, but as an adjunct to education and exercise. There are a number of different types of traction:

- Manual
- Mechanical (Allows for various settings and control but is used in a clinical setting)
- Continuous or intermittent
- Positional
- Gravity-assisted
- Autotraction: A belt is applied to the pelvis with an attached bar at the head or foot of the bed. The athlete pulls (with arms) or pushes the bar (with feet) to control the traction.

Traction may be arranged with the person in prone or supine position, and with either an anterior or posterior pull or bilateral or unilateral pull. Traction is either sustained for a period of time (about 10 minutes) or is intermittent for 10-15 minutes

UTILIZING THERAPEUTIC INTERVENTIONS TO ASSIST PATIENTS IN OBTAINING FULL FUNCTION

Utilizing therapeutic interventions for general medical conditions assists patients to obtain full function because these interventions ensure best patient care available. For example, a patient who suffers from asthma will benefit from participating in regular exercise. The exercise program should be designed to include a gradual warm-up, a steady build-up in exercise time and intensity, a cool-down, and an avoidance of exercise in areas with high pollution. Assurance that asthma medication is taken as prescribed is also beneficial. Implementing all therapeutic interventions available for patients suffering from various general medical conditions, such as in the example, can help patients to participate fully and avoid negative side effects of the general medical condition.

Iliotibial Band Syndrome

Iliotibial band syndrome is a chronic overuse injury common in runners and some cyclists. It is believed to be caused by loose connective tissue that is compressed against the lateral femoral condyle instead of frictional forces that occur during knee flexion and extension. Structural abnormalities common in patients who suffer from iliotibial band friction syndrome include genu varum (bow-legs) and pronated feet (flat feet).

Treatment includes reducing inflammation through ice and Ibuprofen. Thorough stretching must be performed with a focus on stretching the iliotibial band. Proper warm-ups must be performed and the patient should avoid activities that aggravate their condition such as running on inclines. Any structural abnormalities should be corrected such as the use of foot orthotics for flat feet.

Impact of Immobilization on Body Systems

Immobilization negatively impacts various body systems. For example, muscle mass is lost when the muscle is immobilized. The muscle's slow-twitch fibers atrophy the most and their characteristics change to be more like fast-twitch muscle fibers. Neuromuscular control is decreased as the patient's motor units become less efficient at recruiting muscle fibers. Joint surfaces suffer degenerative changes due to lack of compressive forces. Without normal stresses, ligaments and bones become weaker as well.

Minimizing the Effects of Immobilization

There are many steps the athletic trainer can take to decrease the negative effects of immobilization. As much as possible, the patient should exercise without aggravating their injury. Isometric exercises and electrical stimulation can decrease negative affects to the muscles. Continuous passive range of motion, electrical stimulation, and hinged braces can the negative effects of immobilization to the joints. Once a patient no longer requires immobilization, rehabilitative exercises should be performed to strengthen the ligaments and bones. They should be high intensity and short in duration.

Using Graduated Return-To-Play Protocol After a Suffering a Concussion

The graduated-return-to-play protocol is a step-by-step guideline athletic trainers can follow to safely return patients back to physical activity following concussions. The protocol gradually increases activity, allowing assurance that the patient can remain free of concussion symptoms with exercise. Generally, only one step of the protocol should be allowed per day, which should take patients about a week to return to play. The protocol can be begun once patients are completely free of concussion symptoms. Patients must remain asymptomatic to progress in the protocol.

The first day of the graduated return-to-play protocol is complete physical and mental rest, which assists in recovery. During the second day, light aerobic exercise is performed to increase the heart rate and ensure the patient can remain asymptomatic with exercise. The third day non-contact, sport-specific exercises can be performed. The fourth day the patient can progress to more complex sport-specific training drills but still must remain contact-free. If the patient still remains asymptomatic, once receiving medical clearance, they can progress to full contact practice to restore their confidence. Finally, normal game play can be allowed on the sixth day.

Determining If Wounds Require Sutures

Athletic trainers will see many patient wounds and must know when a referral for sutures is advisable. Wounds that require sutures are deep wounds and wounds in which underlying tissues are visible such as fat, vessels, tendons, and bone. If an athletic trainer believes a patient requires sutures, the patient should be referred to a physician as soon as possible, but definitely within 12 hours of the injury. The physician will ultimately determine if sutures are needed. Areas of the body that are placed under high-stress or that take a longer time to heal need sutures that are made of larger material and require more time to heal. Liquid stitches are an alternative to traditional sutures. If the physician decides stitches are not needed they may choose to use steri-strips or butterfly bandages to close the wound.

IMPROVING PROPRIOCEPTION AND KINESTHESIS AFTER AN INJURY

Improving a patient's proprioception and kinesthesis are both essential elements in improving neuromuscular control. To improve these functions, many repetitions of strengthening exercises should be performed in functional movement patterns. The exercises should progress in complexity from simple to more complicated movement patterns, focusing on correct form. As the patient completes several repetitions of the movement patterns, the movements become easier, requiring less concentration, until they become almost automatic. Relearning these movement patterns should be a priority in rehabilitation and can take several months to successfully master.

PSYCHOLOGICAL ASPECTS OF PAIN

The perception of pain is both psychological and physiological, and therefore unique to each individual. It is crucial for the athletic trainer to understand that all pain is real to the patient, regardless of the patient's threshold for pain. Psychological attributes that may increase the perception of pain include anxious and dependent personality types. Also, pain is perceived to be greater at night, when the patient is alone, and when they don't have anything to distract them from their pain. The athletic trainer can take steps to help reduce the patient's pain with several psychological techniques such as reducing muscle tension, diverting attention away from pain, and altering the sensation of pain. Athletic trainers can teach the patient progressive relaxation techniques to reduce muscle tension. Diverting attention away from the pain can be done through imagery and thought stoppage. Using the imagination, the patient can alter their sensation of pain by imagining a pleasant experience, instead of pain.

SCAR TISSUE

Scar tissue is formed when fibroblasts produce collagen fibers, which are laid down in a random manner. The wound's tensile strength is increased proportionally with the collagen fiber production. As the tissues mature, the collagen fibers within the scar can be realigned from the initial random fashion, to a more functional pattern, allowing for functional movement to occur. To facilitate this change, the athletic trainer can have the patient perform exercises that produce stress on the scar within the body part's normal range of motion. The scar will respond to stresses placed on it according to Wolff's law and will become realigned along the lines of the tensile stresses placed on it. Within 3 weeks of the initial injury, a firm scar can be in place while the maturation and healing process may take years to be fully completed.

STRESS FRACTURES

Possible causes for stress fractures include overuse, improper conditioning, inadequate nutrition, and structural abnormalities of the feet. Common foot abnormalities that can lead to stress fractures include flat feet, hypermobile feet, rigid pes cavus, and a shortened metatarsal of the great toe. To prevent stress fractures in athletes with foot abnormalities, orthotics can be used to correct these deviations. Athletic trainers should also ensure athletes are following appropriate training plans that include gradual progression, proper training environments, and suitable amounts of exercise. If a stress fracture does occur, the appropriate amount of rest is needed for the bone to properly heal. If the patient has pain walking, they should not bear weight on the affected limb until they can do so pain-free. Gradual return to play should be implemented when appropriate, keeping bone healing as the priority.

Nerve Healing

If a nerve cell is damaged, the nerve cell itself cannot regenerate. However, if damage occurs to the peripheral nerve, regeneration of the damaged area can occur and result in repaired innervation. This takes place when the axon proximal to the injury starts regeneration. Bulbous enlargements and axon sprouts develop. Only one axon sprout will eventually form a new axon that will restore innervation. The process of regeneration is slow, at around three-to-four millimeters per day. Central nervous system nerves are not as effective as regeneration as are nerves of the peripheral nervous system.

Assessing the Extent of Muscle Injury Using Electromyography

Electromyography (EMG) assesses the electrical activity within a muscle to determine the degree of injury and recovery. EMG can assist in providing a picture of how muscle contractions coordinate during activity. There are two types of EMG:

- **Surface electrode EMG** is non-invasive and uses electrodes on the surface of a muscle to detect the sum of action potentials in the muscle. This type of EMG gives a good overall assessment of muscle function. However, it can pick up electrical activity from adjoining muscles, so it is not as specific as needle EMG.
- **Needle electrode EMG** is an invasive test in which a needle electrode is inserted directly into the muscle. Precise readings of the action potentials of even small muscles can be detected. Because the readings derive from a small area near the electrode, inserting the needle electrode to the correct area is important for accurate readings. Because of its specificity, needle electrode EMG is less useful for overall assessment of muscle function.

Shortwave Diathermy

Shortwave diathermy uses radio waves (27.12 megahertz) to increase the temperature in subcutaneous tissue, and is used along with passive and active range of motion exercises to improve range in painful conditions, such as inflammation of the muscles, tendons, and bursae. The radio waves (eddy currents) are transmitted through a capacitor or inductor in a continuous or pulse waveform. Temperatures increase about 15°C in fatty tissue and 4-6°C in muscular tissue. Shortwave diathermy should not be used over any organs containing fluid, including the eyes, heart, and head, or over pacemakers, as the diathermy may disrupt the settings. Because this treatment may increase cardiac demand, it should be avoided by those with preexisting cardiac conditions and should not be used over malignancies. Additionally, it is contraindicated in areas of inflammation, because heating the tissue increases inflammation. It cannot be used over prostheses, as the metal may heat and damage tissue. Shortwave diathermy should avoid the epiphyses in children, as it may stimulate abnormal growth.

Microwave Diathermy

Microwave diathermy is similar to shortwave diathermy but has a lower rate of heat increase and penetration, so it is used for muscles and joints near the surface rather than deep muscles like the hip. Heat is created by electromagnetic radiation (9.15-14.50 megahertz) and raises temperature in fatty tissues by about 10-12°C and in muscular tissue by 3-4°C. Treatment is usually given for 15-30 minutes per session and is followed by range of motion exercises (passive and active) to increase flexibility. Contraindications are similar to those of shortwave diathermy in that this treatment should not be used where increase in temperature may be detrimental, such as over organs containing fluid, areas of inflammation, and the epiphyses of children. Additionally, it should not be used over prostheses or pacemakers, and should be avoided in those with cardiac disease.

Ultrasound

Ultrasound treats soft-tissue injuries (such as myositis, bursitis, and tendinitis) with sound waves (frequency 0.8-3 megahertz). Ultrasound uses a piezoelectric crystal that vibrates and produces sound waveforms, which are transmitted from the transducer through a gel substance into the tissue. The sound waves bounce off of the bone in an irregular pattern that causes an increase in temperature in the connective tissue (as for instance in the collagen fibers). Temperatures of the tissue may increase up to 43.5°C, increasing local metabolism, neural conduction, and blood flow. Ultrasound is used to decrease both contractures and scarring. During treatment, the transducer passes in a circular motion about the skin surface, staying in contact with the gel medium. If a distal limb is submerged in water, the treatment is given with the head of the transducer 0.5-1 inch from the skin surface. Treatment is followed by range of motion exercises, both passive and active. Contraindications are similar to those of other heat-producing modalities and include peripheral vascular disease, though ultrasound may be used over metal prostheses.

Phonophoresis and Iontophoresis

Phonophoresis uses high-intensity and low frequency ultrasound (at about 20 megahertz) to increase circulation of the skin, for the purpose of administering topical medications like corticosteroids and lidocaine. It is believed that ultrasound allows the medication to better penetrate the underlying tissue to treat inflammation in localized areas, such as for tendinitis and tenosynovitis. Special medicated gels are used instead of the usual gel medium. Preparations include:

- Ketoprofen gel (an NSAID), used for osteoarthritis and musculoskeletal injuries.
- Hydrocortisone gel, a corticosteroid, used for treatment of pain and inflammation.

Iontophoresis is the transdermal administration of ionizable medications, such as NSAIDs or corticosteroids, with a small continuous electrical charge through a special applicator containing medication. Some people find the treatment uncomfortable. Iontophoresis is used for primary hyperhidrosis (excessive perspiration) of the hands and feet, but must be continued indefinitely 1-2 times weekly to control the condition.

Therapeutic Use of Superficial Heat

Superficial heat with externally-applied heat sources penetrates only the superficial layers of the skin (the top 1-2 cm are penetrated after about 30 minutes), but it is believed to relax deeper muscles by reflex, to decrease pain, and to increase metabolism (2-3 times for every 10°C increase in skin temperature). The therapeutic temperature range is 40-45°C. Superficial heat modalities include:

- ***Moist heat packs*** placed on the skin and secured by several layers of towels to provide insulation, applied for 15-30 minutes. ***Paraffin baths***: 52-54° C with the hand, foot, or elbow dipped 7 times, cooled between dippings, and then wrapped with plastic and towels for 20 minutes.
- In ***fluidotherapy***, a hand or foot is submerged for 20-30 minutes in cellulose particles warmed to 38.8-47.8°C by hot air.
- Passive and active range of motion exercises are performed after superficial heat treatment. Contraindications include cardiac disease, peripheral vascular disease, malignant tumor, bleeding, and acute inflammation.
- **Deep heat** differs from superficial heat in that the heat is generated internally using ultrasound, short wave, and microwave diathermy rather than applied to the surface of the skin.

Therapeutic Cold (Cryotherapy)

Cryotherapy is therapeutic cold treatment to cool the surface of the skin and underlying subcutaneous tissues in order to decrease blood flow, pain, and metabolism. The initial response to cold therapy is vasoconstriction for the first 15 minutes but if the tissues are cooled to -10°C, the body responds with vasodilation. Cryotherapy affects sensory response, so the skin will at first feel cold, but will subsequently progress to burning, aching, and finally to numbness and tingling. Treatment is usually given for 15-30 minutes. Treatment modalities include:

- *Ice packs,* such as refrigerated gel packs (-5°C) or plastic bags filled with water and ice chips applied directly to the skin for 10-15 minutes for superficial cooling and 15-20 minutes for greater penetrance.
- A *towel dipped in ice* and water slurry wrapped around the limb to provide cold therapy; this is best used only for emergency situations when ice packs are unavailable, as the towel must be changed frequently since the skin warms it rapidly.
- *Ice massage* is applied directly to the affected area for 5-10 minutes, usually by rubbing the ice in circular motions on the skin surface. An ice massager is easily made by filling a paper cup with water and freezing it with a tongue depressor or Popsicle stick (to use as a handle) inserted into the center. The paper can be torn away from the bottom and sides when the ice is solid. Ice massage is often followed by friction massage.
- *Ice baths* (13-18°C) are used for limbs, such as the lower leg and/or foot or the hand. The body part is immersed for 20 minutes.

Cryotherapy is usually followed by active and passive exercises. Contraindications include impaired circulation or sensation, cardiac disease, Raynaud's disease, and nerve trauma.

Therapeutic Methods of Heating and Cooling

There are a number of different ways to heat (thermotherapy) or cool (cryotherapy) for healing:

- **Conduction:** Conveyance of heat, cold, or electricity through direct contact with the skin, such as with hot baths, ice packs, and electrical stimulation
- **Convection:** Indirect transmission of heat in a liquid or gas by circulation of heated particles, such as with whirlpools and paraffin soaks
- **Conversion:** Heating that results from converting a form of energy into heat, such as with diathermy and ultrasound
- **Evaporation:** Cooling caused by liquids that evaporate into gases on the skin with a resultant cooling effect, such as with perspiration or vapo-coolant sprays
- **Radiation**: Heating that results from transfer of heat through light waves or rays, such as with infrared or ultraviolet light

Therapeutic Whirlpool Baths

Whirlpool baths are used to increase circulation and promote healing. They are tubs with a turbine that mixes air with water; the mixture is pressurized and flows into the tub water to create turbulence. Tubs are usually large enough to accommodate the full body, although smaller, limb-sized whirlpool tubs are available. Water temperature is 95°-104° (adjusted for the individual), and should be deep enough to completely submerge the affected part. The body part should be cleaned with soap and water or a shower should be taken before immersion. If the full body is treated, the athlete should wear a swimming suit. During the whirlpool treatment, the muscles relax from the heat, and range of motion exercises can be done while in the water. Typically, treatments last about 20 minutes, but the athlete should be monitored, especially for the first 5 minutes, as some people become lightheaded and can lose consciousness.

Therapeutic Contrast Baths

Contrast baths (alternating hot and cold) are used in the sub-acute phase of healing (after edema begins to subside) for strains and sprains. It is believed that contrast baths increase the circulation and help to further decrease edema through a pumping action as the vasoconstriction and vasodilation alternate. Two containers are filled with water, one with hot and the other with cold. The hot water should be maintained at about 100°-110° F and the cold at 55°-65° F. The cycle begins and ends with immersion in cold water. Cold water immersions usually last about 1 minute and hot water immersions last 4 minutes (or as ordered by physician). Typically, the affected limb is immersed in the cold water for one minute, removed, and immediately immersed in hot water for 4 minutes. This cycle is repeated 3-4 times.

Therapeutic Use of Vapo-Coolant Sprays

Vapo-coolant sprays (such as Fluori-Methane®) use a cooling mist to decrease pain and muscle spasms and facilitate stretching (cryostretching) of the muscles. They are used primarily for strains of the lower back and cervical area and injuries of the hamstrings. As some sprays are flammable, they must be used in a well-ventilated area away from sparks. Sprays should be used only on intact skin. Coolant sprays only work the superficial tissue, but can facilitate stretching exercises. The spray container should be at least one foot away from the skin surface and held at an angle (about 45°) while spraying in one direction. It's important to spray in a sweeping manner and to keep the spray moving, as focusing on one area could result in frostbite and damage to tissues. After 2-3 sprays, the muscle is manually stretched until warmed. The spray-stretch cycle may be repeated 4 times.

Therapeutic Use of Cervical Traction

Traction stretches the tissue about the spine and relieves pressure on the vertebrae. **Cervical traction** is performed before other therapies to reduce muscle spasms, and is used specifically for cervical disk herniation. Manual traction is usually done with the athlete in the supine position on a bed or table, with the neck flexed at about 20°. The trainer places hands under the occiput or one under the occiput and the other on the forehead, and applies stretch and tension longitudinally (avoiding any twisting). The stretch is held for 1-2 minutes. Mechanical traction is done with a special harness that fits about the back of the head and under the chin, with a rope fed through a pulley and a weight to apply tension. The angle of pull is usually 30°. Traction may be continuous for about 15 minutes, or done intermittently (controlled electronically) with pull for 10-50 seconds followed by relaxation for 5-20 seconds. Mechanical traction may be performed in the sitting or supine positions.

Therapeutic Use of Transcutaneous Electrical Nerve Stimulation

Transcutaneous electrical nerve stimulation (TENS) is applied to peripheral sensory nerve fibers to reduce acute or recurrent pain. TENS machines may be 2-lead or 4-lead, and have adjustments for both frequency (1-20 Hz) and pulse width (50-300 microseconds, 10-50 mA). Stimulation can be intermittent or continuous. TENS units are small and battery-powered, with wires and adhesive electrodes attached so that they can be worn while the person goes about usual activities. The positioning of the electrodes and the settings depend upon the site and type of injury, following guidelines provided by the manufacturer. The TENS machine can be used for several hours, but if used for days at a time, it will be less effective. TENS treatment is contraindicated with demand pacemakers, and should not be used on the head or neck or over irritated skin.

THERAPEUTIC USE OF ELECTRICAL MUSCLE STIMULATION

Electrical muscle stimulation (EMS) uses an electrical stimulation unit that looks similar to a TENS unit, except that the voltage is different (1000-4000 Hz). It is used to relieve muscular spasms and to strengthen and increase the size of the muscle after injury, such as muscle strain, rather than to control pain. It helps to re-educate the muscles and reduce atrophy by targeting peripheral motor nerves (rather than sensory nerves, as does TENS), so electrodes are placed over the muscle's motor points, causing expansion and contraction of the muscles when stimulated. Some athletes, especially body builders, use EMS as an addition to training exercises to stimulate muscle growth and enhance appearance, although EMS cannot substitute for strengthening exercises. It is also used to reduce muscle spasms. Functional EMS is used to stimulate muscles during periods of immobilization or splinting, in order to prevent adhesions of tendons. Russian stimulation uses specific preset EMS parameters to penetrate the muscle deeply and cause strong contractions.

EDUCATING INDIVIDUALS ABOUT MEDICATIONS AND THERAPEUTIC TREATMENT

Athletes should be educated about the use of **medications** to achieve **therapeutic treatment**. Each drug has a specific duration of action: that is, a length of time when the blood level is adequate to provide minimal therapeutic results, based on the drug's half-life (the time required to reduce the blood level of the drug by half). Frequency of administration directly relates to the half-life of the drug. Medications are metabolized at different rates, and when the amount of drug ingested equals that which is metabolized, a steady state has been reached. This is the goal in therapeutic treatment, so it is important that people stay on a regular schedule of medications. In order to reach a steady level of the drug in the blood, medications need to be taken regularly for a period equal to about 5 half-lives. Medications with short half-lives (e.g., 2 hours) reach a steady state fairly soon, within about 3 doses, but those with longer half-lives (e.g., 12 hours) may take 2 or 3 days to reach a steady state.

DETERMINING PATIENTS' FUNCTIONAL STATUS

Determining patients' functional status assists the athletic trainer because it allows for an accurate assessment of patients' functional ability which can guide in decision making about the rehabilitative process and patients' readiness for return-to-activity. For example, if a patient suffers from and ACL sprain determining the patient's function status gives the athletic trainer an idea of an appropriate starting point for rehabilitation as well as appropriate functional goals to work towards. During the rehabilitative process, determining the patient's functional status will help to determine the effectiveness of the rehabilitation towards reaching the patient's goals and can offer insight as to areas for improvement in the plan of care. When the patient is near full recovery, functional testing can assist the athletic trainer in determining if the patient is truly ready for the various demands of their physical activity.

DETERMINING A PATIENT'S READINESS FOR RETURN TO PLAY

There are many considerations that must be considered when determining a patient's readiness for return to play. All members of the sports medicine team involved in the patient's care should be included in the decision, but ultimately it is the team physician's decision on whether a patient is ready for full return to play. There are several considerations to weigh into this decision. For example, the physiological stage of healing, the patient's level of pain, and swelling. Also, the patient's range of motion and strength should be sufficient to protect them from further injury. Neuromuscular control and cardiorespiratory endurance should be at a level consistent with the demands of the patient's sport. Functional testing can show the patient's ability to perform the needed skills of their sport and position. Finally, the patient should be psychologically prepared for the demands of competition, be able to listen to their body, and not be fearful of re-injury.

Personal Boundaries in Assessing and Reassessing Injuries

A Certified Athletic Trainer must always keep **personal boundaries** in mind when assessing and reassessing injuries. Palpation and examination of muscles is a necessary part of rehabilitation and reconditioning, but some athletes are uncomfortable with being touched, and others may have issues related to sexuality or personal space that can affect their perception of touch. There may be gender issues if, for example, the athletic trainer is male and the athlete female. Therefore, the reason for touching a person should always be made clear: "I'm going to feel your hamstring to determine how taut the muscle is during this activity." If possible, it is better to have another person present or to keep a door open during examinations that involve touching. If the athletic trainer feels uncomfortable while examining an athlete, whether because of the athletic trainer's anxiety or the response of the athlete, the examination should be deferred.

Primary, Secondary, and Tertiary Healing

Primary healing (healing by first intention) involves a wound that is surgically closed by suturing, flaps, or grafts to completely cover the wound. Primary healing is the most common approach used for surgeries or repair of wounds or lacerations, especially when the wound is essentially "clean." If a cut is small, cells may bridge the opening and repair the tissue.

Secondary healing (healing by second intention) involves leaving the wound open and allowing it to close through granulation and epithelialization. This approach may be used with contaminated ("dirty") or infected wounds to prevent abscess formation and allow the wound to drain. Tissue fills in from all sides of the wound.

Tertiary healing (healing by third intention) is also called delayed primary closure, because consists of two steps: first, the wound is debrided and allowed to begin healing while open. Later, the wound is closed with suturing or grafts. This approach is common with wounds that are contaminated, such as severe animal bites, or wounds related to mixed trauma.

Reassessing Injuries or Conditions

The **acute inflammatory phase** begins within hours of injury, and lasts 3-5 days in all. It follows the initial vasoconstriction and vasodilation, which releases platelets and other components of blood into the wound. Platelets begin the process of clotting by releasing phospholipids, fibronectin, fibrinogen, and growth factors. Fibrin clots form over blood and lymph vessels, preventing draining and resulting in edema until the wound stabilizes and fibrinolysis takes place, dissolving the clots so that the lymphatics can drain the excess fluid. Within the first 6 hours after injury, neutrophils and polymorphonuclear leukocytes begin to débride the wound; at the end of 1-2 days, these are replaced with large cell mononuclear phagocytes, monocytes, and macrophages, which release growth factors to stimulate cellular activity and healing. Observable signs include erythema, edema, pain, exudate, and increased temperature (from cellular activity). Once the macrophages and other cells complete debridement, proliferation begins and inflammation subsides. Chronic inflammation occurs when macrophages and other large cells persist in the wound, delaying proliferation, because of infection or other irritation.

Reassessing the Status of Ligaments, Muscles, and Tendons

While all types of **tissues** go through similar phases of healing (i.e., hemostasis, inflammation, proliferation, maturation/remodeling) the duration of the process may vary according to tissue type. An understanding of these differences is necessary for reassessing injuries:

- *Ligament*: The inflammatory process begins within 24 hours and persists for about 3 days. Proliferation begins within a few days and continues for about 6 weeks, but remodeling may take up to a year, as collagen is slowly replaced. Usually within 10-12 months, strength is restored.
- *Muscle*: The inflammatory process begins within 6 hours and persists about 10 days. Proliferation begins around days 13-19, followed by remodeling and healing within 1.5 to 6 months, depending upon the degree of injury.
- *Tendon*: The inflammatory phase lasts about 3 days, followed by a long period of proliferation. By about 4 months, remodeling is complete and by 10-12 months, strength should be at 85-95%.

Reassessing the Status of Cartilage

There are 4 different types of **cartilage**, and each has different healing properties:

- *Hyaline/articular cartilage* is found on the spongy bone ends in diarthrodial joints, the nasal septum, and the larynx. It also attaches the ribs to the sternum. This type of cartilage is firm and translucent, and it provides cushioning.
- *Yellow/elastic cartilage* provides structure in the eustachian tube, external ear, and epiglottis. It is elastic enough to stretch and move but strong enough to prevent the collapse of the structures in which it is found.
- *Fibrocartilage* is opaque, white, and very strong, and is rich in type I collagen, so it is similar to tendons in some respects. It occurs in areas of stress and impact, such as between vertebrae and in the symphysis pubis and temporomandibular joints. It also connects some ligaments and tendons.

Most cartilage is comprised of type II collagen, but this is often replaced with type I collagen or scar tissue during healing. Scar tissue forms faster than cartilage can regenerate. Joints must be protected from heavy loads and conformation of the joint maintained for regeneration.

Reassessing the Status of Joints

There are 3 primary types of **joints** in the body:

- *Amphiarthrodial*: a slightly moveable joint, such as the pelvis
- *Synarthrodial*: an unmovable joint, such as the skull
- *Diarthrodial* (synovial): a freely moveable joint, such as the elbow and knee

Diarthrodial joints are the most commonly injured. The capsules of these joints are lined with synovium, a membrane that secretes synovial fluid to lubricate and cushion the joint; however, the synovium does not cover the ends of the bones, which are covered with articular cartilage, and which comprise a collages fiber matrix. There are a number of **diarthrodial joints**:

- *Ball and socket*, with movement in many directions, such as the shoulder and hip joints
- *Hinge,* with movement in one plane, flexion and extension, such as the elbow
- *Biaxial*, with gliding movement, such as the wrist

- ***Condylar***, with movement that rotates as well as flexes and extends, such as the knee
- ***Pivot***: with rotation only, such as the radioulnar area

REASSESSING THE STATUS OF BONES

When **bones** are injured, the inflammatory phase usually lasts 3-4 days. Proliferation begins, and osteoblasts form a soft callus over a 0.5 to 1 month period. Bones usually unite in about 21 days, but the bone is not stable until about the end of the 2nd month. As healing occurs, osteoblasts become chondrocytes, producing cartilage. This cartilage is in turn covered with a fibrous layer by osteogenic cells. Over time, the soft calluses become hard calluses with a cartilage-like appearance, comprised primarily of type I collagen. During the remodeling stage, which may take an additional 3-4 months (total about 6 months), both type I and type II collagen continue to calcify, so that the bone appears more normal in appearance. Normal strength occurs before the remodeling period is completed, usually at about 3 months.

FEMALE ATHLETE TRIAD

Female athletes benefit from exercise, but some may begin to exhibit signs of the **female athlete triad.** This set of conditions requires both education and referral for psychological treatment and counseling, as the condition may be life threatening. The female athlete triad is 3 related conditions that combine to decrease available energy:

- ***Eating disorder:*** Female athletes may suffer from anorexia or other eating disorders, such as binging and purging, or may have a normal intake but exercise excessively without adding nutrition to balance the demands of exercise. They may try to improve performance by losing body fat, and may use laxatives and/or diuretics, putting themselves at increased risk of electrolyte imbalance.
- ***Amenorrhea:*** The body's response to inadequate nutrition and stress causes hormonal changes that lead to menstrual irregularities, including amenorrhea and fertility problems.
- ***Osteoporosis:*** With inadequate nutrition, the metabolic hormones responsible for bone formation are suppressed and menstrual abnormalities decrease estrogen, so bones become brittle.

Healthcare Administration and Professional Responsibility

Evaluating the Goals and Outcomes of the Individual, Stakeholders, and the Organization

Evaluating the goals and outcomes of the individual, stakeholders, and the organization benefits the athletic trainer because it helps the athletic trainer gauge the overall effectiveness of the athletic training program on an individual and organizational level. If the goals of the program are not producing the intended outcomes, then techniques being used can be adjusted to achieve the desired results. It is important for the athletic trainer to ensure all the stakeholders' and organization's goals are being met as this will increase the effectiveness of the program and, therefore, increase its sustainability.

Duties and Responsibilities of the Team Physician

The duties and responsibilities of the **team physician** in providing healthcare are outlined in an informal contract (letter of agreement) that delineates the name of the attending physician, the services the physician will provide to the organization/team, and the availability of the physician. The physician must be a licensed MD or DO in good standing, and must be trained in CPR and provision of care for emergency and traumatic injuries. Specific training in sports medicine is desirable but not required. The agreement should state clearly that the physician is ultimately responsible for decisions regarding the healthcare of the athletes. The physician should agree to meet with the athletic trainer at the beginning of each season to review healthcare plans. The team physician provides counsel regarding transporting injured athletes, but the primary physician makes referrals to specialists and acts as gatekeeper (the person assigned by an insurance company to supervise the athlete's medical care).

Duties and Responsibilities of the Certified Athletic Trainer

The **Certified Athletic Trainer** is responsible for the healthcare of the athlete and for acting in place of the physician in making decisions that are within the scope of responsibility of athletic trainers, assisting both the healthy athlete in order to prevent injury and providing programs to help those who have been injured return safely to play: Duties of the athletic trainer include:

- Preparing the healthcare plan and presenting it to the team physician for consultation and revision as needed.
- Preparing emergency plans.
- Networking with other athletic trainers and healthcare providers.
- Maintaining records and documentation.
- Supervising/managing other staff.
- Ensuring facility safety and making budgetary decisions.
- Working cooperatively with other members of the organization, such as coaches.
- Developing rehabilitation and reconditioning programs for the injured.
- Supervising athletic training exercises.
- Applying bandages, wraps, and braces to prevent injury.
- Massaging and monitoring muscle mass and muscle injury.

Developing a Business Plan

A **business plan** should be composed after a period of planning to determine the type and extent that will fit the needs of the organization. Components may include:

- ***Introduction:*** This should be an overview of the missions, goals, structure, and ownership as well as details about the business. It should include a description of the facilities, needs, equipment, and services that will be rendered.
- ***Marketing:*** This should describe the services, the results of market survey indicating the demand for these services, advertising strategies, and pricing. It may include information about competitors and projections.
- ***Finances:*** This includes capital requirements, the yearly and monthly budget, and estimates of cash flow.
- ***Management:*** This relates to the day-to-day running of the business and includes the organizational structure and personnel issues, such as wages, hiring, supervision, accounting procedures, and record keeping.

Planning and Designing Facilities

The Certified Athletic Trainer, architect, and administration work together during the **planning and designing** of facilities. The overall philosophy and goals of the administration related to the type of facility, use, and population served must be balanced by the athletic trainer's philosophy in relation to the use of the facility in relation to space, flow, staff, lockers, access, and hours. Important issues include:

- ***Space allocation:*** This begins with designation of program areas, activities, and equipment in each area. Square footage is calculated by 2-3 square feet per individual at peak times (not including equipment space).
- ***Special requirements:*** Floor coverings, ceiling types and heights, electrical outlets, door widths, ventilation, workstations, cabinets, plumbing, and wall coverings must be considered.
- ***American with Disabilities Act, Title III:*** Facility planning must include ADA compliance related to necessary ramps, curb cuts, access, telephones, bathrooms, towel dispensers, warning lights, and water fountains.

Planning and Designing Program Areas

There are a number of general considerations, such as color, lighting, ventilation, and electrical outlets for all areas of the facility, but the needs for specific **program areas** must be considered:

- ***Taping***: This is often a busy area, so it must not impede traffic flow and must contain tables, benches, sink, and counter area. Space should be allocated based on peak load. It should be near the entrance for easy access.
- ***Clinical treatment:*** This area contains treatment tables, supply carts, and cabinets, and must provide privacy partitions or curtains while allowing supervision of staff.
- ***Rehabilitation/Training:*** This area houses large equipment and requires exercise space and carpeted exercise floors (wood floors may splinter), usually between 1000 and 1200 square feet.
- ***Hydrotherapy:*** This comprises whirlpools, sink, ice machines and special ventilation to control humidity. The size is determined by the amount and type of equipment. Non-slip flooring and properly elevated and grounded electrical outlets are critical.

- ***Physical examination:*** This area usually includes examining table, x-ray viewing boxes, sink, cabinet, and dry-erase board, and must accommodate a number of people. If suturing is done in this area, then there may be specific lighting requirements (100-200 foot-candle equivalent).
- ***Pharmacy:*** This area, which dispenses prescription drugs, may be available in some facilities. It must be a separate enclosed area that can be secured and that has adequate storage and refrigeration. The Certified Athletic Trainer cannot dispense prescription drugs.
- ***Dental:*** The size is determined by the type of equipment, and must include a sink, counters, and cabinets.
- ***Storage:*** This area, with cabinets and shelving, will vary in size depending upon the extent and types of equipment stored. In areas with 4 distinct seasons, out-of-season equipment may be stored. Temperature and ventilation control may be necessary to protect equipment and materials.
- ***Office:*** This space (one or multiple offices) includes room for desk(s), chairs, and file storage, with windows into the training area to allow line-of-sight supervision.
- ***Locker rooms:*** The number of lockers and showers, as well as the need for separate facilities for male and female athletes, must be considered in the light of peak occupancy. There must be hooks for clothing and towels near the showers, and ventilation must be adequate to control humidity.
- ***Conference room:*** This space is determined by the types of meeting, the number of people that must be accommodated, and the seating arrangement, often a large table with chairs.
- ***Pool:*** If included, it must be ADA-compliant with graduated depths to 7 feet, must be surrounded by non-slip surface with temperature and filtering controls (and space), and must have line-of-sight supervision
- ***X-ray room:*** This space must be lead-shielded and adequate for the type of x-ray equipment used.

MANAGEMENT STYLES

Studies have indicated that the **management styles** of athletic trainers mirror those of people in other professions. There are a number of different leadership styles:

- ***Charismatic:*** Depends upon personal charisma to influence people and may be very persuasive. However, this type of leader may engage "followers" and relate to one group rather than to the organization at large, limiting effectiveness.
- ***Bureaucratic*** (Inspection/production): Follows organization rules exactly and expects everyone else to do so. This is most effective in handling cash flow or managing work in dangerous work environments. This type of leadership may engender respect, but may not be conducive to change.
- ***Autocratic:*** Makes decisions independently and strictly enforces rules, but team members often feel left out of the process and may not be supportive. This type of leadership is most effective in crisis situations but may have difficulty gaining the commitment of staff.
- ***Consultative:*** Presents a decision and welcomes input and questions, although decisions rarely change. This type of leadership is most effective when gaining the support of staff is critical to the success of proposed changes.
- ***Participatory*** (developmental): Presents a potential decision and then makes final decision based on input from staff or teams. This type of leadership is time-consuming and may result in compromises that are not wholly satisfactory to management or staff, but the process is motivating to staff who feel their expertise is valued.

- ***Democratic***: Presents a problem and asks staff or teams to arrive at a solution, although the leader usually makes the final decision. This type of leadership may delay decision-making, but staff and teams are often more committed to the solutions because of their input.
- ***Laissez-faire*** (free rein/impoverished): Exerts little direct control, but allows employees/teams to make decisions with little interference. This may be effective leadership if teams are highly skilled and motivated, but in many cases this type of leadership is the product of poor management skills and little ends up being accomplished.

PERFORMANCE APPRAISAL

Performance appraisal must be documented regularly in order to ensure quality, determine staffing needs, meet legal requirements (such as gender equity), decide promotions, and provide feedback to employees. Performance measures must relate directly to the work performed and must be accurate descriptions of past performance and predictive of future performance in order to be legally valid. Performance appraisal must be uniform across an organization with clear explanations of criteria, and should be objective (with data) when possible. Methods used include:

- ***Comparative:*** Employees are compared against each other and rated from best to worst; however, this always means that some rank low even when all function effectively.
- ***Attributive***: Employees are rated individually on scales of attributes, such as leadership. Attributes should relate to job requirements.
- ***Behavioral:*** Employees are assessed as to how they perform the behaviors necessary for their particular work.
- ***Results:*** Employees are assessed in relation to their abilities to reach the strategic goals established by administration and employees.

CONFLICT RESOLUTION

Conflict is an inevitable result of teamwork, and the Certified Athletic Trainer must assume responsibility for **conflict resolution.** While conflicts can be disruptive, they can produce positive outcomes by forcing team members to listen to different perspectives and to initiate dialogue. The best time for conflict resolution is when differences emerge, but before open conflict and the hardening of positions occur. The leader must pay close attention to the people and problems involved, listen carefully, and reassure those involved that their points of view are understood. The following are basic steps of conflict resolution:

- Allow both sides to present their case without bias, maintaining a focus on opinions rather than individuals.
- Encourage cooperation through negotiation and compromise.
- Maintain the focus, providing guidance to keep the discussions on track, and avoid arguments.
- Evaluate the need for renegotiation, formal resolution process, or third-party intervention.
- Utilize humor and empathy to defuse escalating tensions.

HEALTHCARE FACILITY BUDGETS

A healthcare facility budget is often part of a larger organizational budget, so an understanding of the different **types of budgets** utilized in healthcare management is helpful:

- ***Operating budget***: This budget is used for daily operations and includes general expenses, such as salaries, education, insurance, maintenance, depreciation, debts, and profit. The budget has 3 elements: statistics, expenses, and revenue.

- **Capital budget:** This budget determines which capital projects (such as remodeling, repairing, and purchasing of equipment or buildings) will be allocated funding for the year. These capital expenditures are usually based on cost-benefit analysis and prioritization of needs.
- **Cash balance budget:** This type of budget projects cash balances for a specific future time period, including all operating and capital budget items.
- **Master budget:** This budget combines operating, capital, and cash balance budgets, as well as any specialized or area-specific budgets.

Approaches to Operational Budgeting

Most **facility budgets** will be operational, but there are a number of different approaches that can be used:

- **Fixed/forecast:** Revenue and expenses are forecast for the entire budget period, and budget items are fixed.
- **Flexible:** Estimates are made regarding anticipated changes in revenue and expenses, and both fixed and variable costs are identified.
- **Zero-based:** All cost centers are re-evaluated each budget period to determine if they should be funded or eliminated, partially or completely.
- **Responsibility center:** Budgeting is a cost center (department) or centers, with one person holding overall responsibility.
- **Program:** Organizational programs are identified, and revenues and costs for each program are budgeted.
- **Appropriations:** Government funds are requested and dispersed through this process (when applicable).
- **Continuous/rolling:** Periodic updates to the budget, including revenues, costs, and volume, are calculated prior to the next budget cycle.

Inventory and Purchasing

Inventory is the stock of materials or equipment on hand. Inventories should be tabulated at least once a year. In many cases, reordering is done when inventory of a particular item drops to a certain pre-established count. Just-in-time ordering, however, waits until inventory stock is almost depleted. These types of automatic reordering of supplies are easier with computerized inventories. In some cases, trainers have open accounts that can be used for small purchases without bidding. For larger purchases (especially in public institutions), the trainer should state the items (including brand names when appropriate) to be purchased on a bid form. Then, the bids are sent to prospective bidders (at least 3) in a competitive bid process. The definition of an acceptable varies by organization. Some only accept the low bid, while others accept the best bid (such as those supplying brand names rather than substituting with generic products). Many organizations have private purchase plans that allow them to purchase directly without bids or lease equipment, which is less expensive initially.

Seeking Employment

There are a number of steps involved in **seeking employment** as an athletic trainer:

- **Job search:** This includes review of sports publications, Internet search, convention job notices, and contact with local schools, universities, gyms, and organizations with sports healthcare programs.

- ***Résumé:*** The chronological format with employment and education listed from last to first (reverse order) is most common, but a functional format highlighting training and skills may be more appropriate for those entering the profession. Application: The application form should be filled out electronically or neatly in black permanent ink. It must be complete and include all addenda as required, for instance letters of recommendation or transcripts.
- ***Cover letter:*** This should be well-written, grammatical, and serve as an introduction of the applicant. The applicant may include more information about motivation and interests than may fit on the formal application.
- ***Interview:*** The applicant should answer questions completely, maintain eye contact, and dress, speak, and act professionally.
- ***Letter of appreciation:*** This is sent after the interview.

INTERVIEWS

Interviews are the most important step in gaining employment as an athletic trainer; the request for an interview acknowledges that the person has met the minimum requirements, based on paper screening of the application. In all cases, a professional appearance and demeanor and complete answering of questions is imperative. The applicant should come prepared to ask questions about the job and its benefits. Rehearsing possible interview questions (strong and weak points) or going through mock interviews can provide invaluable practice in maintaining eye contact, shaking hands, and not fidgeting. Some interviews include demonstrations or presentations. If the applicant is given time to plan, these should be carefully planned and practiced so that they appear professional. The applicant should attempt to learn as much as possible about an organization prior to the interview, so that his or her answers can reflect the needs of the organization. If possible, an onsite visit should be made before the interview.

There are 3 primary types of **interviews**:

- ***Screening:*** People are asked questions directly related to experience and skills to determine whether they meet the qualifications for the position. These screening interviews are often conducted by telephone. In some cases, screening takes the form of computerized or written testing. Those who pass the screening interview usually go to the next round of interviews.
- ***Contact:*** These may take place at a variety of locations and usually involve one interviewer who asks questions and observes the applicant to determine the possibility of hiring.
- ***Panel/group/onsite:*** Public institutions, such as universities, often have hiring committees, and interviews are conducted by panels. In other organizations, an interview may be conducted by 2 or 3 people. It's important to look directly at the person asking the question, but to respond to every member of the panel or group, making eye contact with each individually. In some cases, the applicant may have 2 or 3 interviews, each with a different set of people.

TIME MANAGEMENT

Time management is an important function of leaders for managing their own time, modeling time management, and utilizing the time of others effectively. Steps of time management include:

- ***Plan:*** Create goals and establish schedules for yearly, monthly, and daily activities. Plan for each day in advance.
- ***Create task list:*** A daily list should be created/updated, including routine tasks, so that all can be completed.

- ***Prioritize***: Determine the order in which tasks need to be accomplished, beginning with high-priority items.
- ***Minimize paper handling:*** Try to handle papers/tasks once only, instead of shuffling them about and dealing with them repeatedly.
- ***Utilize time effectively:*** Avoid wasting time. Start meetings on schedule and monitor time. Work efficiently, paying attention to necessary details only.
- ***Delegate***: Determine which tasks can be assigned to others.
- ***Utilize computerized technology***: Avoid paper when possible. Keep calendars and lists on the computer for easy updating. Utilize email and the Internet.
- ***Avoid procrastination***: Eliminate time-wasting activities.

Promotion and Public Relations

Athletic trainers are relatively new to the medical and health professions, and many people are unaware of the services they provide. For this reason, athletic trainers should **promote** the profession and title (Certified Athletic Trainer), and plan ways to improve **public relations** and provide information. Trainers should remember to wear professional and appropriate attire when engaged in promotional activities. Activities may include:

- Presentations to physicians and other medical personnel.
- Development of sports teams or groups.
- Websites.
- Advertising: print, radio, TV, or Internet.
- Sponsoring local sports teams, youth recreational activities, and sports events.
- Developing brochures, pamphlets, leaflets, and other educational materials.
- Participating in speaker's bureaus.
- Setting up booths in health fairs.
- Participating in career days at local schools and universities.
- Hosting open-house receptions.

Empowerment

One of the goals of athletic management is to provide staff with the tools people need for **empowerment**. This helps to establish an environment of mutual respect. Empowering others does not mean that management loses authority or the leadership role; rather, sharing responsibilities allows management to work with others to set goals and establish a clear vision for the organization. Empowerment includes encouraging participation in policy making and allowing staff members to take active roles in patient management. Empowerment requires an investment in time and education, so that people are properly trained to assume responsibility and have a clear understanding of the parameters of their authority. Staff members must feel that they have the support of management. Empowerment should be encouraged for patients and families as well, allowing them to participate in decisions about their care as much as possible.

Cultural Diversity

Issues of **cultural diversity** must be an integral and continuous part of the plan of treatment. Individuals vary considerably in their attitudes, so assuming that all members of an ethnic or cultural group share the same values is never appropriate. The individual must be assessed as well as the group. However, basic cultural guidelines should be available to staff, addressing issues such as eye contact, proximity, and gestures. It is important to take time to observe family dynamics and language barriers, arranging for translators if necessary to ensure adequate communication. In patriarchal cultures (such as the Mexican culture) the eldest male may speak for the patient. In some Muslim cultures, females will resist care by males. The attitudes and beliefs of the athlete in relation to care and treatment must be understood, accepted, and treated with respect. In some cases, the use of traditional healers must be incorporated into a plan of treatment.

Leadership Skills

There are a number of **leadership skills** that are needed to facilitate and coordinate the activities of staff members.

- Communicating openly is essential: all members should be encouraged to participate.
- Avoid interrupting or interpreting the point another is trying to make, as this will inhibit the free flow of ideas.
- Avoiding jumping to conclusions, which can effectively shut off communication.
- Active listening means paying attention and asking questions for clarification rather than to challenge other's ideas.
- Respecting others' opinions and ideas, even when opposed to one's own, is absolutely essential.
- Reacting and responding to facts rather than feelings allows one to avoid angry confrontations and defuse anger.
- Clarifying information or opinions stated can help avoid misunderstandings.
- Keeping unsolicited advice out of the conversation shows respect for others and allows them to solicit advice without feeling pressured.

Burnout

There are a number of different theories about **burnout** at work, and a number of ways to categorize the steps involved. All of these theories have a few things in common:

- ***Period of high expectation:*** This is sometimes referred to as the honeymoon period, when the person may have unrealistic expectations and feel very positive about the work and the position.
- ***Changing perception:*** The person begins to realize that expectations are not being met, and that there are problems that cannot be easily resolved. The person may begin to feel disillusioned and frustrated.
- ***Chronic fatigue and escape:*** The person begins to lose sleep and change behaviors, sometimes indulging in self-destructive behaviors, such as substance abuse or risk-taking. The person may become depressed and critical of the work and of other employees.
- ***Despair and exhaustion:*** This final phase of burnout usually occurs after 3-4 years, but it can have a profound impact on the person's emotional and physical health, sometimes resulting in suicide or stroke. Employees in this stage become very pessimistic and lose hope.

Factors Contributing to Occupational Stress

There are a number of factors that contribute to **occupational stress** for athletic trainers:

- ***Overload:*** Sometimes trainers are simply overwhelmed by the amount and difficulty of the work that needs to be done. Trainers often try to cope by working harder and faster or putting in extra hours, but this only increases stress.
- ***Organizational role:*** Frustration often occurs if the trainers are unsure of their roles or what the organization expects. Trainers may be caught between others in conflict, such as coaches and athletes.

- ***Job security:*** It can be difficult to advance in this field, since there are few high-status jobs and few jobs in administration. The trainer may be at the mercy of an unsupportive supervisor. Women, especially, may have limited opportunities in some sports fields.
- ***Lack of input:*** Trainers may be left out of the decision-making loop, leading to increasing frustration.

COPING WITH OCCUPATIONAL STRESS AND PREVENTING BURNOUT

There are a number of methods to cope with occupational stress and **prevent burnout** at work:

- ***Work schedule:*** Sticking to a reasonable workweek is very important, so trainers should review the employment regulations related to work hours and breaks and avoid putting in extra hours.
- ***Interests:*** Trainer must develop outside interests and take time for family and friends to keep life in balance.
- ***Time management:*** Trainers should review processes to determine if they are making the best use of time and must seek ways to make work more time-efficient.
- ***Job description:*** Trainers should review their job description (or request one) to determine if it is reasonable or needs revision.
- ***Dialogue:*** Trainers must communicate with others. Supervisors or other personnel may be unaware of work-related problems.
- ***Assistance:*** Trainers may need counseling, mediation, or other assistance to help them to put work into proper perspective.

PROFESSIONAL NETWORKING

Networking, creating a network of contacts throughout the sports industry and healthcare community, not only helps a trainer to find employment but also provides valuable professional resources. Networking should begin with professors and instructors while the trainer is still a student. The trainer can cooperate with others involved in clinical tasks or research, gaining experience and credibility. Equipment salesmen are invaluable resources that can provide the trainer with information about the current trends. One of the most effective ways to network is to become involved in national organizations, such as the National Athletic Trainer's Association, and to participate in conferences through attendance and conference presentations. The trainer should make an effort to maintain periodic contact with those in an informal network by telephone, mail, or email.

ADDRESSING RISKS AND ORGANIZATIONAL NEEDS BY DEVELOPING, REVIEWING, AND REVISING POLICIES

Developing, reviewing, and revising policies that address risks and organizational needs benefits the athletic trainer because it can help the athletic trainer to be more effective in managing risks and meeting the needs of the organization. To manage the risks inherent with physical activity, specific policies should be put into place so that unnecessary risks are not being taken and unavoidable risks have specific plans set in place to properly manage them. For example, a lightning policy should be developed, reviewed, and revised to keep up-to-date with best practices. Policies should be developed to ensure organizational needs are being met and should be revised as the needs of the organization change. For example, if organizational expansion occurs, it is possible that more sports and athletic facilities will be added, therefore increasing the needs of the organization. New policies will need to be collaboratively developed to ensure risks are minimized and emergency action planning is in place for all sports and athletic facilities.

Human Resource Best Practices

Employing the most qualified personnel helps to ensure the success of athletic training programs. Therefore, consideration and effort should be put into recruiting, hiring, and retaining the best personnel possible. Federal laws mandate many human resource policies and must be followed. To comply with the Equal Employment Opportunity Commission when recruiting and hiring applicants, all qualified applicants must receive equal consideration for the position they are applying for regardless of their race, nationality, gender, religion, or sexual preference. Job descriptions, chain of command, and a code of conduct should be well developed and in writing. Regular performance evaluations should be performed that focus on strengths, as well as weaknesses, and a collaborative plan should be developed to improve any weaknesses.

Liability and Negligence

Liability is legal responsibility for harm caused to another person. Negligence is failure to provide the reasonable care that someone with similar training would provide. When an athletic trainer is sued, the lawsuit usually is for a claim of negligence. For the defendant to be found guilty of negligence, the plaintiff must prove four things. They are that the defendant had a duty to provide care to plaintiff, proper care was not given, the injury was caused directly by the defendant not providing reasonable care, and damage resulted. An example of a possible lawsuit for negligence would be if an athletic trainer did not provide proper advanced emergency medical care for an injured patient, moved them from the playing field, and in so doing caused further injury to occur.

Statutes of Limitation

Statutes of limitation provide a set amount of time that a plaintiff can sue for damages that resulted from negligence. The athletic trainer should be aware of the statutes of limitations for the state in which they practice, as they vary from state to state. Most statutes of limitation are for a period of one to five years. The statute of limitation begins once the negligent act is committed or once the plaintiff becomes aware of the damage that occurred from the negligent act. However, in some states special considerations for minors exist that extends the statutes of limitation up to three years after the person turns 18 years old. The athletic trainer must keep all medical documentation at least until the statute of limitation expires for the population for which they provide care.

Reducing the Risk of Litigation

There are many steps athletic trainers should take to reduce the risk of litigation. Good working relationships should be established with all involved parties including athletes, parents, coaching staff, administrators, and the team physician. Emergency action planning should be established, reviewed, and followed. The athletic training clinic should be carefully supervised and thorough documentation should be kept that includes safety measures being taken, injury evaluations, and all rehabilitation. Confidentiality must be maintained, professional liability insurance should be in place, and directions from the team physician must be followed.

Athletic trainers must not allow themselves to be pressured into allowing an injured patient to compete before the patient is physiologically and psychologically prepared to compete. Athletic trainers cannot dispense prescription drugs and extreme caution must be followed in administration of non-prescription drugs if allowed by the state. If caring for minors, the athletic trainer should obtain consent-to-treat from parents or guardians prior to the start of activity. Athletic trainers must know the limitations of their scope of practice and perform only the actions they are allowed to within their state.

Requirements to Become a Certified Athletic Trainer

The National Athletic Trainers' Association Board of Certification has developed requirements that must be successfully completed for a person to become a certified athletic trainer. This includes successful completion of a CAATE-approved, entry-level athletic training education program, practical experience in the clinical setting, and a passing score on the national BOC exam. A candidate in their last semester of their athletic training education program can take the BOC exam if their Program Director confirms that they are within one semester of graduating. BOC certification gives the athletic trainer the credential ATC (Athletic Trainer Certified) and is usually required to obtain a license or certificate to practice athletic training in the state in which they reside.

Continuing Education Requirements to Maintain Certification

To maintain national certification, athletic trainers must earn a minimum of 50 continuing education units (CEUs) during a two-year cycle. Ten of those CEUs must be approved evidence-based-practice courses. Many CEUs available to athletic trainers including approved evidence-based courses can be found on the Board of Certification's (BOC) website. Athletic trainers must also have current CPR and AED certification. The BOC's website lists accepted CPR and AED certifications for athletic trainers. CEUs can be earned in a variety of ways such as attending conferences, seminars, online study courses, and writing research articles for professional magazines. Athletic trainers must also be aware of their specific state requirements they need to follow to maintain their state athletic training licensure, certification, or registration. These requirements vary by state and can be found on the website of the organization that manages the athletic training profession of that state.

NCAA's Drug-Testing Policy

The NCAA has enacted drug-testing policies to protect athletes and ensure a fair and level playing field. Random, mandatory drug testing of athletes is performed during the year as well as during and after NCAA championship competitions. All NCAA athletes must sign a consent form stating they will comply with the drug-testing program. If an athlete is selected to complete a drug test, they must show identification and then urinate in two specimen containers while being directly observed. The specimen containers are then sealed and sent to a NCAA laboratory that performs the drug testing. If the first specimen tests positive for banned substances, the second specimen will then be tested for confirmation. If an athlete has a positive drug test, they will be banned from participation in the NCAA for at least a year and must comply with continued drug testing to return to competition once their suspension has ended.

Corporate Drug-Testing Program

Athletic trainers may manage drug-testing programs in various employment settings such as corporations and clinics. These drug-testing programs can range from performing basic pre-employment drug screenings to full-service drug testing programs in compliance with federal requirements. Drug-testing programs ensure safety is kept as a priority at the workplace by ensuring employees do not work under the influence of drugs or alcohol. They also deter drug users from applying for and obtaining employment with the company. To maintain legal defensibility, only federally certified laboratories should be used to screen for drugs and if a positive test is found, it must be verified by a medical review department.

Purchasing, Budgeting, and Inventorying Supplies

Athletic training program budgets vary considerably, however, several practices can be employed to ensure good fiscal management is a priority. For example, organizational goals and immediate needs should be considered to ensure purchases stay in line with the present needs of the organization. Budget and purchasing records should be kept to assist the athletic trainer in predicting what supplies will be needed. When making purchases, either a direct buy or a competitive bid can be used. When using a competitive bid, vendors offer price quotes for the supplies needed by the athletic training program. Usually the vendor offering the lowest bid gets the business, which can save the athletic training program considerable funds.

There are different categories for supplies used in athletic training clinics. Expendables are items that cannot be reused, such as athletic tape and gauze. Non-expendables are supplies that can be reused, such as ankle braces and compression wraps. Equipment is items that can be used for many years, such as athletic training kits and ice machines.

Designing an Athletic Training Clinic

The design of athletic training clinics varies based on the needs of the organization, the scope of the athletic training program, and the number of athletes that will receive care. If an athletic trainer is given the opportunity to assist in the design of an athletic training clinic, they should work with the architects to ensure the best layout to serve the patient population is developed. All areas of the athletic training clinic should be able to be supervised by the athletic training staff to ensure patient safety. If possible, several types of areas should be considered within the plan.

A taping and bandaging area could be included and should have taping tables, stools, a sink, storage cabinets, and all needed supplies. An electrotherapy area could be designed for electrical modalities and should have grounded outlets and a locking storage cabinet for equipment and supplies. A hydrotherapy area could be developed for whirlpools and the floors should be sloped toward a floor drain. Electrical outlets in this area should have ground fault interrupters, be four-to-five feet above the ground, have spring-locked covers, and water spray deflectors. An area for rehabilitative exercises could be designed and should have room for all the needed exercise equipment and space for patients to safely perform therapeutic exercises.

Commission for Accreditation of Athletic Training Education

The Commission for Accreditation of Athletic Training Education (CAATE) serves as the accrediting agency for athletic training education programs and has served in this capacity since 2006. CAATE accreditation ensures athletic training education programs meet national educational standards to provide quality education. Ensuring athletic training education programs comply with CAATE standards has had many positive affects for the field of athletic training. For example, advancements have been made in the incorporation of athletic training in nontraditional settings and improvements in insurance billing have been made as well. In 2015, it was decided that future entry-level athletic training education programs will be master's degree programs.

Maintaining a Profitable Business

To maintain a profitable business, much planning, implementation, evaluating, and revising must be done. Ultimately, businesses must ensure a positive accounts-payable-to-accounts-receivable ratio is achieved and maintained, which signifies more money is being made than is being paid out in expenses. Other important business planning includes establishing organizational goals, developing plans to achieve those goals, determining a working budget, and developing long-term financial planning. Contracts can be created with insurance companies to improve business. Billing systems that comply with current third-party reimbursement regulations must be established and maintained. Beyond all these measures, quality patient care must be of top priority in all healthcare business endeavors.

Long-Range Planning vs. Strategic Action Plan

Long-range planning identifies end goals, such as where the organization plans to be in 5 or 10 years. These long-range goals help to establish the direction of strategic action plans. Long-range planning implies a certain degree of stability (such as a dependable source of income and adequate staffing) and must be balanced by planning that considers the dynamics of change.

Strategic action planning recognizes the reality of changes and provides a plan for informed response. Strategic action planning identifies organizational purpose, effective use of resources, organizational focus, base measurements, efficiency efforts, staff cohesion, and team building. Strategic action planning must consider:

- Internal and external forces.
- Analysis of history and performance.
- The range of functions and possible extent of integration.
- Personnel and management issues.
- Effective research and planning models.
- Creative approaches to problem solving.

Components of a Strategic Action Plan

The **strategic action plan** may vary from one organization to another, but there are common elements in most plans:

- *Assessment:* This includes lists of both the strengths of the organization as well as areas that have the potential for improvement. Internal (funding, support) and external (competition, economy) threats to the organization must be considered, as well as opportunities,
- *Vision/Policy statement:* This incorporates the goals of long-range planning, determining where the organization wants to be in 5-10 years.
- *Mission statement*: This describes the overall purpose of the organization and delineates its role.
- *Value statement:* This outlines the standards by which the organization establishes values, such as complying with NATA standards.
- *Goals and objectives:* These indicate desired and measurable outcomes in a specified period of time (usually 1-3 years).
- *Action plans:* These are the specific steps that must be taken to meet the goals and objectives, in keeping with the mission and value statements.

Emergency Care Plan

Each organization needs an **emergency care plan** that outlines exactly the care that must be provided in any emergent event, including response to natural/environmental disasters as well as medical emergencies like cardiac arrest. The care plan should cover these areas:

- *Materials and equipment:* This includes the number and location of emergency kits, consent and transfer forms, and maps that indicate access, exits, and locations of keys or other equipment.
- *Identification of emergency response team:* Key personnel as well as qualifications, lines of authority, and individual responsibility must be delineated. Roles include team physician, facilitator or supervisor, care providers, traffic coordinator (to manage observers), EMS contact person, and emergency vehicle monitor/escort.

- ***Procedures****:* Detailed procedures for dealing with different types of emergencies must be outlined, in addition to plans for contacting team members and a list of the type of information that can be divulged.
- ***Contingency plans:*** This includes planning for out-of-town emergencies or alternate plans if key personnel are absent.

RISK MANAGEMENT

Risk management is an organized and formal method of decreasing liability, financial loss, and harm to athletes, staff, or others by performing an assessment of risk and implementing risk management strategies. Risk management must address security, fire, and emergency plans. Decreasing risk involves stopping an activity, sharing risk, or evaluating/revising activity. Risk management focuses first on preventing injury and ensuring adequate supervision:

- ***Risk identification*** begins with an assessment of processes to identify and prioritize those that require further study to determine risk exposure.
- ***Risk analysis*** requires a careful documenting of process, utilizing flow charts, with each step in the process assessed for potential risks. This may utilize root cause analysis methods.
- ***Risk prevention*** involves instituting corrective or preventive processes. Responsible individuals or teams are identified and trained.
- ***Assessment/evaluation*** of corrective/preventive processes is ongoing to determine whether the processes are effective or require modification.

DETERMINATION OF NEGLIGENCE IN RISK MANAGEMENT

Risk management must attempt to determine the burden of proof for acts of **negligence**, including compliance with duty, breaches in procedure, degree of harm, and cause. Negligence indicates that *proper care* has not been provided, based on established standards. *Reasonable care* provisions establish the rationale for decision-making in relation to providing care. State regulations regarding negligence may vary, but all have some statute of limitation (time limit allowed for suing).

There are a number of different types of negligence:

- ***Negligent conduct*** is when an individual fails to provide reasonable care or to protect/assist another, based on standards and expertise.
- ***Gross negligence*** is willfully providing inadequate care while disregarding the safety and security of another.
- ***Contributory negligence*** is when the injured party contributes to his/her own harm.
- ***Comparative negligence*** attempts to determine what percentage amount of negligence is attributed to each individual involved.

RISK ISSUES

There are a number of **risk issues** about which the Certified Athletic Trainer must be aware:

- ***Statute of limitation:*** Each state specifies the length of time after injury when a person can file suit for negligence/malpractice. The period is usually 1-3 years where Certified Athletic Trainers are licensed and covered by malpractice laws, but there may be no statute of limitation in other states. If the athlete is a minor, in most states, the statute of limitation is "tolled": that is, it is delayed until age 18 or a specific age set by the law. Trainers should maintain all records to the maximum year covered by a statute of limitation.

- **Assumption of risk:** This assumes that the athlete knew about the dangers of an activity before participating, and was fully informed of ALL risks and outcomes, such as those involved in returning to play after injury.
    - *Express:* Athlete agrees in advance not to hold the trainer/facility liable for injury.
    - *Implied:* Athlete has witnessed an event, is aware of dangers, and participates.

STANDARD OF CARE AND SCOPE OF PRACTICE

Standard of care refers to the minimum level of care that must be provided to an athlete/patient. Certified Athletic Trainers are professionals who must, at minimum, have a bachelor's degree in athletic training, and the American Medical Association and the American Hospital Association have recognized Certified Athletic Trainers by providing CPT and UB billing codes. However, states vary in **scopes of practice** (that is, the services the athletic trainer is allowed to provide), and the scope of practice of a particular state may not include all of those competencies that are required by the National Athletic Trainer's Association. Those states that require licensure to practice have a qualifying exam, while those that mandate registration require evidence that standards of eligibility have been met. The Board of Certification (BOC) provides examinations to certify athletic trainers in 7 direct standards and 8 service program standards. BOC certification is different from state certification, although many states have contracted to use the BOC examination.

ESTABLISHING THAT THE STANDARD OF CARE HAS BEEN PROVIDED

There are a number of criteria for establishing that the **standard of care** has been provided:

- Standards of care should be in keeping with the usual practice of professionals within the local area.
- The trainer must act with an adequate level of skill in providing care, but success can never be guaranteed.
- When there are multiple accepted treatment options, the trainer may choose among them.
- Specialists, such as orthopedists, are expected to perform at a higher level and are held to higher standards than non-specialists.
- Lack of experience does not excuse errors, as those newly certified or licensed are held to the same standards as those who are experienced in the profession.
- Courts may determine which standards are negligent.
- With the exception of emergency treatment, trainers must always ensure that the athlete has made informed consent and has been apprised of all risks.

MANAGEMENT OF TRAINING FACILITIES

Management of training facilities includes management of people, the facility, and the equipment. There are issues that must be resolved:

- Establishing policies (basic principles) and procedures (action process), and providing these in written form in a manual for standardization.
- Determining the population to be served. In some cases, the organization (such as a school) will determine the population, but in other cases population may derive from referrals or companies. This population must be considered when establishing policies and procedures.
- Establishing guidelines for use of the facility, such as maintaining standards through confidentiality, standard precautions, and respect for the individual. This includes establishing rules of conduct and access to the training facility.

- Establishing standard operating procedures for treatment, documentation, and billing.
- Supervising human resources issues, such as hiring, firing, training, sexual harassment, lines of authority, and scheduling personnel.

PRINCIPLES OF ADULT LEARNING THAT FACILITATE TEACHING, TRAINING, AND MAKING PRESENTATIONS

Part of a Certified Athletic Trainer's professional responsibility is to teach, train, and make presentations. There are some **principles of adult learning** that a trainer should consider when planning strategies for teaching:

- **Practical and goal-oriented:**
    - Provide overviews, summaries and examples.
    - Use collaborative discussions with problem-solving exercises.
    - Remain organized, with the goal in mind.
- **Self-directed:**
    - Allow active involvement; ask for input.
    - Allow different options for achieving the goal.
    - Give the students responsibility.
- **Knowledgeable:**
    - Show respect for their life experiences/education.
    - Validate their knowledge and ask for feedback.
    - Relate new material to information with which they are familiar.
- **Relevancy-oriented:**
    - Explain how information will be applied on the job.
    - Clearly identify objectives.
- **Motivated:**
    - Provide certificates of professional advancement and/or continuing education credit when possible.

APPROACHES TO TEACHING

There are many **approaches to teaching**, and the athletic trainer must be prepared to present and coordinate a range of educational workshops, lectures, discussions, and one-on-one instruction. Planning time for instruction and workshops should be considered part of the job description. All types of classes may be needed, depending upon the purpose and material:

- *Educational workshops* are usually conducted with small groups, allowing for maximal participation. They are especially good for demonstrations and practice sessions.
- *Lectures* are often used for more academic or detailed information that may include questions and answers but limits discussion. An effective lecture should include some audiovisual support.
- *Discussions* are best with small groups, so that people can actively participate. This is a good setup for problem solving.
- *One-on-one instruction* is especially appropriate for targeted instruction in specific areas.
- *Computer/Internet modules* are good for independent learners.

Required Critical Reading Skills to Evaluate Research

There are a number of steps in **critical reading** that an athletic trainer must use to evaluate research:

- *Consider the source* of the material. If it is in the popular press, it may have little validity compared to something published in a juried journal.
- *Review the author's credentials* to determine if he or she is an expert in the field of study.
- *Determine the thesis*, or the central claim of the research. It should be clearly stated.
- *Examine the organization* of the article, whether it is based on a particular theory, and the type of methodology used.
- *Review the evidence* to determine how it is used to support the main points. Look for statistical evidence and sample size to determine if the findings have wide applicability.
- *Evaluate* the overall article to determine if the information seems credible and useful and should be communicated to others on the staff or put into practice.

Practicing Within Local, State, and National Regulations

Practicing within local, state, and national regulations will protect the athletic trainer by ensuring that best available care is being provided to patients, unnecessary risks are not being taken, and risk of litigation is reduced. There are many rules and regulations that govern the practice of athletic training to establish the appropriate scope of the field of athletic training and to set the standard for how emergency situations prevalent in the field of athletics are managed. Following these local, state, and national guidelines safeguards the athletic trainer and the patients the athletic trainer provides service for. For example, changes have been made detailing the best plans of care for patients suffering from concussions. Following these regulations ensures patients receive the best care available and protects the athletic trainer because they are acting within the nationally accepted guidelines for concussion management.

Organizations Responsible for Establishing Standards of Athletic Training and Sports Safety

There are a number of **organizations** that have established standards and guidelines that are used by Certified Athletic Trainers to ensure ethical, quality care and safety:

- The **National Athletic Trainer's Association** establishes guidelines related to the scope of practice of the athletic trainer, as well as a code of ethics.
- **The National Safety Council** educates people to prevent accidental injury and death, and compiles statistics regarding sports injuries. Education is coupled with supporting statistics, such as the number of people receiving head injuries from sports, and how many lives could be saved with helmets.
- **OSHA** provides regulations regarding safety in the workplace, including proper hygiene for training rooms and equipment.
- The **Hockey Equipment Certification Council (HECC)** sets standards for hockey equipment, such as facemasks.
- The **Commission on Accreditation of Rehabilitation Facilities (CARF)** sets standards for organizations engaging in rehabilitation.

Primary and Secondary Insurance Coverage

There are a number of different types of **insurance** coverage that may be available for training staff and athletes. There may be exclusions for injuries/conditions not covered by the policy, such as overuse syndromes, or for pre-existing conditions. Riders may be added to a policy to override exclusions, with an accompanying increase in premium. Insurance includes:

- ***Primary*** insurance pays all of the costs of injury to a preset dollar or percentage amount (often 80%) of what is considered usual, customary and reasonable (UCR), usually with no deductible. However, premiums are often high, and justifying expenses may require considerable paperwork. Some primary insurance plans include a deductible or co-payment for some types of care, such as doctor or emergency room visits. This insurance may be the athlete's or may be required for the athlete by the school or organization.
- ***Secondary*** insurance pays remaining expenses after the primary insurance benefit. Usually, there are deductibles that must be paid. Typically, the athlete/family carries the primary policy, although some schools provide insurance for athletes.

TYPES OF MANAGED CARE USED TO PROVIDE HEALTHCARE SERVICES

There are a number of different **models** for managed care to provide healthcare services:

- ***Exclusive provider organization (EPO):*** Healthcare providers deliver services at discounted rates to enrolled individuals. Some providers may be prohibited from caring for those not enrolled, and enrollees are only reimbursed for care within the network.
- ***Health maintenance organization (HMO):*** With an HMO, there is a prepaid contract between healthcare providers, payors, and enrollees for specified services in a specified time period, provided by a list of providers, usually representing a variety of specialties.
- ***Point of service plans (POS):*** This is a combination HMO and PPO structure, in which people can receive service within the network but also can opt to seek treatment outside the network in some situations.
- ***Preferred provider organizations: (PPO):*** These are healthcare providers who have agreed to be part of a network that provides services to an enrolled group at reduced rates of reimbursement. Care received outside of the network may be only partially covered.

INFORMED CONSENT AND WAIVERS

Certified Athletic Trainers must be proactive in **reducing risk** and must have a thorough understanding of issues related to informed consent and waivers:

- ***Informed consent:*** Athletes involved in rehabilitation or post-injury reconditioning should sign an informed consent outlining all possible complications that may result from the injury, the rehabilitation, or the reconditioning exercises, as well as return to play. They should be provided an estimate of time for recovery.
- ***Waivers:*** This type of document may be signed by the athlete or a parent or guardian (if the athlete is a minor) and waives the right to sue in return for services/participation. Waivers don't shield the trainer from misconduct or negligence. Waivers should include the responsibilities of the athlete, such as reporting injury immediately.

HEALTH INSURANCE PORTABILITY AND ACCOUNTABILITY ACT

HIPAA regulations are designed to protect the rights of individuals regarding the privacy of their health information. The athletic trainer must not release any information or documentation about an athlete's condition or treatment without consent, as the individual has the right to determine who has access to his or her personal information. Personal information about the athlete is considered protected health information (PHI), and consists of any identifying or personal information about the athlete, such as health history, condition, or treatments in any form, and any documentation, including electronic, verbal, or written. Personal information can be shared with the parents (of a minor), spouse, legal guardians, or those involved in the care of the athlete, such as physicians, without a specific release. However, the athlete should always be consulted if personal information is to be discussed with others present, to ensure there is no objection. Failure to comply with HIPAA regulations can make a trainer liable for legal action.

PROFESSIONAL RELATIONSHIPS WITH EXTERNAL AGENCIES

The athletic trainer must initiate and facilitate involvement with **external agencies,** because many of these have direct impact on athletic care:

- Industry contacts should include other facilities with a shared interest in patient care or medical supply companies. It's important for trainers to have a dialog with companies about their products and equipment in order to determine future needs.
- Payors have a vested interest in containing health care costs, so providing information and representing the interests of the patient is important.
- Community groups may provide resources for athletes and families, both in terms of information and financial assistance.
- Political agencies are increasingly important, as new laws are created regarding standards of care or scope of practice.
- Public health agencies are partners in health care with other facilities and must be included, especially in issues related to communicable disease, which may impact athletes.

NATIONAL ATHLETIC TRAINERS' ASSOCIATION (NATA) CODE OF ETHICS

The NATA code of ethics establishes guidelines athletic trainers must follow to maintain high standards and professionalism in the field of athletic training. The code of ethics is general in nature, contains four principles, and represents the spirit in which athletic trainers should make decisions and conduct themselves for the betterment of the profession.

The first principle states that athletic trainers will respect the rights, welfare, and dignity of all people. This includes not discriminating, providing the best care possible, and protecting patient confidentiality. The second principle states that athletic trainers will follow the laws and regulations that direct the field of athletic training. This includes following all local, state, and federal laws as well as NATA rules and regulations. The third principle states that high standards in patient service will be achieved and maintained. This includes providing only the services that athletic trainers are qualified to provide and participating in continuing education opportunities. The fourth principle states that athletic trainers must not engage in behaviors that reflect negatively on the profession. This includes positioning the needs of the patient over financial gain and maintaining professionalism.

The National Athletic Trainer's Association (NATA) has established a **Code of Ethics** governing the ethical behavior of athletic trainers. **Principles** include:

- **Members shall respect the rights, dignity and welfare of all.**
  - Members must provide competent care, preserve confidentiality, and avoid discrimination.
- **Members shall comply with the laws and regulations governing the practice of athletic training.**
  - Members must abide by all applicable laws and NATA rules and regulations, report illegal or unethical practices, and avoid and/or seek rehabilitation for substance abuse.

- **Members shall maintain and promote high standards in their provision of service.**
  - Members must represent their services correctly, provide only services for which they are qualified, make referrals, participate in continuing education, educate others, and promote ethical conduct in research.
- **Members shall not engage in conduct that could be construed as a conflict of interest or that reflects negatively on the profession.**
  - Members must conduct themselves professionally and avoid exploiting NATA or patients or profiting from sports gambling.

BOARD OF CERTIFICATION (BOC) STANDARDS OF PROFESSIONAL PRACTICE

The **Board of Certification (BOC),** formerly part of the National Athletic Trainer's Association but now independent, has certified athletic trainers since 1989 and has established Standards of Professional Practice, which consist of two parts: Practice Standards (7) and Codes of Professional Responsibility (6). *Practice Standards* include the following:

- Service is provided with direction of a physician.
- Preventive measures are used with all patients.
- Emergency and immediate care must meet common standards.
- Evaluation and diagnosis include patient input and assessment of function.
- Strategies must ensure that treatment, rehabilitation, and reconditioning are appropriate, goal-directed, outcome-based, and include assessment.
- Treatment is terminated when optimal improvement has been reached.
- Record keeping includes documenting all services provided, including details regarding health of the patient.

CODES OF PROFESSIONAL RESPONSIBILITY

As part of the Standards of Professional Practice, the **Board of Certification (BOC)** has established *Codes of Professional Responsibility* with which all trainers must comply. *Codes* include:

- *Patient responsibility:* Trainers must provide care without discrimination, protecting patients from harm, taking action against incompetent or illegal healthcare providers, maintaining confidentiality, communicating clearly and openly, showing respect for the individual, and exercising professional judgment.
- *Competency:* Trainers must strive to improve, obtain continuing education, and comply with BOC policies/requirements.
- *Professional responsibility:* Trainers must comply with all regulations and requirements of the BOC, uphold standards of practice, collaborate with others, report violations, avoid criminal acts, report criminal convictions, and cooperate with BOC investigations.
- *Research:* Trainers must conduct research in an ethical manner following standards of research.
- *Social responsibility:* Trainers serve as positive professional role models in the community.
- *Business practices:* Trainers conduct business in an ethical manner and carry liability insurance.

Services Provided by BOC to State Regulatory Agencies

The **Board of Certification (BOC)** provides a number of **services** to state regulatory agencies:

- Board of Certification (BOC) examination and State Athletic Trainer Examination Program (SATEP) examination for use as state certification examinations
- Online verification and search for Certified Athletic Trainers both within and outside of a state
- Publication of disciplinary actions taken against a Certified Athletic Trainer by the BOC or the state
- Mailing lists according to the specifications of the state
- Contact information and links related to standards of practice for individual states
- Processing of license applications for Certified Athletic Trainers based on state requirements
- Online reporting and accounting of continuing education
- Information for the public about state regulatory board actions
- Customer service and call centers to provide assistance

Professional Practice and Discipline Committee

The **Professional Practice and Discipline (PPD) Committee** is responsible for disciplinary actions related to those who fail to uphold the BOC Standards of Professional Practice. The board has jurisdiction over any BOC Certified Athletic Trainers or those applying for BOC exams. The board reviews allegations against individuals, conducts an investigation, and imposes appropriate sanctions. Actions include:

- ***Conducting investigations if aware of violations or upon receiving an official complaint***. Investigation procedures include conducting an initial review of charges and notifying the person filing the complaint (complainant) and the person about whom the charges are made (respondent) in writing. Confidentiality is maintained during this period, and there are 15 days (with a possible extension to 30 days) allowed for both to respond in writing.
- ***Determination of probable cause***: After reviewing all materials, the PPD Committee either deems there is insufficient evidence to proceed and dismisses charges or processes a charge against the individual.
- ***Processing a Charge letter***: Allegations against the individual are outlined along with descriptions of the standard or code that was purportedly violated. This letter describes the rights of the individual and is transmitted by certified or tracked mail to ensure receipt. The respondent has 30 days (which may be extended to 45 days) to respond in writing. The respondent may request a hearing if he or she wishes to dispute the charges.
- ***Default/failure to respond***: Failure to respond is considered admission of guilt by default.
- ***Consent***: If the respondent admits or fails to dispute charges, then the PPD Committee shall request a Consent Agreement.

Consent Agreements

The **Professional Practice and Discipline (PPD) Committee** may enter into a formal legally binding **Consent Agreement** any time within the investigation of charges against an individual. The Consent Agreement, as well as any modifications made at a later time, must be approved by the PPD Committee, the director, and the individual respondent. By signing the agreement, the person acknowledges that the charges are correct and forfeits appeal within the BOC or the judicial system. The Consent Agreement details the allegations, the codes or practices that were violated, and the action, including suspension or revocation of certification (permanent), to be taken against the individual. The Consent Agreement outlines the degree of confidentiality. In most cases, Consent Agreements are confidential, but in some cases, publication may be indicated for the public good.

CRIMINAL ACTION AND PROFESSIONAL DISCIPLINE

The Certified Athletic Trainer has a duty to report convictions of **criminal actions or professional discipline** (such as suspension of license) to the BOC's Professional Practice and Discipline (PPD) Committee in writing within 10 days, including an original or authenticated copy of court proceedings indicating conviction or letter of disciplinary action from a governmental or regulatory agency:

- *Crimes* include all criminal actions EXCEPT misdemeanor traffic violations, not involving alcohol or drugs.
- *Serious crimes* includes all felonies and misdemeanors regarding public health, provision of health care, athletics/sports, or education, including use of weapons, sale or distribution of controlled substances, and any attempt to influence the outcome of sports events or profit by gambling
- *Professional discipline* includes any type of disciplinary action.

Upon receiving proof of actions against the individual, the PPD will begin an investigation and file a complaint against the respondent, who has no right of hearing if actions are admitted or proven, with appropriate action, such as revocation of certification.

RIGHT TO A HEARING

According to the guidelines/procedures of the **BOC Professional Practice and Discipline (PPD) Committee**, if an individual wishes to refute allegations put forth in a charge, the person can request a **hearing** as long there is no Consent Agreement or proof of conviction of a crime or professional disciplinary action. Hearings are held orally, by conference call, or in person in Omaha, Nebraska (BOC headquarters). Request for the hearing is made through the Hearing Panel, comprised of 3 Certified Athletic Trainers and 2 members of the public. The Hearing Panel schedules the hearing and notifies the respondent of the time, date, and method of communication. During the hearing, an audio recording or transcript is made. The hearing is conducted much like a court case, with examination of evidence, testimony, and cross-examination of witnesses. The Panel renders a decision in writing and sends the respondent a certified letter stating the decision.

APPEAL PROCESS

According to the guidelines/procedures of the **BOC Professional Practice and Discipline (PPD) Committee**, a respondent can **appeal** the decision of the Hearing Panel, but not a Consent Agreement, within 30 days of receiving the decision. The individual must outline the justification for the appeal and desired action. The Executive Director of the BOC may file a response with the appeal, which is sent to the Appeals Panel (comprised of 3 directors). This panel makes a decision without an oral hearing, although written material may be submitted. The Appeals Panel renders a decision in writing, which is sent to the respondent in a certified letter. The Appeals Panel may affirm or reverse PPD Committee decisions, refer the matter back to the PPD Committee for consideration, make modifications in the decision, or vacate a prior finding of guilt by default because of failure to respond to allegations.

Disciplinary Actions

The **BOC Professional Practice and Discipline (PPD) Committee** may impose a number of different **disciplinary actions**:

- **Revocation of certification:** Serious permanent disciplinary action that is made public.
- **Suspension of certification:** Period of up to 5 years. Suspension is made public. Emergency suspensions may be imposed if there is a threat to the public health.
- **Eligibility denial:** Denies the applicant the right to apply for certification permanently or for a prescribed period of time.
- **Censure (private):** Written censure that is not made public.
- **Censure (public):** Written censure that is made public.
- **Probation:** Includes specific restrictions or conditions to be met; may be for up to 3 years, with a required annual report by the respondent.
- **Sanctions:** May include extra training, classes, continuing education (CE) courses, payment of delinquent fees, and annual reports of continuing education courses.
- **Delinquent status:** Relates to failure to complete CE or pay fees, and may include restrictions for up to 6 months, during which fees must be pain and/or CE completed.

Impairment

The **BOC Professional Practice and Discipline (PPD) Committee** takes actions to sanction or restrict the activities of Certified Athletic Trainers who suffer **impairment** as a result of substance abuse (drugs and/or alcohol); or personality (disruptive), psychological, or physical impairment, including loss of mental ability through aging or loss of motor skills. All Certified Athletic Trainers must be capable of performing with competence and safety. The Certified Athletic Trainer must report impairment of others so that early intervention, especially in the event of substance abuse, may be instituted. Sanctions may include mandatory participation in rehabilitation programs. Restrictions may be imposed to ensure that the trainer can practice safely, or certification may be suspended or revoked. If courts or governmental agencies have mandated testing, then the results may be required by the BOC. Monitoring of a restricted trainer must be instituted, and may be conducted by an employer or governing person.

BOC's Certification Statuses

Certification may be defined in a number of different ways:

- **Active**: Certification is current and in good standing.
- **Administrative**: Review is pending, but trainer/applicant still in good standing and may perform duties.
- **Delinquent**: Trainer is not in good standing because of failure to pay dues or complete continuing education but may continue to perform duties for up to 6 months.
- **Resigned**: Trainer does not plan to continue practice and resigns.
- **Inactive**: Trainer chooses to suspend certification and may not be considered a Certified Athletic Trainer during the period the certification remains inactive.
- **Administrative suspension:** Suspension takes place if delinquent fees or continuing education is not completed within 6 months. Those on suspension may not be considered Certified Athletic Trainers.
- **Disciplinary suspension:** Trainer is not in good standing and may not practice for up to 5 years because of disciplinary action or danger to the public.
- **Emergency suspension**: Certification is suspended because of danger to the public.
- **Revoked:** Certification is lost permanently.

Reinstatement

Athletic trainers who have been inactive may apply to the Board of Certification (BOC) for **reinstatement** by applying and meeting any requirements necessary, such as continuing education. Those who have been suspended for periods of less than 1 year are automatically reinstated if the suspended trainer files an affidavit within 30 days certifying that all conditions have been met. Those who were suspended for periods more than 1 year must file a formal petition with the PPD Committee within 6 months, certifying that all conditions related to disciplinary actions have been met. Also, the applicant must meet all requirements for recertification, including continuing education and payment of fees. The BOC conducts an investigation and renders a decision about reinstatement. If reinstatement is denied, the trainer may petition a second time; if that reinstatement is denied, the certification is revoked. If there are extenuating circumstances, such as illness, the BOC may allow a third petition.

Recertification Requirements

There are a number of Board of Certification (BOC) requirements that must be met for an athletic trainer to obtain **recertification**:

- Professional practice is keeping with the BOC Standards of Professional Practice.
- Annual fee for recertification is included with membership dues for those who are members of NATA but is billed separately for those who are not members.
- Emergency cardiac care (ECC) certification must be current, and topics covered must include adult and pediatric CPR, second rescuer CPR, AED, barrier devices, and airway obstruction. No CEUs are granted for ECC. Online courses may only be used if an instructor tests the practice portion.
- Continuing education units (CEUs) must be completed, currently 75 CEUs within each 3-year period. These CEUs must meet established criteria and must increase the knowledge necessary for professional practice as a Certified Athletic Trainer.

Continuing Education Unit Requirements

The BOC has currently established a rotating schedule for reporting **continuing education units (CEUs)** and, by 2009, all trainers will be on a 3-year cycle, with 75 CEUs required for each reporting period. CEUs may be reported via the Internet (free) or by mail ($25 processing fee). There are 4 categories of CEUs that can be used to meet requirements:

- *BOC-approved programs:* These include workshops, seminars, conferences and BOC-approved home study courses. Up to 75 CEUS may be earned in this category.
- *Professional development:* This includes a variety of activities, such as serving as an examiner (5 CEUS per exam to total of 10/year), taking initial emergency medical technician training, participating in conferences, authoring material related to the field, serving as a home-study reviewer, and writing exam items. These activities can earn varying degrees of units to a total of 50 CEUS.
- *College/university studies (post-certification):* Courses at colleges and universities can be used for CEUs as long as the course content falls within the professional domain of the Certified Athletic Trainer, the course assigns credits, and official transcripts are available. These courses can earn 10 CEUs/credit hour or 25 CEUs per year for medical residency, to a total of 75 CEUs.

- ***Individualized activities:*** This category includes attending non-BOC sponsored programs and events when topics fall within the domains of the Certified Athletic Trainer. CEUs are limited to a maximum of 20. Each category of CEUs requires a different type of documentation to prove participation, and the trainer should refer to the guidelines to ensure that the activity is approved, and that proper documentation is received, so that the activity can be counted towards CEUs.

ROLE DELINEATION STUDY

The Board of Certification (BOC) publishes the results of role delineation studies, with updates every 5 years. The current report, *Role Delineation Study, 5th ed.* is in effect until 2011. The purpose is to ensure that current training standards reflect the range of practice of the Certified Athletic Trainer. It identifies the tasks that an entry-level athletic trainer must perform and the type of knowledge necessary to perform those tasks. The study has established the domains that are tested as part of the certification exam. These include:

- ***Prevention:*** This domain includes knowledge of anatomy and physiology and an understanding of risks, such as those associated with head injuries or return to play issues, and the need to educate athletes in order to prevent injury.
- ***Clinical evaluation and diagnosis.*** This includes understanding the mechanics and pathophysiology of injury, recognizing signs and symptoms, evaluating injuries, and conducting appropriate testing.
- ***Immediate care:*** This includes knowledge of life-saving techniques and the ability to plan and execute an emergency action plan.
- ***Treatment, rehabilitation and reconditioning:*** This includes extensive knowledge of body function, structure, and healing, with the ability to use exercise, assistive devices, and therapeutic modalities to promote healing and recovery.
- ***Organization and administration:*** This includes a solid understanding of organizational needs and the ability to manage resources and risks.
- ***Professional responsibility:*** This includes the recognition that practice must be professional and ethical, complying with standards, such as the BOC Standards of Professional Practice and NATA Code of Ethics.

NATA, BOC, AND CAATE

The National Athletic Trainer's Association (NATA), founded in 1950, is the national professional association for athletic trainers. It has been active in establishing consistent standards for Certified Athletic Trainers across the United States and increasing recognition and acceptance of the profession. It was instrumental in the American Medical Association's recognition of athletic training as a healthcare profession in 1990.

The Board of Certification (BOC) was originally part of NATA but is now a separate non-profit certification board that provides certification and recertification for athletic trainers, based on compliance with Standards of Professional Practice.

The Commission on Accreditation of Athletic Training Education (CAATE) is the agency that accredits over 350 athletic training programs in the United States. This commission operates in collaboration with other agencies, such as NATA, the American Orthopedic Society for Sports Medicine, the American Academy of Family Physicians, and the American Academy of Pediatrics.

INSTRUCTING OTHERS OF CHANGES IN POLICIES, PROCEDURES, AND/OR WORKING STANDARDS

Changes in policy, procedures, and/or working standards are common, and the athletic trainer is often responsible for educating the staff about them. This communication should be performed in an effective and timely manner:

- *Policies* are usually changed after a period of discussion and review by administration and staff, so all staff should be made aware of policies under discussion. Preliminary information should be disseminated to staff regarding the issue during meetings, or through printed notices.
- *Procedures* may be changed to increase efficiency or improve patient safety, often as the result of surveillance and data about outcomes. Procedures changes are best communicated in workshops with demonstrations. Posters and handouts should be available as well.
- *Working standards* are often changed because of regulatory or accrediting requirements; this information should be covered extensively in a variety of different ways (for example, discussions, workshops, and handouts) so that the implications are clearly understood.

WORLD FEDERATION OF ATHLETIC TRAINING AND THERAPY AND THE NATA INTERNATIONAL COMMITTEE

The **World Federation of Athletic Training and Therapy (WFATT)** is a coalition of national healthcare organizations involved in sports, exercise, and treatment. The National Athletic Trainer's Association (NATA) is a founding member of WFATT. Member organizations include those from Asia, Africa, Europe, and North America. The WFATT promotes global standards and opportunities for the exchange of information and research and conducts ongoing surveys, such as Global Practice Analysis.

The **NATA International Committee** provides information and assistance to members who are employed, living, or stationed (as in the military) outside of the United States. The NATA International Committee also supports WFATT activities. The NATA International Committee provides information about opportunities for international internships, continuing education opportunities (such as Category D or attendance at WFATT conferences), overseas employment (through the Council of Employment), and international liability insurance.

MAINTAINING LIABILITY INSURANCE

All athletic trainers should be covered by **liability insurance**, starting from the time they are students. Most universities require insurance, and many provide it at a low cost during training. There can be tremendous costs associated with legal action, even if a suit is dismissed. Some employers provide liability insurance, but the trainer must look carefully at the benefits provided by the policy; in some cases, the benefits may not be adequate, and policies may contain restrictions that affect the type of service the trainer can provide. In some cases, the trainer may want to carry private liability insurance in addition to that provided by the employer. Self-employed trainers are especially vulnerable, as they can lose their business. Some policies do not cover the trainer for any volunteer activities, so this must be clarified. While Good Samaritan laws may protect a trainer in the case of providing emergency care, this is not adequate protection.

APPROPRIATE DOCUMENTATION PROCEDURES

Using appropriate documentation procedures will help the athletic trainer because documentation provides written proof of the care being provided to patients and helps the athletic trainer to recall pertinent details about patients' injuries. Athletic trainers should document injury evaluations, plans of care, write updates on patients' improvements using progress notes, and document all treatments given. This can be achieved with SOAP notes, progress notes, and daily treatment logs. Medical documentation is protected by HIPAA laws for patient privacy and must be followed. In cases of litigation, medical documentation can be used to demonstrate that thorough and appropriate care was given to the patient by the athletic trainer.

Progress Evaluation

A progress evaluation is a physical evaluation, more limited in scope than the off-the-field evaluation. It focuses on how the patient is progressing through the healing process. The progress evaluation should cover pertinent aspects of the patient's history, observations, palpations, and special tests focusing on any positive or negative changes from previous evaluations.

During the history portion, the athletic trainer should ask the patient how their pain is compared to the last time they saw them and if treatments seemed to help or hurt the healing process. The observation portion should look for any observable changes such as increased or decreased swelling or muscular guarding. During the palpation portion, the athletic trainer will palpate looking for any changes such as increased or decreased pain or a change in the texture of swelling. When the athletic trainer performs special tests, they look for changes such as increased pain, instability, or a change in range of motion. Progress evaluations should be documented in the patient's medical records. Athletic trainers can use progress evaluations to evaluate the plan of rehabilitation and adapt it if necessary to meet the patient's needs.

Electronic Medical Record vs. Electronic Health Record

An electronic medical record (EMR) is an electronic medical document that contains information such as a patient's medical history, immunizations, allergies, and lab test results. EMRs are used to document specific medical visits and are more limited in scope than an electronic health record (EHR). An EHR is an electronic medical document, more long-term in scope, detailing the overall health of the patient. The two types of documentation can be differentiated by looking at the terms *medical* and *health*. *Medical* signifies current medical treatments, while *health* is broader in scope, encompassing the overall health of an individual.

Benefits of having electronic records include the ability for healthcare providers to more easily share and review medical documents between multiple facilities that provide care to the patient, increasing the quality of patient care. However, the portability of these documents creates patient privacy issues. Healthcare providers must ensure they comply with HIPAA laws respecting patient privacy.

Injury Reports and Patient Treatment Logs

An injury report is a detailed report documenting information about an injury that has occurred. Injury reports include information such as the type of injury, how the injury occurred, when the injury occurred, and where. Injury reports also document actions that were taken to care for the injured patient as well as any treatments offered. Injury reports should be completed as soon as possible, filed in the patient's medical records, and filed in the athletic trainer's office as well. Injury reports can be used as legal documents during possible litigation to demonstrate how an injury occurred and what care was given.

Patient treatment logs are daily records that document all services provided by the athletic training clinic. Every service the athletic trainer provides should be recorded. Patient treatment logs can also be used in possible litigation to establish what care was given to patients.

Computer Software Programs That Improve Services Provided

There are many computer software programs that can be highly beneficial to athletic trainers. When selecting software to meet organizational needs, athletic trainers should consult professionals, ensure the software is compatible with their computer systems, and take steps to confirm patient confidentiality is maintained. Many software programs have been created specifically to document athletic injuries such as SportWare. This software can make the injury documentation process more streamlined and offer the athletic trainer statistical data about the injuries their patients suffer. Other software can be used to keep track of inventory, budgeting, and schedules, increasing efficiency and effectiveness of the athletic training program.

Diagnostic Codes and Procedural Codes

A diagnostic code is a 6-digit code that identifies a patient's injury or illness for which they are seeking treatment. All the various diagnostic codes are listed in a book titled, *International Statistical Classification of Diseases and Related Health Problems.* When requesting payment from an insurance provider for athletic training services provided, the diagnostic code must be included on the insurance form. A procedural code is a numeric code that identifies what services the patient received that the athletic trainer is billing for and must be included on the insurance form. These procedural codes can be found in *Current Procedure Terminology Code* (CPT) that is developed by the American Medical Association.

Ruling Made by Centers for Medicare & Medicaid Services Affecting Billing Abilities

The ruling made by the Centers for Medicare & Medicaid Services (CMS) negatively affects athletic trainers' ability to bill for their services as it states CMS will no longer pay for therapy provided by an athletic trainer for patients who have Medicare or Medicaid insurance. While other insurance companies do not have to follow this ruling, many generally follow the practices of Medicare and Medicaid. The NATA has attempted to have this ruling reversed or modified without any success yet. Despite setbacks, the NATA continues to keep the reimbursement capability of athletic trainers by third-party payers as a priority.

Third-Party Reimbursement and Coding

Third-party payment from insurance carriers for services provided by Certified Athletic Trainers varies from state to state because of differences in licensure. Athletic trainers who receive third-party reimbursement are able to offset their salaries or, if working independently, obtain an income. Third-party payment is recognition of the athletic trainer as a healthcare professional, but some athletic trainers feel it is unethical to charge for services that traditionally have been provided for free. In reality the costs associated with care have always existed but have been paid by the organization. With increasing costs and a need to economize, third-party reimbursement has become much more important. Reimbursement requires the use of different **codes**:

- **International Classification of Disease (ICD)**: Used to code for diagnosis
- **Diagnostic-related group (DRG)**: Used to classify a disorder according to diagnosis and treatment
- **Current procedural terminology (CPT)**: Used to define those licensed to provide services
- **Universal billing (UB)**: Used to describe services

Record Keeping

There are a number of different methods of **record keeping,** but the most important issue is making daily documentation: that is, recording any injuries, treatments, or responses. Written records cannot be left where the public has access to them, but must be secured (in a locked cabinet or room) or, if electronic, password protected. Accurate record keeping is critical, because records may be used in court if a legal action is taken. Generally, if an action is not documented, it is, for legal reasons, considered to have not been done. However, failing to document an error doesn't mean the error didn't happen; rather, it compounds the error and increases liability. Errors are usually documented as incident reports on special forms that describe what happened, how it happened, the action taken, and when the physician was notified. It is illegal to manipulate or falsify documentation to cover errors or to increase profit (such as charging insurance companies for treatments not provided).

MEDICAL RECORDS

It is very important that medical records be clear and not subject to interpretation. **Guidelines for charting** include:

- Use only standardized vocabulary and approved lists of abbreviations and symbols, so that other medical personnel, such as physicians, can understand the documentation. It is best to use few abbreviations, as they can be easily misinterpreted.
- Avoid the use of subjective terms, such as tired, angry, confused, and irrational. Instead, use objective descriptions, like Athlete yawning every few seconds, or quote directly, Athlete shouting, "Treatment is not helping." The use of negative terms may be cited in court to establish bias.
- Never chart in advance of giving treatment.
- Chart within 1-2 hours of treatment, noting the time of treatment.
- Use blue or black permanent ink for written documentation, writing neatly or printing in block form, and draw lines through spaces.
- Do not erase or use whiteout, and indicate any late entries or corrections. Draw a line through errors, write "error," and sign.

FORMATS FOR MEDICAL RECORD DOCUMENTATION

Different **methods of documentation** are used for an athlete's medical records:

- *Narrative*: This charting format provides a chronological report of the athlete's condition, treatment, and responses. It is an easy method of charting but may be disorganized and repetitive. Also, if different people are making notes, they may address different issues, making it difficult to get an overall picture of the athlete's progress.
- *SOAP (subjective data, objective data, assessment, and plan of action):* This problem-oriented form of charting includes establishing goals, expected outcomes, and needs, and then compiling a numbered list of problems. A SOAP note is made for each separate problem.

    S = Subjective: Client's statement of problem.
    O = Objective: Trainer's observation.
    A = Assessment: Determination of possible causes.
    P = Plan: Short – and long – range goals and immediate plan of care.

If there are multiple problems (edema, pain, restricted activity, etc.,), this charting can be very time-consuming, as each element of SOAP must be addressed. SOAP notes may be extended to ***SOAPIER*** (including ***intervention, evaluation, and revision***.)

Continuation of **methods of documentation**:

- *PIE (problem, intervention, evaluation):* This problem-oriented form of charting is similar to SOAP, but less complex. It combines use of flow sheets with progress notes and a list of problems. Each problem is numbered sequentially, and a PIE note is made for each problem at least one time daily (or during treatment, depending on the frequency).
- *Focus/DAR (data, action, response):* This type of focused charting includes documentation about health problems, changes in condition, and athlete concerns or events, focusing on data about the injury, the action taken by the trainer, and the response. The written format is usually in 3 columns (D-A-R) rather than the traditional narrative linear form. A DAR note is used for each focus item.
- **Charting by exception:** This form of charting was developed in response to problem-oriented charting, in an attempt to simplify charting. It includes extensive use of flow sheets and intermittent charting to document unexpected findings and interventions. However, because of the focus on interventions, those problems that require no particular intervention (such as increased discomfort after a particular exercise) may be overlooked, and charting may not be adequate for legal challenge because lack of charting may be construed as a lack of care of evaluation.
- *Computerized:* All record keeping is done electronically, usually at point of care. Computer terminals must be placed where others cannot read notes being written, and access must be password protected. These systems may include clinical decision support systems (CDSS), which provide diagnosis and treatment options based on symptoms. Computerized charting has some advantages: it is legible, tamper-proof, and tends to reduce errors, as many systems signal if a treatment is missed or the wrong treatment is given.
- *Flow sheets:* These are often a part of other methods of charting and are used to save time. They may be used to indicate completion of exercises or treatments. They usually contain areas for graphing data and may have columns or rows with information requiring checkmarks to indicate a completed action or observation.
- *Critical pathways:* These are specific multi-disciplinary care plans that outline interventions and outcomes of diseases, conditions, and procedures. Critical pathways are based on data, literature, and best practices. The expected outcomes, sequence of interventions, and the timeline needed to achieve the outcomes are all delineated. There are many different forms that appear similar to flow sheets but are more complex and require more documentation. Any variance from the pathway or expected outcomes must be documented. Critical pathways are increasingly used to comply with insurance limitations to ensure cost-effective timely treatment.

Insurance Terminology

Allowable charge: The highest payment amount an insurance company will disburse for medical services provided. Allowable charges vary by insurance company and individual policies.

Claim: A form requesting payment for medical services provided sent to an insurance company. A claim form must include the name and address of the insured individual, procedural codes, diagnostic codes, and the date services were provided.

Deductible: The payment amount the insured person must meet out-of-pocket yearly before the insurance company begins to pay for services.

Gatekeeper: A patient's primary care physician who must provide a referral for a patient to seek specialty services.

Participatory provider: A healthcare professional whom has a contract with the insurance company agreeing to charge only the insurance company's allowable charge for procedures.

SAID principle: An acronym standing for specific adaptations to imposed demands. This principle states that the body will adapt to whatever stresses are placed upon it over time.

Hypertrophy: The increase in the cross-sectional diameter of a muscle. Hypertrophy typically occurs with weight training.

Atrophy: The decrease in the cross-sectional diameter of a muscle. Atrophy occurs with immobilization and lack of physical activity.

Concentric contraction: A muscular contraction that results in the shortening of muscle fibers, also referred to a positive contraction. An example of this is the up-phase of a bicep curl.

Eccentric contraction: A muscular contraction that results in the lengthening of muscle fibers, also called a negative contraction. An example of this is the down-phase of a bicep curl.

Metabolic heat production: Heat that is produced through metabolism. The higher the intensity of a workout it, the higher the resulting metabolic heat production will be.

Conductive heat exchange: An exchange of heat through physical contact that can result in either a heat loss or a heat gain.

Convective heat exchange: An exchange of heat through contact with air or water that moves around a person. Convective heat exchange can result in either a heat loss or a heat gain depending on the temperature of the air or water.

Radiant heat exchange: The transfer of heat through radiant energy that could result in either a heat loss or heat gain. Exposure to sunshine results in radiant heat gain while the body emits radiant energy on a cloudy day, resulting in a radiant heat loss.

Evaporative heat loss: Heat that is lost during the evaporation of sweat because heat is taken during the evaporation process.

Clonic: A muscle spasm that alternates quickly between an involuntary muscle contraction and relaxation.

Tonic: A continuous involuntary muscle contraction that lasts over a period of time. Both clonic and tonic muscle spasms can lead to a strain of the contracting muscle and can be very painful.

Crepitus: A cracking sound produced within the body by a pathology. Crepitus is common in joints after a patient suffers a severe sprain to that joint. A meniscus tear in the knee usually produces crepitus as well.

Tendinosis: The degeneration of a tendon that may include microtears. Tendinosis usually results from overuse.

Ecchymosis: A blue or purple discoloration of the skin caused by bleeding underneath the skin. Severe ecchymosis is usually present after a patient is hit by a baseball traveling at a high speed.

Pathomechanics: Abnormal mechanical forces that are applied to the body due to a structural abnormality within the body that leads to overuse injuries. Pathomechanics resulting from foot abnormalities, inflexibility, and weak musculature can lead to iliotibial band syndrome (ITBS).

Symptom: Subjective factors a patient reports which are relative to the injury but cannot be physically observed by the examiner. Symptoms a patient may report after a head injury include dizziness, headache, and sensitivity to light.

Sign: An abnormality related to the injury that can be physically observed by the examiner. Possible signs of a concussion include loss of balance and decreased cognitive function. These signs can be measured using the Sport Concussion Assessment Tool 3 (SCAT 3).

Syndrome: Multiple abnormalities that when combined, signify a certain injury or disease.

Sequela: A new condition that emerges from an existing injury or illness. An example of this would be osteoarthritis that develops after a patient suffers from a severe sprain.

Ischemia: A decreased flow of blood to an area of the body. A blockage to the heart can cause ischemia.

Cryokinetics: A simultaneous combination of cold therapy and active exercise. This treatment can be used to regain normal range of motion while the affected body part is numb from cryotherapy.

Proprioception: A patient's ability to sense how the various joints of their body are positioned. Proprioception should be improved during the rehabilitative process.

Apophysis: A naturally occurring protrusion on a bone.

Exostosis: A bony outgrowth that is benign and usually covered by cartilage.

Patella alta: A leg alignment abnormality in which the patella is situated more superior than normal when the patient is standing.

Patella baja: A leg is a leg alignment abnormality in which the patella is situated more inferior than normal when the patient is standing.

Genu valgum: A leg alignment abnormality in which the patella is situated more medial than normal when the patient is standing, commonly called knock-knees.

Genu varum: A leg alignment abnormality in which the patella is situated more lateral than normal when the patient is standing, commonly called bow-legs.

Genu recurvatum: is a leg alignment abnormality in which the knees are hyperextended when the patient is standing.

Coup injury: An injury to the brain on the same side as the impact occurred.

Countercoup injury: An injury to the brain on the opposite side as the impact occurred. For example, if a soccer player hits the back of their head on the turf and the brain moves within the skull and is injured on the front of the brain, this is a countercoup injury.

Epistaxis: Is a nosebleed and can occur in various physical activities, but is most often seen in wrestling. To control epistaxis, have the patient pinch the bridge of their nose and look down.

Diplopia: Double vision, most often occurs with a head injury

Auricular (pinna) hematoma: An injury to the ear that occurs from shearing forces to the ear and results in a hematoma. This condition is commonly referred to as cauliflower ear and is most often seen in wrestling and boxing.

Malaise: Feelings of discomfort a patient feels when sick. Patients suffering from the flu and common cold frequently report feelings of general malaise.

Photophobia: Sensitivity to light, this is a common symptom of a head injury.

Embolus: A collection of matter that is stuck together. An example of this is as a blood clot.

Benign: Describes a condition that is of no threat to a patient's health. A benign tumor is not cancerous and not life threatening.

Amenorrhea: The absence of a menstrual cycle. Amenorrhea is a common sign for patients who suffer from the female athlete triad.

NATA Practice Test

Want to take this practice test in an online interactive format?
Check out the bonus page, which includes interactive practice questions and much more: **mometrix.com/bonus948/athtraining**

1. The Occupational Safety and Health Administration (OSHA) mandates that any employee who is at risk for exposure to blood-borne pathogens must be offered a vaccination for which of the following conditions?

   a. Hepatitis A
   b. Hepatitis B
   c. Hepatitis C
   d. Human immunodeficiency virus (HIV)
   e. PPD

2. Which of the following is TRUE regarding the National Collegiate Athletic Association (NCAA)-mandatory medical examination of student athletes?

   a. The medical examination must be conducted by the team physician.
   b. The student athlete may participate in conditioning or limited practices prior to the completion of the medical examination.
   c. The student athlete will require an updated medical examination each year only if his or her health condition changes.
   d. The medical examination must be conducted within six months prior to participating in any type of conditioning, practice, or competition associated with the team.
   e. The medical examination must be conducted within one month prior to participating in any type of conditioning, practice, or competition associated with the team.

3. Which of the following scenarios is illegal based on National Collegiate Athletic Association (NCAA) guidelines?

   a. A football player with an artificial leg
   b. A basketball player's wrist covered with a half-inch of foam and tape
   c. A pole-vaulter using a forearm cover
   d. A softball pitcher with a neutral-colored cast on her non-pitching arm
   e. A volleyball player with newly pierced ears who has taped her ears in preparation for a game

4. Which of the following symptoms may be indicative of the female triad in a female athlete?

   a. Stress fracture
   b. Difficulty concentrating
   c. Frequent urination
   d. Cold intolerance
   e. Significant weight loss

5. A urinalysis may be useful in detecting which of the following? Choose all that apply.
   a. Alterations in hydration
   b. Urinary tract infection
   c. Bone Issues
   d. Hypoglycemia
   e. Drug use

6. Which of the following would NOT contribute to the development of a heat-related illness during exercise?
   a. Use of alcohol
   b. Use of hats or bandanas
   c. Obesity
   d. Age greater than 65 years
   e. Frequent water breaks

7. Which of the following best describes the recommended percentage of total calories from protein, fat, and carbohydrates for most physically active adults?
   a. 10% protein, 20% fat, 70% carbohydrates
   b. 20% protein, 30% fat, 50% carbohydrates
   c. 10-15% protein, 30% fat, 55-65% carbohydrates
   d. 25-30% protein, 10% fat, 60% carbohydrates
   e. 30% protein, 30% fat, 40% carbohydrates

8. The athletic trainer for a high school football team is giving an informational presentation on concussions in high school football to the players and parents. Which of the following points should be included in this presentation?
   a. Symptoms of a concussion can include headache, dizziness, irritability, and a reduced reaction time.
   b. It is imperative that a concussion be identified and treated to allow time for the brain to heal.
   c. It's acceptable to wait 24 hours before reporting the onset of fuzzy vision and light sensitivity after receiving an elbow to the head during practice.
   d. An athlete is typically able to return to playing football within 24 hours of a concussion.
   e. There is a risk of additional brain damage or death if a concussion does not heal sufficiently and another concussion occurs during this time.

9. A collegiate athletic trainer is giving an information presentation to student athletes on the effects of alcohol on athletic training. Which of the following points should be included in this presentation?
   a. Alcohol provides empty calories at approximately 150-200 calories per drink.
   b. The body processes alcohol in a way similar to fat converting alcohol to fatty acids which can lead to weight gain.
   c. Alcohol can lead to dehydration.
   d. Alcohol interferes with the quality of sleep an athlete receives.
   e. The effects of alcohol can last for a few days leading to a reduction in reaction time and decreased ability to concentrate.

10. An athlete who is trying to gain weight should consume how many additional calories per day?

　a. 250 calories
　b. 500 calories
　c. 750 calories
　d. 1000 calories
　e. 1500 calories

11. A basketball player who weighs 250 pounds (114 kg) is eating a regular, balanced diet. He is trying to build muscle and has started supplementing his diet with a commercial protein shake. What is a good range of daily total protein intake for this athlete?

　a. 90-100 grams
　b. 100-135 grams
　c. 135-195 grams
　d. 230-340 grams
　e. 250-300 grams

12. What are some of the dangers of using anabolic steroids?

　a. Stunted growth in teenagers
　b. Infertility for men only
　c. Potential enlargement of the heart
　d. High cholesterol levels
　e. Violent or aggressive behavior

13. Which of the following findings on a female student athlete's pre-participation examination would most likely impact her ability to begin training with the cross-country team?

　a. A blood pressure of 118/70 mm Hg
　b. A heart rate of 60 beats per minute
　c. A history of asthma that is controlled on medication
　d. A hemoglobin level of 25%
　e. A body mass index of 18

14. A 60-year-old man with cardiovascular disease has been medically cleared to begin an exercise program. What test would be an appropriate measure of cardiovascular endurance?

　a. Sprint test
　b. Vertical jump test
　c. One-mile run test
　d. Harvard step test
　e. One-repetition maximum test

15. Which of the following are methods used for assessing body composition?

　a. Edgren test
　b. Skinfold analysis
　c. Body mass index
　d. Underwater weighing
　e. Bioelectrical impedance

16. A 25-year-old man is training for his first marathon. He was diagnosed with type 1, insulin-dependent diabetes when he was 18 years old. He is done stretching and is getting ready start his run. He appears sweaty, shaky, and sluggish, but he brushes it off saying he didn't sleep well last night. Which of the following is the most appropriate initial response to this situation?

   a. Accept his explanation and allow him to run.
   b. Suggest he take a dose of insulin before running due to high blood sugar.
   c. Ask additional questions about his most recent insulin dose and meal, due to low blood sugar.
   d. Prevent him from running until his blood glucose level has been checked and treated accordingly.
   e. Call 911.

17. During a high school basketball training camp, a young boy complains of knee pain after landing from a jump shot. He reports hearing a popping sound when the injury occurred. Which of the following is the most likely explanation?

   a. Fractured tibia
   b. Anterior cruciate ligament (ACL) tear
   c. Sprained knee
   d. Herniated disc
   e. Jumper's knee

18. Which of the following injuries are common in long distance runners?

   a. Rotator cuff injury
   b. Shin splints
   c. Stress fracture of the lower leg or foot
   d. Iliotibial band friction syndrome
   e. Achilles tendonitis

19. Which of the following is an indication that an athlete is suffering from a chronic injury instead of an acute injury?

   a. Dull ache when the body is at rest
   b. Sudden and sharp pain
   c. Swelling and extreme tenderness
   d. Inability to perform weight-bearing activity on a lower extremity
   e. Inability to perform full range of motion in the affected extremity

20. What is the medical term that describes a dangerous increase in pressure within the muscles?

   a. Fracture
   b. Compartment syndrome
   c. Tendonitis
   d. Bursitis
   e. Muscle strain

21. While lifting weights, an athlete experiences lower back pain on one side of the body. What tests should the athletic trainer perform to assess for lumbar disc herniation?
    a. X-ray of the spine
    b. Straight leg raise (SLR) test
    c. MRI
    d. Heel-toe walk
    e. Electrostimulation

22. A 60-year-old woman is experiencing mild pain and tenderness in her wrist, but is able to move it through full range of motion. She reports no obvious trauma to the area. She has a history of diabetes, controlled with diet and medication. She has fractured her wrist twice in the past 10 years. What are the potential diagnoses based on this clinical evaluation?
    a. Osteoarthritis
    b. Carpal tunnel syndrome
    c. Wrist dislocation
    d. Wrist fracture
    e. Tendonitis

23. What is the difference between a sprain and a strain?
    a. There is no real difference between the terms.
    b. A strain hurts more than a sprain.
    c. A strain is pain in the muscle, and a sprain is overstretched or torn ligaments.
    d. A sprain is common in areas like the ankle, knee, or wrist, whereas a strain is common in the back, legs, or neck.
    e. A strain will not show any bruising.

24. Which of the following statements is true regarding the initial treatment of a strain or sprain?
    a. An individual with a strain or sprain should go immediately to the emergency room or call 911.
    b. An individual with a sprain should wear a splint, cast, or elastic bandages to reduce swelling.
    c. An individual with a sprain or a strain should go to a physician for further evaluation.
    d. An individual with a strain or sprain should try to walk it off and reassess it in a couple hours.
    e. An individual with a strain or sprain should take pain medication such as acetaminophen or ibuprofen.

25. During a high school varsity football practice, the temperature is 95°F. One of the linebackers is complaining of nausea, lightheadedness, and fatigue. He has a headache and vomited approximately 30 minutes earlier. What should be done to initiate treatment?
    a. Have him go inside where there is air conditioning.
    b. Provide a pain reliever for the headache.
    c. Provide 4 ounces of water or sports drink every 15 minutes.
    d. Use a fan to help cool the skin, and apply cool compresses on pulse points.
    e. Provide salt tablets to help replace lost electrolytes.

26. Which of the following is NOT an appropriate step to take when initiating treatment for cold injury to the feet?
 a. Remove any wet clothing and have the individual elevate the feet to reduce swelling.
 b. Have the individual place the feet near a space heater to help gradually thaw the feet.
 c. Avoid rubbing the feet because this may damage the tissue.
 d. Put cotton between the toes to avoid friction.
 e. Call for emergency medical services immediately if there is evidence of deep cold injury.

27. During soccer practice, a player falls against the goal post and has a large laceration on his arm that is bleeding. Which of the following is the most appropriate immediate treatment of the injury?
 a. Either you or the injured player apply a clean bandage and press the wound while someone else retrieves the first-aid kit and gloves.
 b. Apply a tourniquet above the laceration.
 c. Have the goalie apply pressure to the wound using a clean cloth while retrieving a pair of gloves.
 d. Apply pressure on the femoral artery.
 e. Apply a splint to the arm to help control the bleeding.

28. If an athlete with sickle cell disease experiences chest or abdominal pain and pain in the joints, he or she may be at immediate risk for which of the following complications?
 a. Kidney failure
 b. Seizures
 c. Dehydration
 d. Rhabdomyolysis
 e. Hypotension

29. What piece of equipment is most likely to be carried by an athletic trainer to be used in conjunction with cardiopulmonary resuscitation (CPR)?
 a. Positive pressure ventilator
 b. Bag valve mask resuscitators
 c. Oxygen tank
 d. Oropharyngeal airway tube
 e. Pocket mask

30. In the initial treatment of an athlete with a suspected spinal cord injury, which of the following is NOT an appropriate step to take?
 a. Ensure open airway and adequate breathing and circulation.
 b. Stabilize the neck with a soft cervical collar.
 c. Use a shovel stretcher if available.
 d. Ask the athlete to move the neck through normal range of motion.
 e. Stabilize the neck with a rigid collar.

31. A cheerleader falls during a competition. Upon examination, her tibia bone is protruding. What are appropriate steps to take in the immediate treatment of her fracture?
   a. Move her to a safe place.
   b. Immobilize the leg.
   c. Have her lay flat and cover her with a blanket.
   d. Provide an over-the-counter pain reliever.
   e. Apply sterile dressing to the wound.

32. An athlete with known diabetes mellitus has a hypoglycemic reaction during an athletic event. What should be done to begin treatment?
   a. Have the athlete drink water.
   b. Have the athlete drink a quart of orange juice and return to the game.
   c. Have the athlete eat a sandwich.
   d. Administer glucagon.
   e. Have the athlete drink 4 ounces of juice or soda, then reassess in 15 minutes.

33. A female student athlete may have an eating disorder. She has experienced significant weight loss, and a few of her teammates have approached the athletic trainer with concerns regarding her use of laxatives and restrictive eating. The athletic trainer discusses this issue with the coach. What is the most appropriate plan for addressing this situation with the student-athlete?
   a. Do not allow her to participate in training or competition until she receives a full medical examination.
   b. Call her parents and tell them to deal with this issue immediately.
   c. Make a direct referral to an eating disorder specialist or counselor on campus.
   d. Ask one of her teammates to talk to her about the health concerns, and if she is receptive, refer her to a health care specialist.
   e. Privately approach her and express concerns regarding her health, avoiding the topic of eating habits or weight, and arrange a medical examination.

34. A tennis player experiences a moderate hamstring strain. A week later, he is ready to begin rehabilitation. Which of the following is the most appropriate suggestion for the first week in rehabilitation?
   a. Rest, Ice, Compression, and Elevation (RICE) protocol
   b. Static stretches 5 times per day
   c. Running on the treadmill for 20 minutes at a time
   d. Ice to the hamstring muscle
   e. Light sports massage to the hamstring muscle

35. What are the best rehabilitation exercises after a back injury?
   a. Flexibility exercises
   b. Jogging
   c. Walking
   d. Core muscles exercises
   e. Stationary bicycle

36. What are the reported benefits of massage therapy for rehabilitation following a sports injury?

   a. Relief from spasms
   b. Decreased cell metabolism
   c. Increased cell metabolism
   d. Improved blood flow
   e. Increased nerve excitability in surrounding tissues

37. Magnetic therapy devices are available in which of the following forms?

   a. Pills
   b. Wraps
   c. Mattress pads
   d. Shoe inserts
   e. Necklaces

38. A foam roller is an example of what type of therapeutic modality?

   a. Myofascial release
   b. Deep massage
   c. Electromagnetic therapy
   d. Static therapy
   e. Thermotherapy

39. A college athlete has a recurrent stress fracture in her foot due to long distance running. A bone density test reveals a T-score of 2.2, indicating osteopenia. A registered dietitian recommends a high-calcium diet. Which of the following foods are good sources of calcium?

   a. Yogurt
   b. Cheese
   c. Tofu
   d. Dark green, leafy vegetables
   e. Whole grains

40. An athlete is recovering from a fractured clavicle. He no longer requires the use of a sling and is beginning rehabilitation. Which of the following exercises are appropriate to begin strengthening the clavicle?

   a. Bicep curls and triceps extensions with weights
   b. Bicep curls and triceps extensions without weights
   c. Shrugs
   d. Internal and external rotation using exercise bands
   e. Free weights

41. An athlete asks for advice on how to rehabilitate a knee injury while at home, without the use of equipment. What exercises is NOT recommended for strengthening the knee?

   a. Straight leg raise
   b. Side lying abduction
   c. Standing hamstring curl
   d. Gluteal contractions
   e. Toe raises

42. An athlete gets hit in the mouth by a softball and loses a front tooth. A teammate has located the tooth. Which of the following are appropriate next steps?
    a. Scrub the tooth to remove the dirt, and then reinsert it into the socket.
    b. Put the tooth into saline solution or an emergency tooth preservation kit.
    c. Place the tooth in a cup of cold whole milk.
    d. Wrap the tooth in clean gauze and give it to the athlete's parents.
    e. Ask the athlete to hold the tooth in the mouth, between the cheek and gum.

43. When measuring an athlete's agility during rehabilitation for a knee injury, which of the following tests might be used?
    a. Harvard Step Test
    b. Cooper Agility Test
    c. Edgren Side Step Test
    d. Vertical Jump Test
    e. T-test

44. A ball-and-socket joint, such as the shoulder, of is capable of which of the following types of range of motion?
    a. Dorsiflexion and plantarflexion
    b. Flexion and extension
    c. Internal and external rotation
    d. Abduction and adduction
    e. Pronation and supination

45. An athletic trainer suspects that a 19-year-old female gymnast might have an eating disorder. She reveals that she is being treated by student health services, but does not disclose the reason. The athletic trainer calls student health services and talks to the physician, but the physician declines to provide any information regarding the athlete's medical condition. What gives the physician this right?
    a. Family Educational Rights and Privacy Act (FERPA)
    b. Health Insurance Portability and Accountability Act (HIPAA)
    c. Occupational Safety and Health Administration (OSHA)
    d. Academy of Nutrition and Dietetics (AND)
    e. Title IX

46. Which of the following are required of athletic trainers?
    a. Following Board of Certification (BOC) practice standards
    b. Obtaining federal licensure
    c. Following Health Insurance Portability and Accountability Act (HIPAA) requirements
    d. Following Family Educational Rights and Privacy Act (FERPA) requirements
    e. Graduating from an accredited program with a minimum of an Associate's Degree in Athletic Training

47. Which of the following regulatory agencies requires athletic trainers working with professional sports teams to document any injury received by a player?
   a. Joint Commission (JCAHO)
   b. Occupational Safety and Health Administration (OSHA)
   c. Commission on Accreditation of Rehabilitation Facilities (CARF)
   d. National Collegiate Athletic Association (NCAA)
   e. National Football League (NFL)

48. Which of the following is NOT an appropriate way to record information in an athlete's medical record?
   a. Document care in pencil.
   b. Date all entries and legibly sign the entry with name and title.
   c. Document only the care that was actually provided.
   d. Erase or white-out any mistakes in documentation.
   e. Write entries in the chronological order that the care occurred.

49. Which of the following is NOT considered part of the operating budget for the athletic training room in a high school?
   a. Band-Aids
   b. Whirlpool
   c. Slings and splints
   d. Taping bench
   e. Povidone-iodine

50. Which of the following are recommendations provided by the National Collegiate Athletic Association (NCAA) for lightning safety?
   a. One person should be designated to monitor the weather before and during sporting events and practices.
   b. Be aware of the location of the closest safe structure where teams and spectators can seek shelter if necessary.
   c. Cancel sporting events at the first sound of thunder.
   d. If the time between lightning and thunder is thirty seconds or less, the athletic site should have already been evacuated and all individuals relocated to a shelter.
   e. If thunder is heard but the sky is blue, there is no immediate danger and play can continue until lightning is seen.

Answer Key and Explanations

1. B: The Occupational Safety and Health Administration (OSHA) is mandated by law to offer the hepatitis B vaccination to any employee who is at risk for being exposed to blood-borne pathogens. Hepatitis B is a virus that is spread through direct contact with bodily fluids, such as blood from an infected individual. Individuals who are at high risk for contracting the hepatitis B virus include health care workers, athletic trainers, and any workers who have the potential to be exposed to blood. Additionally, OSHA requires that a plan be in place that outlines the procedure for dealing with exposures, including training, staff responsibilities, proper documentation, and the use and availability of personal protective equipment. Any potential biohazardous waste needs to be disposed of in proper containers lined with special red biohazard bags.

2. D: The National Collegiate Athletic Association (NCAA) mandates that all student athletes undergo a complete medical examination within six months of starting any type of required preseason conditioning, practice, or competition. This mandate includes student athletes who are starting their first season of NCAA eligibility and transfers. This medical examination must be completed prior to the start of the academic year and covers the academic year and summer. Student athletes are then required to receive an updated medical examination each academic year. Appropriate documentation must be submitted and retained for the athletes' entire college career. The examination may be completed by the team physician or family physician. It may also be completed by a nurse practitioner or physician assistant working under the direction of a licensed medical doctor.

3. A and E: The National Collegiate Athletic Association (NCAA) has rules for each sport and athletic trainers need to be informed and knowledgeable about these rules because the use of illegal equipment poses a risk for injury to student athletes. Many rules pertain to the mandatory use of protective equipment, such as helmets, to prevent injuries. Artificial limbs are considered illegal for football players because of the potential to cause harm to other players. A basketball player can play with certain injuries involving the arm area, as long as the material used to cover the injury is soft and not likely to cause harm. A pole-vaulter may use a forearm protector. In softball, various types of casts and splints are allowed, but they must be well padded for the protection of all players. The pitcher must wear a cast that is neutral in color so it does not distract other players. All jewelry is prohibited in volleyball and jewelry must not be taped.

4. A, B, C, D, and E: The *female triad* is term used to describe disordered eating that leads to the development of amenorrhea and osteoporosis. The disordered eating (DE) does not have to be a fully diagnosed eating disorder, such as anorexia nervosa, but the female triad begins with DE. Disordered eating typically involves not eating enough calories in an attempt to be thin. Weight loss is the first clue. Significant weight loss can lead to amenorrhea, which is when menstruation stops. When this occurs for a prolonged period, it can lead to loss of bone mass or osteoporosis due to lack of estrogen. Osteoporosis can be further complicated by inadequate calcium intake. Other symptoms of DE may include dehydration, frequent urination, cold intolerance, inability to focus, and dental problems. It is important to monitor the menstrual cycles of female athletes, and to focus on health and nutrition rather than weight and body size.

5. A, B, and E: A urinalysis is typically a part of the pre-participation physical examination (PPE). As part of the PPE, legal permission is not required unless the urinalysis is being done as part of a drug testing program. A urinalysis can provide information on the presence of a urinary tract infection with an elevated white blood cell count. Blood or nitrates in the urine may also indicate infection, and an elevated urine specific gravity may indicate dehydration. A urinalysis can detect issues with the kidney or liver, but is not commonly used to screen for bone issues. It can also detect the presence of glucose or ketones, both of which may signal diabetes. A urinalysis does not detect hypoglycemia.

6. E: There are many factors that will increase the chance of developing a heat-related illness while exercising. These factors include being older than 65 years or a very young child. Obesity is a risk factor, as well as the presence of a medical condition that may further stress the body. The use of alcohol is a risk factor because alcohol causes dehydration. Wearing the wrong type of clothing is a risk factor. Hats or other types of headwear are not recommended during exercise because this prevents heat from escaping. Loosely fitting, light weight clothing should be selected. Frequent water breaks are recommended to keep well hydrated. Athletes from different climates should also become acclimated to a new climate prior to exercise to prevent heat-related illness.

7. C: It is important for everyone to eat a well-balanced, nutritious diet, but it is especially important for athletes or those who are physically active. Proper nutrition helps to effectively fuel the body and maximize endurance. The amount of calories required by each athlete varies greatly based on body size, gender, activity level, and age. For most physically active adults, the appropriate percentage of calories is 55-60% from carbohydrates, 10-15% from protein, and no more than 30% from fat. The majority of carbohydrates should be complex carbohydrates from whole grains breads and cereals, rather than simple sugars. All carbohydrates break down to glucose and are used by the muscles for energy. Glucose that is not used for energy is stored as glycogen for use when needed. Protein is used for building muscle and repairing cells. Fat is also used as a source of energy as well as protecting organs and preventing excessive heat loss.

8. A, B, and E: A *concussion* is a brain injury that occurs in response to a blow to the head. This can happen when a player's head has direct contact with another player, a hard surface, or a piece of equipment. Concussions can be extremely dangerous and in some cases can result in permanent brain damage or death. Each athlete will experience a concussion in a different way. Loss of consciousness does not need to occur with a concussion. In football, it is important to discourage any head or helmet contact between players. This includes stepping on another player's head, elbowing to the head, or any type of hitting. Symptoms of a concussion are wide ranging but can include confusion, disorientation, vision trouble, headache, nausea, reduced reaction time, and imbalance. It is extremely important for an athlete not to ignore these symptoms. The brain needs time to rest and heal. Additional injuries are likely if a concussion does not heal.

9. A, B, C, D, and E: Alcohol can have a significant and lasting effect on athletic performance. The effects of one night of drinking can last as long as three days and can affect overall performance and reaction time. Alcohol is considered a source of empty calories because it does not provide vitamins or minerals. The body processes alcohol similar to how it processes fat, which can lead to excessive fat deposition and weight gain. Alcohol interferes with the quality of sleep, which can also impact performance and lead to fatigue. Alcohol dehydrates the body; this can be dangerous for athletes because, due to stress and environmental conditions, they require more fluids to keep hydrated. Alcohol can increase the risk of injury while playing a sport and also impacts the body's ability to recover following an injury. Alcohol can also lead to long-term health issues.

10. B: Many sports, such as football, basketball, and rugby, require or encourage athletes to gain weight in order to maximize performance. Weight gain must be done gradually. If accomplished too quickly, the resultant weight gain will be in the form of adipose tissue rather than lean body mass. Lean body mass consists of muscle tissue, bones, and connective tissue. An increase in body fat will negatively affect performance. In order for the body to gain weight, an additional 500 calories per day must be consumed above what is expended. A rate of weight gain of approximately 1.5% per week is a good goal. This increase in caloric intake should be coupled with a weight-training program to help build lean body mass.

11. C: Protein is an extremely important nutrient, especially for athletes. Protein helps to build and repair muscle tissue and plays a role in many other functions within the body. A normal person requires approximately 0.8 grams per kilogram of protein per day. An athlete has a slightly higher protein requirement of approximately 1.2-1.7 grams per kilogram per day. For the basketball player described in the question, this would be approximately 135-195 grams per day. The majority of athletes can meet their protein requirements through a normal diet. There is no scientifically sound evidence showing that extremely high levels of protein will help build muscle faster. Excessive amounts of protein in the diet will make the kidneys have to work harder to metabolize the protein and may cause the body to lose water in this process. Too much protein can also impact the bones. The athlete's normal diet should be evaluated by a dietitian to determine if additional protein is required.

12. A, C, D, and E: The use of steroids is illegal without documented medical necessity. Steroids can have dangerous side effects, especially for teenagers. Stunting of growth is one important side effect. The bones mature faster than normal, sending a signal to the body to stop growing. Steroid use can lead to infertility in both men and women. In men, there can be a loss of sperm and a reduction in testicle size. In women, steroid use can lead to disruption of the menstrual cycle. Steroids can lead to enlargement of the heart, certain types of cancer, muscle aches, and hair loss. Steroids can cause elevations in blood cholesterol levels that can lead to heart disease. Steroids can also lead to a change in behavior, characterized by violence, mood swings, and aggression. Most athletes in college, Olympic, and professional sports will need to undergo drug testing to monitor for steroid abuse. Athletes found to be abusing steroids face legal consequences.

13. D: Evaluating a pre-participation examination should be done in conjunction with the athlete's physician. There are a number of conditions that would prohibit an athlete from competition; however, it is at the physician's discretion to make this decision. A history of asthma would not necessarily prohibit and athlete from training or competing if it is well managed and medication is available. The blood pressure noted is in the optimal range, which is a systolic reading less than 120 mm Hg and a diastolic reading less than 80 mm Hg. A normal heart rate is 60-100 beats per minute (BPM) and some athletes in superb physical condition may have a heart rate as low as 40 BPM. The hemoglobin level, however, is low, with a normal range of 34.9-44.5% for adult women and 38.8-50% for adult men. Hemoglobin is a type of protein found in red blood cells that helps transport oxygen. A low hemoglobin level can lead to heart problems, because the heart may try to work harder to pump more oxygen throughout the body.

14. C and D: The main purpose of fitness testing is to determine a baseline level of fitness. This can help designate the most appropriate exercises to perform. In order to test cardiovascular endurance, the Harvard step test and the run test are used. The Harvard step test involves the use of steps that are 20 inches high. The participant steps up and down at a rate of 30 steps per minute until reaching exhaustion, which is defined as the point at which the participant is not able to keep the pace for 15 seconds. At this point, the heart rate is monitored at one-, two-, and three-minute intervals. The results are converted to the number of heartbeats in the recovery period and are evaluated on a range of poor to excellent based on score. The run test measures endurance on a timed test of nine, 10, or 12 minutes or a distance test of 1.0 or 1.5 miles, depending upon age and fitness level.

15. B, D, and E: *Anthropometry*, the measurement of an individual's height and weight, is commonly done in fitness testing. However, what is important is the assessment of body composition, which cannot be done with a scale. Body weight is composed in part of adipose (or fat) tissue and muscle. Many athletes have an increased level of muscle mass. Methods used to assess this are skinfold analysis, underwater weighing, and bioelectrical impedance. BMI is an equation that has been determined to be ineffective at correctly assessing body composition and is no longer recommended as a diagnostic tool. Skinfold analysis is completed using skinfold calipers that directly measure the thickness of the skin when gently pulled away from the body at certain points. Equations are then used to convert those measurements into body compositions. Underwater weighing involves the use of lung volume, the individual's weight when measured underwater, and an equation. Bioelectrical impedance measures the electrical resistance between electrodes placed on various points on the body. Body fat will resist electricity, and body fat percentage can be calculated based on this data.

16. C and D: *Hypoglycemia* (low blood sugar) is a common side effect of insulin because blood glucose stability is dependent on so many different factors. These factors include insulin dosage, timing and composition of meals, exercise level, and more. Signs of a hypoglycemic reaction include shaking, sweating, and hunger. Later signs can include confusion, fatigue, appearing intoxicated, and seizures that can lead to unconsciousness. Exercise has a direct effect on blood glucose levels as well. Hypoglycemia is commonly seen and can occur before, during, or after exercise. High levels of exercise can accelerate a low blood sugar reaction. It is important to monitor blood glucose levels prior to exercising to determine if a snack or meal is needed. An athletic trainer needs to be familiar with the signs of hypoglycemia, especially if working with individuals with a known history of any type of diabetes.

17. B: An injury to the anterior cruciate ligament (ACL) is common in individuals participating in basketball, skiing, soccer, and football. Injury to the ACL typically involves a hit to the side of the knee, landing from a jump, hyperextending the knee, pivoting the knee, or a quick change in direction when running. The common symptom that helps to distinguish this injury is a popping sound made at the time of injury. This sound occurs as the ACL is torn either partially or completely. Significant knee swelling will occur within a few hours of injury. Initial treatment should include elevating the leg so the knee joint is above the heart, applying ice, and administering pain relievers such as ibuprofen. The individual should be directed to obtain medical care from a licensed physician.

18. B, C, D, and E: Athletic trainers who work with long-distance runners need to be aware of injuries common to this sport. Most injuries involve the hip, leg, or foot. *Shin splints* typically refers to pain that involves the area of the tibia. It can be related to muscle, bone, or the attachment of the muscle to the bone. A *stress fracture* is a microscopic break that is caused by repetitive force on an area such as the foot, lower leg, tibia, or fibula. *Achilles tendonitis* is inflammation of the large tendon that is located in the back of the ankle. *Iliotibial band friction syndrome* is pain in the knee that worsens with running or stepping up or down stairs. It is commonly referred to as *runner's knee*.

19. A: An acute injury is one that is considered to have occurred recently due to some type of trauma. A chronic injury is one that is due to overuse or due to a condition that has been present for a period of time. Symptoms of an acute injury include sudden and severe pain and swelling, tenderness, or extreme weakness. Full range of motion in the affected area may not be possible. There may be an obvious visible break or dislocation of a bone. Weight-bearing activity will likely not be possible with an acute injury. Chronic injuries, on the other hand, typically will have symptoms of a dull, achy pain when the body is at rest or not engaged in any particular activity. Swelling may also be present. Pain with either type of injury should not be ignored.

20. B: *Compartment syndrome* is the medical term used to describe an extremely painful condition that occurs when pressure in the muscles increases to a dangerously high level. Compartment syndrome can be acute or chronic, but an acute case is considered a medical emergency. It can occur with acute trauma to a muscle because the fascia (or thick tissue) that surrounds and separates muscle groups is not able to expand. This increase in pressure or swelling within the fascia stops the muscle and nerve cells from receiving oxygen and nutrients and can lead to permanent nerve damage. Chronic compartment syndrome can be caused by activities that utilize repetitive movements, such as running. The symptoms of this syndrome include loss of sensation to the area, severe pain, and weakness. The skin will appear pale. On physical examination, the individual will experience pain in the area if the muscle compartment is squeezed or attempt is made to move the area.

21. B and D: The athletic trainer is not qualified to do many medical tests such as x-ray or MRI. If needed, these types of tests will most likely be done by a licensed physician or medical professional. Though electrostimulation *as a treatment* is within the scope of practice for an athletic trainer, it would not be performed *as a test*. The athletic trainer can do a couple of simple tests during a physical examination to try to assess the lower back pain. The first is straight leg raise (SLR) test. The individual should lie flat on his back and try to lift the leg straight up. The knee should remain straight. If pain is felt down the leg and below the knee, a herniated disc is very likely. A second test to assess weakness is the heel-toe walk. Inability to do this type of walk may signal nerve compression in the spine, caused by a herniated disc. A referral to a physician is needed in this case. Treatment typically involves rest and anti-inflammatory medication for pain relief. Sometimes physical therapy or steroid injections may be recommended.

22. A, B, and E: There are many possible causes of wrist pain. It is unlikely to be due to a fracture or dislocation because this would result in a higher level of pain and inability to move through full range of motion. *Osteoarthritis* is a possibility, given her age and history of wrist injuries. *Tendonitis* and *carpal tunnel syndrome* are also possible. These types of injuries are typically caused by repetitive motion that uses the wrist for a long period of time without a break such as playing tennis, using a computer, driving cross country, or playing a string instrument. Additional information should be obtained about recent activities. Treatment can vary based on actual diagnosis but involves pain relievers such as acetaminophen or ibuprofen.

23. C and D: A *sprain* and a *strain* are similar injuries, but there are some differences. They are similar because both injuries cause pain and may cause some swelling and bruising. A strain is more serious than a strain. A sprain can occur when the ligaments have been overstretched or torn, causing a mild to severe sprain. A sprain will typically cause pain immediately and the individual may not be able to put any pressure on the injured area at all. Sprains will usually involve wrists, knees or ankles. A strain is pain in a muscle that has been stretched too far. The most common areas for strains are the back, legs, or neck. Strains are more likely to occur if an individual does not properly warm up before engaging in certain activities.

24. B, C, and E: If an individual might have a strain or a sprain, he or she should be advised to refrain from using the affected part of the body. A physician can better assess the injury and an x-ray may be required. Referral to an emergency room or a call to emergency medical services is not usually necessary, although some patients may choose to be seen in an urgent care facility. A sprained area will most likely require some type of support, such as a splint, cast, or elastic bandage. An area with a strain will require rest. Both types of injuries will benefit from some type of pain relief medication, such as acetaminophen or ibuprofen. A strain will usually heal within a week, whereas a sprain may take as long as four weeks to heal.

25. A, C, and D: The student athlete is showing signs of heat exhaustion. Some of the early symptoms are dizziness, lightheadedness, extreme sweating, nausea, muscle cramps, weakness, and fatigue. Late symptoms include headache, nausea and vomiting, and dilated pupils. As heat exhaustion progresses, it can lead to irrational behavior and loss of consciousness. Immediate treatment consists of moving the individual to a cooler place and elevating feet. A fan can be used to help lower body temperature and cool cloths can be placed on the skin at various pulse points such as the neck, armpits, or groin. The individual should begin to slowly rehydrate with cool water or sports beverages with approximately 4 ounces every 15 minutes. Pain relievers should not be administered. Salt tablets should not be given because these may cause harm. If the individual does not show signs of recovery or begins to show signs of shock or seizure, emergency care should be sought.

26. B: Cold injury is most likely to occur in the hands, feet, nose, and ears. There are varying degrees of cold injury, with frostbite being less severe. Deep cold injury is less common in athletics. Cold injury can cause extensive tissue damage if not treated appropriately. The most important point to remember is to prevent gradual thawing of the area or to warm the area if there is a risk of the area refreezing. Rewarming of a deep cold injury should occur quickly (within 15-30 minutes) using a warm water bath. The individual should not be placed close to a heat source, such as a space heater. Wet clothing should be removed. In the case of cold injury to the feet, cotton should be placed between the toes to prevent friction and the area should not be massaged because this may cause tissue damage. Individuals with frostbite or deep cold injury will often require hospitalization for a couple days to ensure the area is healing and there is no infection.

27. A: At any sign of blood, universal precautions should be the first step in treatment. Universal precautions will help to stop the spread of blood-borne infection. If the player is conscious and able to apply pressure to the wound on his own, he should be given a sterile or clean bandage and begin to apply pressure while the athletic trainer puts on gloves. If he is not able to do this on his own and the athletic trainer is not able to put on gloves right away, the trainer must make sure to use enough bandages to prevent blood from saturating the bandage and to prevent direct contact with blood. A tourniquet is a last-ditch effort to stop bleeding and is not routinely indicated. Pressure on the femoral artery will not help stop the bleeding for an arm injury because the femoral artery is located in the groin area. A splint is required in the case of a broken bone to help immobilize the area as well as to help stop the bleeding.

28. D: Sickle cell disease is a hereditary disease commonly seen in individuals of African or Mediterranean descent. It involves abnormally shaped red blood cells that are severely affected by low oxygen levels. Sickle cell crisis involves extreme pain in the bones and joints. Symptoms include abdominal or chest pain, shortness of breath, rapid heart rate, fever, and fatigue. In some cases, a sickle cell crisis can progress to rhabdomyolysis. This can cause damage and even death to muscle tissue. If rhabdomyolysis occurs and is not treated, kidney failure can result. An athlete with sickle cell disease should ensure adequate hydration before, during, and after exercise. This helps to keep the urine diluted enough to flush out the dangerous toxins that may be present, to prevent damage from occurring. Athletes with sickle cell disease should be monitored closely at all times.

29. E: The ability to provide emergency care during sporting events is essential. The certified athletic trainer is able to handle some basic care until first responders arrive on the scene. The *pocket mask* is the piece of equipment most likely to be carried by an athletic trainer. This device is used to assist with delivering oxygen to an individual who requires resuscitation. The mask is placed over the individual's mouth to act as a shield during resuscitation. Oxygen, if available, can also be delivered. Emergency care providers such as emergency medical technicians (EMTs), paramedics, or physicians will have additional equipment such as tubes to open up the airway, bag-valve mask resuscitators and oxygen tanks. It is imperative that an athletic trainer provide only the level of emergency care for which he or she has been trained, and to let emergency responders take over when they arrive on the scene.

30. B and D: In the case of a suspected spinal cord injury, it is imperative that the neck and spine be immobilized to prevent additional damage. The first step is to always ensure that the individual is breathing. The ABCs—airway, breathing and circulation—should be verified. The neck should be stabilized with a cervical collar of the rigid type, not a soft collar. The individual should not be moved if possible and when ready for transfer, a scoop type or shovel stretcher should be used. It is best to wait for first responders to assist with treatment but it is important to know how a possible spinal cord injury should be handled.

31. B, C, and E: Emergency medical services should be called immediately because of the protruding bone. After making sure the individual is breathing appropriately, initial treatment should begin. The point at which the tibia punctured the skin should be covered with a sterile dressing to prevent infection. The leg should be appropriately immobilized to prevent additional damage to nerves or circulation. Ice can be applied to help prevent swelling. The individual should lie flat and be kept warm using a blanket to help prevent shock. Administration of pain relievers should be delayed until additional medical help arrives, due to the potential for surgery due to the open fracture.

32. E: Hypoglycemia is defined as a blood sugar level less than 70 mg/dL. Symptoms of hypoglycemia include shaking, cold sweats, blurry vision, headache, hunger, irritability, and weakness. Most individuals with diabetes will be able to recognize the initial symptoms and will know they need to address the issue immediately. If untreated, this can lead to seizures, unconsciousness, or coma. Treatment typically consists of 4 ounces of juice or soda, five or six hard candies, or about a tablespoon of sugar. Then wait 15 minutes to see if the blood sugar rises. If it does not, additional help may be needed. Once the blood sugar is in the normal range, a healthy snack should be eaten to help sustain the blood sugar level. It is important not to over-treat a hypoglycemic reaction with too much sugar, because this can cause additional issues if the blood sugar is too high.

33. E: The most important step for beginning to deal with a student athlete who is suspected of having disordered eating is to make the initial contact non-threatening. This needs to be done by a person of authority, such as the athletic trainer or any of the coaching staff. The athlete should be approached in private and should not be made to feel uncomfortable or embarrassed. Discussions about her weight or disordered eating should not be brought up at this time. Instead, the focus should be on her health and well-being. She should be advised that a medical examination is being arranged and it is not optional. She will not be allowed to participate in the sport until the issue is addressed. A referral to a health care provider specializing in disordered eating may be necessary. This health care professional may also need to talk to the team about the issue, although confidentiality will prevent this person from directly discussing the athlete.

34. B and E: Initial treatment of a moderate hamstring strain should include the RICE protocol: rest, ice, compression, and elevation. After a week, however, the athlete should begin to start rehabilitation at some level. Static stretches, like the hamstring stretch, are most appropriate. Strengthening the hamstring muscle should also commence and this can be accomplished using a resistance band. Range of motion exercises that gently begin to work the injured muscle— such as light jogging, stationary bike or water activities—can gradually begin. These activities should only last a few minutes with a goal of building endurance. Running or excessive use of the injured hamstring should wait until there is no pain with previous exercises. After gentle exercise, ice should be reapplied.

35. A, C, and D: It is important to begin rehabilitation as soon as possible following a back injury to hasten the healing process. Resuming cardiovascular type exercise is an important step. Walking is one of the best exercises to start with because it keeps the spine straight. The individual can walk for a certain amount of minutes, based on tolerance, and gradually build up from there. The use of an upright bike is not indicated due to spine position, but a recumbent bike may be an option. Flexibility or stretching exercises of the hip and leg muscles are also important. If the individual is able to maintain or improve flexibility, it will allow less movement of the spine. Strengthening exercises for the core muscles of the back and abdomen are also indicated. The individual should be advised to work on pulling their belly button inwards towards the spine and hold the muscles tight while remembering to breathe.

36. A, C, and D: Massage is an example of a manual therapeutic modality that involves pressing and manipulating various parts of the body through the skin, muscles, tendons, and ligaments. The form of massage can vary from light touch to deep pressure techniques. In sports, massage is used to help treat or prevent injury to specific muscles. There are many reported benefits to massage therapy, including relief of spasms or muscle pain, improvement in blood flow (which also promotes healing), and increased cell metabolism. This means that cells are regenerating in the affected area. Other reported benefits include helping to restore full range of motion. Athletic trainers should be suitably trained in massage techniques in order to prevent injuries such as nerve damage, bleeding, and temporary paralysis.

37. B, C, D, and E: Magnetic therapy is used as part of the treatment and rehabilitation plan for various types of sports injuries. There is not a solid base of medical research to support this theory; however, it is unlikely to cause harm and many individuals are able to feel the benefits. There are many types of devices used in magnetic therapy, including wraps for areas like the knee or elbow, necklaces, shoe inserts to help with foot pain, and mattress pads to assist with larger areas like the back. The magnets placed in these devices are static magnets and come in various degrees of strength, which is measured in gauss and tesla units. Magnets may be unipolar or alternating polar. Magnets are placed in certain positions on the body based on the desired effect. Uses of magnetic therapy include relief of pain from arthritis, fibromyalgia, chronic muscle pain, lower back pain, carpal tunnel syndrome, and many other reported uses.

38. A: A foam roller is a device used in myofascial release. It can be used by athletes to perform self-massage for soft tissues in various muscle groups. An athletic trainer may perform this modality, but would likely use their own hands. Soft tissues include muscle, tendons, ligaments, and the fascia. Foam rollers come in various sizes. The athlete can roll the device over an area 10 times to help loosen up an area that may be tight. Common areas include lower and upper back, hamstring, gluteus, hip rotators, and shoulders. It can also be used to warm up or cool down following exercise. The benefits of this therapeutic modality include improving range of motion of various joints, relieving muscle pain and soreness, and helping to maintain the normal function of the muscle length.

39. A, B, C, and D: Calcium is an important mineral in bone growth and repair. It has many other functions in the body as well, including regulation of blood pressure and blood clotting. A bone density test is a test that uses x-rays to determine the presence of osteoporosis and the overall risk of fracture. Osteoporosis is the thinning of the bones over time and osteopenia is the condition in which the bones have started to thin but have not progressed to the more advanced form of osteoporosis. Risk factors for osteoporosis include poor calcium intake, poor overall eating habits, low body weight, smoking, female gender, Caucasian or Asian ethnicity, and certain medications. Increasing calcium in the diet is one way to help treat osteopenia. High-calcium foods include dairy products, tofu, and dark green leafy vegetables. Weight-bearing exercise is also recommended, as well as refraining from smoking or excessive alcohol use.

40. B and C: A fractured clavicle or collarbone can take up to 12 weeks to fully heal, depending upon the age of the individual. When entering the rehabilitation phase, the main goals are to maximize flexibility in the shoulder, to improve range of motion, and to strengthen the muscles surrounding the collarbone area including the shoulders, upper arms, upper back, and chest. After initial treatment with immobilization using a sling, the athlete is gradually able to increase the level of activity in the shoulder. Initially, Codman's exercises are utilized, which consist of bending at the waist and allowing the arms to move like a pendulum. Next, the athlete can progress to additional strengthening exercises if no pain is present. These exercises are biceps curls, shoulder shrugs, triceps extensions, and arm raises done without the use of weights. As healing progresses, the use of elastic bands followed by weights can be incorporated. Returning to full activity requires verification by x-ray that the fracture is completely healed.

41. D: Following knee injury, there are a number of exercises that can be done to strengthen the knee without the use of equipment. These include straight leg raises, side lying abduction, standing hamstring curl, and toe raises. Stretching exercises include calf stretch, quadriceps stretch, hamstring stretch, and iliotibial band (ITB) stretch. Single-leg exercises include step up and down exercises, single-leg wall slide, and single-leg squats. Gluteal contractions work the gluteal muscle. The goal is to regain muscle strength using both legs. Additional exercises utilizing equipment can be incorporated when the athlete is at the training facility.

42. B, C, D, and E: If any athlete sustains an injury to the mouth that results in a tooth being knocked out, the best chance of saving the tooth is to replace the tooth in its socket within 30 minutes. The tooth should only be handled by its crown, not the roots. The tooth should be gently rinsed off with water but not scrubbed. If possible, the athletic trainer should assist the athlete in repositioning the tooth in the socket and have the athlete hold it in place with her fingers. If it is not possible to replace the tooth, the tooth should be placed in an emergency tooth preservation kit, cold milk, or saline solution. If none of these options is available, the tooth should be placed in the athlete's mouth between the cheek and gum. The main point is to keep the tooth moist at all times. Emergency dental services should be obtained for additional treatment.

43. C and E: *Agility* is defined as the ability to start and stop as well as to change directions. Agility in sports is important and regaining agility following an injury is a goal of rehabilitation. Testing for agility requires an individual to accelerate and decelerate quickly, which can be difficult when recovering from a knee or ankle injury. Results of agility testing should be compared with other individuals in similar situations. One test for agility is the Edgren Side Step Test. This test measures how well an individual can sidestep in three-foot increments in a 12-foot area, then change direction and sidestep back to the other side. The other test for agility is a T-test. This test utilizes cones set up in a T formation with 10-yard spacing. The individual runs 10 yards forward, 5 yards to the left, then 10 yards over to the right, then back to center and back steps to the first cone.

44. B, C, and D: A ball-and-socket joint is a type of joint in which a ball moves within a socket so that rotary movement is allowed in almost any direction. Examples of this type of joint are the shoulder and hip. The range of motion seen in ball-and-socket joints are *flexion and extension* (bending and straightening), *abduction and adduction* (pulling away from the midline and bringing back), and *internal and external rotation. Pronation and supination* are seen in the forearm when twisting the palm to face up or down. *Dorsiflexion and plantar flexion* are seen in the foot when the foot is bent upwards or downwards. *Eversion and inversion* are another set of terms applying to the foot when the sole is rotated away or toward the median. During rehabilitation, one of the goals is to increase range of motion in ball-and-socket joints in order to return to as close to pre-injury status as possible.

45. B: The Health Insurance Portability and Accountability Act (HIPAA) is a federal law enacted in 1996 to protect the privacy of consumers in matters pertaining to health information. The law has other purposes besides privacy: it covers health care providers, health insurance plans, and health care clearinghouses. Unless a written release is signed specifically stating that personal health information may be provided to athletic trainers or coaching staff, the physician is not obligated to comply with the request. Given that the athlete is over the age of 18, even her parents would not be able to obtain information unless written authorization is provided. Many schools now require student athletes to sign releases authorizing release of medical information to certain individuals in order to participate in a sport. HIPAA is a confusing law in regards to college athletics, but it is important to understand the role of an athletic trainer.

46. A and C: To become an athletic trainer, an individual must graduate with a bachelor's degree from an accredited institution. Next, the individual must pass the examination offered by the Board of Certification (BOC) to become certified in athletic training (ATC). In order to work in most states, the individual must apply and meet the requirements for registration, licensure, or certification. This is state-based and not a federal requirement or law. Athletic trainers will be affected by the Health Insurance Portability and Accountability Act (HIPAA) but likely not the Family Educational Rights and Privacy Act (FERPA), as this is a law that deals with privacy of student education records. Athletic trainers are also required to follow the BOC practice standards and code of ethics. In order to become recertified, continuing education guidelines must be followed.

47. B: Documentation is an important part of an athletic trainer's job for many reasons. In professional sports, the Occupational Safety and Health Administration (OSHA) requires athletic trainers to document any injuries received by players. If the athletic trainer works for a facility that is associated with a hospital, clinic, or rehabilitation hospital, requirements for documentation requirements may be set by the Joint Commission (formerly JCAHO) or Commission on Accreditation of Rehabilitation Facilities (CARF). Documentation is important because it provides legal protection. This provides written evidence that care was provided. Documentation also helps the athletic trainer to remember what treatments have been performed with a player and also helps improve communication with other professionals involved in the athlete's care. In some cases, documentation is part of insurance reimbursement.

48. A and D: The medical record is considered a legal document and care must be taken when entering information. Only permanent ink should be used, never pencil or erasable ink. Mistakes should never be erased and entries should not be altered in any way. Each entry should have the time, date, signature, and title of the person providing the documentation. Only factual and objective information can be entered. The care should be written in chronological order. The player's response to treatment should be documented. Appropriate and approved medical terminology should be used. Any change in condition, including progress, should be documented. Records should be securely stored so access is restricted to protect privacy.

49. B and D: A budget is a financial plan that dictates how the athletic training room will function for a certain period of time. An operating budget includes the items needed for the day-to-day operations and is typically written for a one-year period. A capital budget includes items that are required for the long-term operations. A capital budget is projected for five to 10 years. The money for these two budgets is separate from each other. Typical items in the operating budget for an athletic training room include first-aid supplies, various instruments needed such as scissors, and products needed for the different modalities such as flexi-wrap, heat packs, and ice bags. All the various types of tape needed would be included in the operating budget. Items for the capital budget would be more expensive items such as a taping bench or whirlpool.

50. A, B, and D: The development of a lightning safety plan is a necessary part of athletics. One person should be designated to monitor the weather and also to make the decision about suspending or cancelling an event. The nearest safe shelter location should be defined. This includes the nearest building that people normally use for business (i.e., not a shed or bathroom facility) or a vehicle with a hard roof. The presence of thunder with a blue sky can still be a source of danger because lightning can strike from as far as 10 miles away. The flash-to-bang (or lightning to thunder) count should be no less than 30 seconds. Once the 30 second count is reached, everyone should be already in a safe shelter or location. This is the equivalent of the storm being about six miles away. At least 30 minutes should elapse between the last flash of lightning and the last clap of thunder before resuming the sporting event.

How to Overcome Test Anxiety

Just the thought of taking a test is enough to make most people a little nervous. A test is an important event that can have a long-term impact on your future, so it's important to take it seriously and it's natural to feel anxious about performing well. But just because anxiety is normal, that doesn't mean that it's helpful in test taking, or that you should simply accept it as part of your life. Anxiety can have a variety of effects. These effects can be mild, like making you feel slightly nervous, or severe, like blocking your ability to focus or remember even a simple detail.

If you experience test anxiety—whether severe or mild—it's important to know how to beat it. To discover this, first you need to understand what causes test anxiety.

Causes of Test Anxiety

While we often think of anxiety as an uncontrollable emotional state, it can actually be caused by simple, practical things. One of the most common causes of test anxiety is that a person does not feel adequately prepared for their test. This feeling can be the result of many different issues such as poor study habits or lack of organization, but the most common culprit is time management. Starting to study too late, failing to organize your study time to cover all of the material, or being distracted while you study will mean that you're not well prepared for the test. This may lead to cramming the night before, which will cause you to be physically and mentally exhausted for the test. Poor time management also contributes to feelings of stress, fear, and hopelessness as you realize you are not well prepared but don't know what to do about it.

Other times, test anxiety is not related to your preparation for the test but comes from unresolved fear. This may be a past failure on a test, or poor performance on tests in general. It may come from comparing yourself to others who seem to be performing better or from the stress of living up to expectations. Anxiety may be driven by fears of the future—how failure on this test would affect your educational and career goals. These fears are often completely irrational, but they can still negatively impact your test performance.

Elements of Test Anxiety

As mentioned earlier, test anxiety is considered to be an emotional state, but it has physical and mental components as well. Sometimes you may not even realize that you are suffering from test anxiety until you notice the physical symptoms. These can include trembling hands, rapid heartbeat, sweating, nausea, and tense muscles. Extreme anxiety may lead to fainting or vomiting. Obviously, any of these symptoms can have a negative impact on testing. It is important to recognize them as soon as they begin to occur so that you can address the problem before it damages your performance.

The mental components of test anxiety include trouble focusing and inability to remember learned information. During a test, your mind is on high alert, which can help you recall information and stay focused for an extended period of time. However, anxiety interferes with your mind's natural processes, causing you to blank out, even on the questions you know well. The strain of testing during anxiety makes it difficult to stay focused, especially on a test that may take several hours. Extreme anxiety can take a huge mental toll, making it difficult not only to recall test information but even to understand the test questions or pull your thoughts together.

Effects of Test Anxiety

Test anxiety is like a disease—if left untreated, it will get progressively worse. Anxiety leads to poor performance, and this reinforces the feelings of fear and failure, which in turn lead to poor performances on subsequent tests. It can grow from a mild nervousness to a crippling condition. If allowed to progress, test anxiety can have a big impact on your schooling, and consequently on your future.

Test anxiety can spread to other parts of your life. Anxiety on tests can become anxiety in any stressful situation, and blanking on a test can turn into panicking in a job situation. But fortunately, you don't have to let anxiety rule your testing and determine your grades. There are a number of relatively simple steps you can take to move past anxiety and function normally on a test and in the rest of life.

Physical Steps for Beating Test Anxiety

While test anxiety is a serious problem, the good news is that it can be overcome. It doesn't have to control your ability to think and remember information. While it may take time, you can begin taking steps today to beat anxiety.

Just as your first hint that you may be struggling with anxiety comes from the physical symptoms, the first step to treating it is also physical. Rest is crucial for having a clear, strong mind. If you are tired, it is much easier to give in to anxiety. But if you establish good sleep habits, your body and mind will be ready to perform optimally, without the strain of exhaustion. Additionally, sleeping well helps you to retain information better, so you're more likely to recall the answers when you see the test questions.

Getting good sleep means more than going to bed on time. It's important to allow your brain time to relax. Take study breaks from time to time so it doesn't get overworked, and don't study right before bed. Take time to rest your mind before trying to rest your body, or you may find it difficult to fall asleep.

Along with sleep, other aspects of physical health are important in preparing for a test. Good nutrition is vital for good brain function. Sugary foods and drinks may give a burst of energy but this burst is followed by a crash, both physically and emotionally. Instead, fuel your body with protein and vitamin-rich foods.

Also, drink plenty of water. Dehydration can lead to headaches and exhaustion, especially if your brain is already under stress from the rigors of the test. Particularly if your test is a long one, drink water during the breaks. And if possible, take an energy-boosting snack to eat between sections.

Along with sleep and diet, a third important part of physical health is exercise. Maintaining a steady workout schedule is helpful, but even taking 5-minute study breaks to walk can help get your blood pumping faster and clear your head. Exercise also releases endorphins, which contribute to a positive feeling and can help combat test anxiety.

When you nurture your physical health, you are also contributing to your mental health. If your body is healthy, your mind is much more likely to be healthy as well. So take time to rest, nourish your body with healthy food and water, and get moving as much as possible. Taking these physical steps will make you stronger and more able to take the mental steps necessary to overcome test anxiety.

Mental Steps for Beating Test Anxiety

Working on the mental side of test anxiety can be more challenging, but as with the physical side, there are clear steps you can take to overcome it. As mentioned earlier, test anxiety often stems from lack of preparation, so the obvious solution is to prepare for the test. Effective studying may be the most important weapon you have for beating test anxiety, but you can and should employ several other mental tools to combat fear.

First, boost your confidence by reminding yourself of past success—tests or projects that you aced. If you're putting as much effort into preparing for this test as you did for those, there's no reason you should expect to fail here. Work hard to prepare; then trust your preparation.

Second, surround yourself with encouraging people. It can be helpful to find a study group, but be sure that the people you're around will encourage a positive attitude. If you spend time with others who are anxious or cynical, this will only contribute to your own anxiety. Look for others who are motivated to study hard from a desire to succeed, not from a fear of failure.

Third, reward yourself. A test is physically and mentally tiring, even without anxiety, and it can be helpful to have something to look forward to. Plan an activity following the test, regardless of the outcome, such as going to a movie or getting ice cream.

When you are taking the test, if you find yourself beginning to feel anxious, remind yourself that you know the material. Visualize successfully completing the test. Then take a few deep, relaxing breaths and return to it. Work through the questions carefully but with confidence, knowing that you are capable of succeeding.

Developing a healthy mental approach to test taking will also aid in other areas of life. Test anxiety affects more than just the actual test—it can be damaging to your mental health and even contribute to depression. It's important to beat test anxiety before it becomes a problem for more than testing.

Study Strategy

Being prepared for the test is necessary to combat anxiety, but what does being prepared look like? You may study for hours on end and still not feel prepared. What you need is a strategy for test prep. The next few pages outline our recommended steps to help you plan out and conquer the challenge of preparation.

STEP 1: SCOPE OUT THE TEST

Learn everything you can about the format (multiple choice, essay, etc.) and what will be on the test. Gather any study materials, course outlines, or sample exams that may be available. Not only will this help you to prepare, but knowing what to expect can help to alleviate test anxiety.

STEP 2: MAP OUT THE MATERIAL

Look through the textbook or study guide and make note of how many chapters or sections it has. Then divide these over the time you have. For example, if a book has 15 chapters and you have five days to study, you need to cover three chapters each day. Even better, if you have the time, leave an extra day at the end for overall review after you have gone through the material in depth.

If time is limited, you may need to prioritize the material. Look through it and make note of which sections you think you already have a good grasp on, and which need review. While you are studying, skim quickly through the familiar sections and take more time on the challenging parts.

Write out your plan so you don't get lost as you go. Having a written plan also helps you feel more in control of the study, so anxiety is less likely to arise from feeling overwhelmed at the amount to cover.

STEP 3: GATHER YOUR TOOLS

Decide what study method works best for you. Do you prefer to highlight in the book as you study and then go back over the highlighted portions? Or do you type out notes of the important information? Or is it helpful to make flashcards that you can carry with you? Assemble the pens, index cards, highlighters, post-it notes, and any other materials you may need so you won't be distracted by getting up to find things while you study.

If you're having a hard time retaining the information or organizing your notes, experiment with different methods. For example, try color-coding by subject with colored pens, highlighters, or post-it notes. If you learn better by hearing, try recording yourself reading your notes so you can listen while in the car, working out, or simply sitting at your desk. Ask a friend to quiz you from your flashcards, or try teaching someone the material to solidify it in your mind.

STEP 4: CREATE YOUR ENVIRONMENT

It's important to avoid distractions while you study. This includes both the obvious distractions like visitors and the subtle distractions like an uncomfortable chair (or a too-comfortable couch that makes you want to fall asleep). Set up the best study environment possible: good lighting and a comfortable work area. If background music helps you focus, you may want to turn it on, but otherwise keep the room quiet. If you are using a computer to take notes, be sure you don't have any other windows open, especially applications like social media, games, or anything else that could distract you. Silence your phone and turn off notifications. Be sure to keep water close by so you stay hydrated while you study (but avoid unhealthy drinks and snacks).

Also, take into account the best time of day to study. Are you freshest first thing in the morning? Try to set aside some time then to work through the material. Is your mind clearer in the afternoon or evening? Schedule your study session then. Another method is to study at the same time of day that you will take the test, so that your brain gets used to working on the material at that time and will be ready to focus at test time.

STEP 5: STUDY!

Once you have done all the study preparation, it's time to settle into the actual studying. Sit down, take a few moments to settle your mind so you can focus, and begin to follow your study plan. Don't give in to distractions or let yourself procrastinate. This is your time to prepare so you'll be ready to fearlessly approach the test. Make the most of the time and stay focused.

Of course, you don't want to burn out. If you study too long you may find that you're not retaining the information very well. Take regular study breaks. For example, taking five minutes out of every hour to walk briskly, breathing deeply and swinging your arms, can help your mind stay fresh.

As you get to the end of each chapter or section, it's a good idea to do a quick review. Remind yourself of what you learned and work on any difficult parts. When you feel that you've mastered the material, move on to the next part. At the end of your study session, briefly skim through your notes again.

But while review is helpful, cramming last minute is NOT. If at all possible, work ahead so that you won't need to fit all your study into the last day. Cramming overloads your brain with more information than it can process and retain, and your tired mind may struggle to recall even previously learned information when it is overwhelmed with last-minute study. Also, the urgent nature of cramming and the stress placed on your brain contribute to anxiety. You'll be more likely to go to the test feeling unprepared and having trouble thinking clearly.

So don't cram, and don't stay up late before the test, even just to review your notes at a leisurely pace. Your brain needs rest more than it needs to go over the information again. In fact, plan to finish your studies by noon or early afternoon the day before the test. Give your brain the rest of the day to relax or focus on other things, and get a good night's sleep. Then you will be fresh for the test and better able to recall what you've studied.

STEP 6: TAKE A PRACTICE TEST

Many courses offer sample tests, either online or in the study materials. This is an excellent resource to check whether you have mastered the material, as well as to prepare for the test format and environment.

Check the test format ahead of time: the number of questions, the type (multiple choice, free response, etc.), and the time limit. Then create a plan for working through them. For example, if you have 30 minutes to take a 60-question test, your limit is 30 seconds per question. Spend less time on the questions you know well so that you can take more time on the difficult ones.

If you have time to take several practice tests, take the first one open book, with no time limit. Work through the questions at your own pace and make sure you fully understand them. Gradually work up to taking a test under test conditions: sit at a desk with all study materials put away and set a timer. Pace yourself to make sure you finish the test with time to spare and go back to check your answers if you have time.

After each test, check your answers. On the questions you missed, be sure you understand why you missed them. Did you misread the question (tests can use tricky wording)? Did you forget the information? Or was it something you hadn't learned? Go back and study any shaky areas that the practice tests reveal.

Taking these tests not only helps with your grade, but also aids in combating test anxiety. If you're already used to the test conditions, you're less likely to worry about it, and working through tests until you're scoring well gives you a confidence boost. Go through the practice tests until you feel comfortable, and then you can go into the test knowing that you're ready for it.

Test Tips

On test day, you should be confident, knowing that you've prepared well and are ready to answer the questions. But aside from preparation, there are several test day strategies you can employ to maximize your performance.

First, as stated before, get a good night's sleep the night before the test (and for several nights before that, if possible). Go into the test with a fresh, alert mind rather than staying up late to study.

Try not to change too much about your normal routine on the day of the test. It's important to eat a nutritious breakfast, but if you normally don't eat breakfast at all, consider eating just a protein bar. If you're a coffee drinker, go ahead and have your normal coffee. Just make sure you time it so that the caffeine doesn't wear off right in the middle of your test. Avoid sugary beverages, and drink enough water to stay hydrated but not so much that you need a restroom break 10 minutes into the test. If your test isn't first thing in the morning, consider going for a walk or doing a light workout before the test to get your blood flowing.

Allow yourself enough time to get ready, and leave for the test with plenty of time to spare so you won't have the anxiety of scrambling to arrive in time. Another reason to be early is to select a good seat. It's helpful to sit away from doors and windows, which can be distracting. Find a good seat, get out your supplies, and settle your mind before the test begins.

When the test begins, start by going over the instructions carefully, even if you already know what to expect. Make sure you avoid any careless mistakes by following the directions.

Then begin working through the questions, pacing yourself as you've practiced. If you're not sure on an answer, don't spend too much time on it, and don't let it shake your confidence. Either skip it and come back later, or eliminate as many wrong answers as possible and guess among the remaining ones. Don't dwell on these questions as you continue—put them out of your mind and focus on what lies ahead.

Be sure to read all of the answer choices, even if you're sure the first one is the right answer. Sometimes you'll find a better one if you keep reading. But don't second-guess yourself if you do immediately know the answer. Your gut instinct is usually right. Don't let test anxiety rob you of the information you know.

If you have time at the end of the test (and if the test format allows), go back and review your answers. Be cautious about changing any, since your first instinct tends to be correct, but make sure you didn't misread any of the questions or accidentally mark the wrong answer choice. Look over any you skipped and make an educated guess.

At the end, leave the test feeling confident. You've done your best, so don't waste time worrying about your performance or wishing you could change anything. Instead, celebrate the successful completion of this test. And finally, use this test to learn how to deal with anxiety even better next time.

> **Review Video: Test Anxiety**
> Visit mometrix.com/academy and enter code: 100340

Important Qualification

Not all anxiety is created equal. If your test anxiety is causing major issues in your life beyond the classroom or testing center, or if you are experiencing troubling physical symptoms related to your anxiety, it may be a sign of a serious physiological or psychological condition. If this sounds like your situation, we strongly encourage you to seek professional help.

Additional Bonus Material

Due to our efforts to try to keep this book to a manageable length, we've created a link that will give you access to all of your additional bonus material:

mometrix.com/bonus948/athtraining